Toward a Caring Curriculum:
A New Pedagogy for Nursing

Toward a Caring Curriculum: A New Pedagogy for Nursing

Em Olivia Bevis and Jean Watson

Pub. No. 15-2278

nln

National League for Nursing

ISBN 0-88737-440-9

Printed in the United States of America

Contents

v

Contributors

Em Olivia Bevis, MA, RN, FAAN, is Nursing Educational Consultant, Bluffton, South Carolina, and Adjunct Professor of Research, Georgia Southern College, Statesboro, Georgia.

Joyce P. Murray, EdD, MSN, RN, is Associate Professor and Head, Department of Nursing, Georgia Southern College, Statesboro, Georgia.

Jean Watson, PhD, RN, FAAN, is Dean and Professor, School of Nursing, University of Colorado Health Sciences Center, Denver, Colorado.

Preface

So here we are with a dream to build, hopes to fulfill, visions to realize, and a future to construct.

Em Olivia Bevis (p. 64)

Past debates on education have focused on whether it was designed for the individual or society, as an avenue for personal growth and enlightenment or as a means of socialization and enculturation into the status quo, as a progressive or conservative force. Whatever positions may be held on these and other issues, Bowers (1987) argues there are more points of agreement than disagreement among contemporary theorists of education. Identifying the works of John Dewey, Paolo Freire, Carl Rogers, and B.F. Skinner as representative of educational variations of liberalism, Bowers further argues *against* their commonly held assumptions which include the following:

> that education contributes to a progressive form of social change, that the power and authority of the individual must be progressively strengthened either through skill development or consciousness raising . . . , that a critical form of rational thought must replace more traditional forms of cultural authority, and that educated judgment enables the individual to stand for truth, and thus above the partisan use of power. (p. 17)

In contrast to these liberal theories, Bowers (1987) suggests that we "de-center" the individual. He advances the idea and working concept of the individual as a social-cultural being embedded in interdependencies.

Education, for Bowers, is "developing a conceptual basis for a discourse that allows us to consider the full inter-relatedness of individuals and community" (p. 137). Bowers also proposes that such a reformed view of the individual and a post-liberal theory of education are necessary conditions for strengthening the relationship between the individual and community.

Hegelian scholar J. Glenn Gray (1984), in *Re-Thinking American Education*, makes a similar case about education's function relative to the relationship between individuals and their world. In Gray's view, "education understood in its full philosophic sense is a search for the meaning and purpose of individual and collective existence" (p. 74). Education can "help to reconcile the individual and his world" (p. 37) and "develop individuality in community" (p. 67). Gray is even stronger in his argument for education as the necessary and critical step for the advancement of societies that more accurately reflect their holistic natures in contrast to distorted fragments. "*Only* to the degree that we become educated," Gray states, "do we gain relationships of depth and intimacy to the encompassing world" (p. 35).

Education, then, is the process whereby individuals re-unite with their realities, by looking through the abstractions that present themselves as real, by probing the apparent but false separations and differences for real connections that exist. No doubt, such education is closer to what we need as we prepare for the emerging realities of our lives.

However, regardless of how it is resolved and no matter which realities are legitimized and which are not, there is a prevailing danger: the way the current debate is framed. A focus on which books to read, what information to possess and use, and which skills to perfect—even if they are different, new, and technologically sophisticated—will lead to a place as problematic as where we now find ourselves. It will lead again to a place where, according to Greene (1986), "There is little sense of agency, even among the brightly successful; there is little capacity to look at things as if they could be otherwise" (p. 438).

While new ideas might replace old ideas, while existing power relationships might be equalized or reversed, a preoccupation with "what to teach" distorts the relationship between students and their worlds and distracts all involved from the development of freedom and health.

In a recent essay, "The Loss Is A Gain," psychologist Robert Coles (1988) tells about a black student from the South who was at Yale in 1957 and who struggled with the chasm between the supposed benefits and opportunities of his Ivy League education and the reality of the price to be paid. The young man felt the loss of his essential relationships acutely and was skeptical of whether being "accepted" by the dominant culture was any progress worth having.

> I go home—not to Atlanta (that's a place of convenience), but to Fitzgerald, Georgia, where my grandparents still live, and I'm with my people again. I'm not with some sociologist's *idea* of my people, or an economist's *idea* of how they live, or a psychologist's *interpretation* of their attitudes; I'm with each and every one of *them,* my kin. (p. 8)
>
> All those urban studies authorities and rural studies authorities, all those people full of *ideas*—about the black personality and black culture and black history and black this and black that. They're doing to us what they did to the white man (equal justice under the law)! They're dissecting us, analyzing us, folding us into their theories. They're changing the way we think about ourselves. But they miss the most important thing: our soul. I don't mean soul food; I don't even mean soul music . . . .
>
> I cringe sometimes: I know all I've gained up here, but there will be some days when I feel the loss deep inside, and I want with all my heart and soul to go back and sit with my grandmother and pray to Him, the God Almighty of my memory. (p. 9)

There ought be no list of what to teach because education for the new age is not about content, *it is about soul, it is about process.* Similarly, there ought be no list of how to recognize an educated individual because education for the emerging order is not about either individuals or their worlds; it is about the relationships between the two. It is not about what was, or even, solely, about what can be; it is about the relationships between the two—between what was and what can be. It is about uncovering the entire complexity of real connections between apparently unrelated phenomena, and in that uncovering it is the creating of new connections, new possibilities.

Education for the new age is about how to create and extend an educational community that will foster three fundamental feelings for all involved: a sense of agency, a sense of responsibility and accountability, and sense of connection. Education is the process that Greene (1988) describes in the *Dialectic of Freedom:*

> It is through and by means of education many of us believe that individuals can be provoked to reach beyond themselves into their intersubjective space. It is through and by means of education that they may become empowered to think about what they are doing, to become mindful, to share meanings, to conceptualize, to make varied sense of their lived worlds. (p. 12)

This work by Em Olivia Bevis and Jean Watson is within the tradition of education as an emancipatory project. Indeed, they have created the wondrous phrase, "the elegance of liberation." Within such an approach to education, there are to be spaces and places where teachers and students can together: explore, know and create their relationships to the whole, to their histories, their present contexts and future possibilities. They will refuse to accept as given the separations that divide us from each other, and each from the whole. They will connect what has been disconnected and they will disrupt relationships of power, domination, and submission in a manner that respects and extends the reality of our interdependence.

Patricia Moccia, PhD, RN, FAAN

REFERENCES

Bowers, C.A. (1987). *Elements of a post-liberal theory of education*. New York: Teachers College Press.

Coles, R. (1988). *Harvard diary. Reflections on the sacred and the secular*. New York: Crossroads.

Gray, J.G. (1984). *Re-thinking American education. A philosophy of teaching and learning* (2nd edition). Connecticut: Wesleyan University Press.

Greene, M. (1986). In search of a critical pedagogy. *Harvard Educational Review, 56* (4), 427–441.

Greene, M. (1988). *The dialectic of freedom*. New York: Teachers College Press.

Editor's Preface

With the 1990s almost upon us, nursing philosophy and theory and nursing education have come to a cross roads. Critical and ethical thinking, creativity in approaches to care, liberating curriculum from restrictive methodologies, grounding education in the realities of practice are areas of significant concern. Preeminently, however, it is caring that must be reoriented toward a new vision of the whole person, body, mind, and heart alike, and pervade the curriculum structure and form its ethical content. It is no longer sufficient for nursing to concern itself with anything less. It is no longer sufficient for nurses to be anything less than what this vision entails. But to create such nurses is no minor task. It relies upon the intelligence and will of educators to constantly test limits, accepted and traditional paradigms, and the professional status of the nurse in a more and more technologically sophisticated industry. It also relies upon educators to understand their own limitations, hesitancies, and fears when faced with the need to enhance expertise in this most *human* perspective, the whole person. For this is the perspective in which nursing will come into its own. Yet it is precisely this perspective that remains to be systematically explored beyond, for example, behaviorist landmarks.

This book has been written with that aim in mind. Nursing educators and future educators will find here a new beginning. Nursing students, as well, will benefit from the arguments proposed and conclusions reached. Although nursing began as a modern profession over 100 years ago, the full realization of its mature development encourages us still.

Allan Graubard
Editor, National League for Nursing

Acknowledgments

The impossibility of our acknowledging and thanking all those whose time, efforts, help, good wishes, and ideas contributed to this book is clear. Since the early 1980s, the two of us have shared concerns about the state of nursing curriculum. Those discussions and interactions, the criticism, reading, dreaming, seeking, and work resulted in the ideas expressed in this volume. Each of us made a private journey as well as the one we made together, so each of us has her own special acknowledgments to make.

Em Olivia Bevis . . .

The following persons have my deepest respect and thanks:

Gerald Firth—Chairman of the Department of Curriculum and Supervision at the University of Georgia—for his caring. He came to the office of a stranger, someone he knew only by reputation, and asked me to enroll at the University of Georgia in the doctoral program in Curriculum and Instruction. He has never failed to give support and to exhibit concern for my growth and welfare. His was genuine caring of the highest order, that which compels action on behalf of one who is unknown. His action has had more impact than I can describe.

John Newfield—teacher extraordinaire—for his introduction to the nonbehaviorist curriculum writers. He introduced me to Lawrence Stenhouse, Joseph Schwab, Maxine Green, Paulo Freire, Dwaine Huebner, Michael Apple, Elliot Eisner, and others. I felt like a child turned loose in Santa's storeroom, and sugar plum fairies did indeed dance in my head.

Mary Compton, a warm, intelligent, inspirational, loving guide and coach, who keeps me straight and consistent (relatively), and tries to dampen my hyperbole without drowning my song. The gods smiled on me when they gave me Mary.

Verle Waters—my always and forever friend and best critic—whose perception of nursing education is the clearest of them all, and, I believe, the most real. Her views have a moral and philosophical consistency and a scholarly base that enhances her dreams and visions. Her impact on my thinking has, through the years, been substantial.

Joyce Murray—dear friend and colleague—who struggled through this with me. She really knows how to be a friend and how to make caring live. Our dialogue sometimes becomes surrealistic; of such things reality is tempered.

All my teachers over the years who never knew whether to point with pride or view with alarm.

James Edison Bevis and Willie Bullock Bevis—my mother and father—who both died while this book was being written. My educational heritage comes from them, both teachers in elementary schools all of their lives. They never stopped going to school, learning, and growing. I grew up with discussions about Dewey, Hutchins, and Thorndike at breakfast, dinner, and supper. I did not know how much of these discussions became as much a part of my nourishment as the food I ate until I too became a teacher and found the names and ideas of these educators to be old friends. My sister and two brothers and I were very fortunate to be part of James' and Willie's lives.

Julian Friedman—loving husband and friend—who reads everything I write, making excellent suggestions, offering criticisms, and entering into intelligent discussions. His enthusiasm for the project never flagged though it has cost us much of our time together. Thank you for all those wonderful trips to Pritchardville.

Esther and Sheldon Friedman . . . the children . . . just because.

Jean Watson . . .

I offer my deepest thanks and appreciation to all the faculty and students who have been associated with the University of Colorado School of Nursing since 1973, when I first joined the school as a new faculty member. Since that time, exploration of many of the ideas set forth in this book have occurred at the University of Colorado in various degrees, at different points in time and at different levels, ranging from individual teaching–learning experiments to total system changes. As Dean of the School of Nursing during the writing of this work, I was always energized and inspired by the openness and willingness of faculty and students to be a part of the transformation that is occurring in nursing education and practice. But my thanks do not do justice to the hard work and dedication of the entire University of Colorado School of Nursing, to go beyond being a part of the transformation, but, indeed, to making it happen.

Special gratitude to Marilyn Stember, Juanita Tate, Sally Phillips, and Jurate Sakalys who are not only educators of excellence, but administrators supreme who have the profound ability and enthusiasm to contribute to the implementation of many of my idealistic goals and ideas and sometime creative unleashing that was often overly challenging for us all. Nevertheless, they were always there for me and for the School of Nursing faculty, students, and clinical affiliates with a firmness, stability, and commitment to excellence. In addition, the faculty were always open to experimentation with new and creative ideas that were untried and utterly new in nursing. As a result, many successes have been forthcoming. Perhaps more importantly than the successes were the failures and the openness to keep experimenting and moving with a vision of openness for the betterment of the nursing profession. Such experimentation that has occurred in the school during these past several years is exceedingly rare and largely unsurpassed for a major, traditional, institutionalized system of nursing education today. The privilege of being a part of making some of the ideals and ideas in this book more attainable has been a precious, once-in-a-life-time happening for me. For all of these reasons and many more, I am blessed. I hope this book will inspire many more faculty, students, and administrators to reach beyond what is not yet, but perhaps ought to be, and keep the flow of teaching–learning and living open and alive with new hope and courage for nursing's future.

We are grateful to Allan Graubard, our editor, whose competence made a great deal of difference in the finished text.

Finally, we acknowledge and thank the staff at the National League for Nursing (NLN) for their commitment to progressive, even revolutionary ideas; for their aggressive leadership in renewing the League as a force for scholarship, excellence, and educational sanity; for bringing healing to the ranks of educators from associate of arts, diploma, and baccalaureate and higher degrees; and for helping make nursing a human centered force in a technology focused, reductionistic, materialistic health system, and for helping us restore the passionate urgency to the moral ideal of nursing which is caring.

To *Julian Richard Friedman*
  We share our time and space
  We make our own music
  We dance in the sea and give each other
    Gifts of falling stars
      Birdsongs
        And laughter.

                                        EOB

As always, my love and devotion to *Douglas, Jennifer*, and *Julie,* whose spirit and light are always with me; and now the new loves in my life, *Miguel,* my new son-in-law, and baby dragon boy *Demitri,* my 15-month old grandson, who awaits me to come join him and his mother, Jennifer, right now, while Doug and Julie are biking in the mountains of Colorado. Thank you, thank you for all of it.

                                        MJW

Seeking Truth

The art of it lies
In creating the blanks:
The open spaces
With no traces of thought
To mar the empty
Stealing away of mind and
Feeling.
It is an act requiring reverence,
Kneeling
Before the God within;
Seeing without looking
In the soundless void
Where The God has been
But is not seen.
Where Being is all
And meaning must wait its turn.

Em Olivia Bevis

Introduction

PURPOSE

It is the purpose of this work to create a new curriculum-development paradigm for nursing education. This new model is designed to enable nursing graduates to be more responsive to societal needs, more successful in humanizing the highly technological milieus of health care, more caring and compassionate, more insightful about ethical and moral issues, more creative, more capable of critical thinking, and better able to bring scholarly approaches to client problems and issues and to advocate ethical positions on behalf of clients. In short, any new paradigm for nursing education must be able to graduate the skilled, compassionate scholar-clinicians necessary for the remaining years of the 20th century and the beginning of the new millennium.

To be effective, the alternative paradigm must accomplish what has been made difficult or impossible by the current model:

1. It must liberate both students and faculty from the authoritarian restraints of empiricist/behaviorist models as represented by specified behavioral objectives and the teacher roles and functions necessitated by these objectives.

2. It must acknowledge students as equal partners in the educational enterprise so that it restructures the way faculty and students relate to each other.

3. It must define curriculum as interactions between and among students and teachers with the intent that learning take place.

4. It must facilitate the structuring of learning differently so that

the learner is actively engaged in scholarly pursuits, and through this it must support abandoning the dominance of lecture in nursing education.

5. It must help faculty humanize the educational process so that the curriculum is not dominated and driven by a surfeit of content.

6. It must support an alliance of students, teachers, and clinicians in the educational enterprise.

7. It must restructure the focus of learning so that experiences are clinically grounded.

8. It must provide practical guidelines to faculty without restricting individuality, creativity, and style.

9. It must acknowledge the wide variety of ways of knowing and must legitimize those things that are not empirically verifiable.

10. It must eliminate the education-based class and caste system in nursing by acknowledging and valuing the contributions of all nurses and by making higher levels of nursing education more easily accessible.

11. It must offer a criticism model for assessing learning.

THE PROBLEM

The Tylerian/behaviorist curriculum-development paradigm has prescribed nursing curriculum and the direction of nursing educational thought for the last 35 years. Changing this, the current model, will not be an easy task. Not only must a viable alternative be offered, but a national effort must be mounted to deinstitutionalize the behaviorist model. This will be difficult because, in an effort to create criteria for ensuring the quality of nursing educational programs, state-approval bodies and the national accrediting agency have adopted Tylerian/ behaviorist curriculum products as criteria for approval and accreditation. This institutionalized behaviorism is the nation's tacitly agreed-upon version of truth in curriculum.

The slide from utility to dogma is an easy one to understand. First comes the argument about the merits of various curriculum-development models. That argument is part of the classical argument regarding research methodology. It is, in fact, a dispute about the nature of reality and about how we come to know that reality. It cannot be reduced to overly simplistic strings of differences as if believing one thing inevitably leads one to believe all the others in that string. The fluidity of the searching mind and its willingness and ability to conceive of all things as possible finally focuses on some things it believes as more possible or more useful than others. In this way, openness to possibilities can imperceptibly begin its slide into dogma. As a system of belief develops and becomes researched, it evokes priests and acolytes, disciples and true believers. The system increasingly tolerates decreasing levels of deviation until it becomes a new orthodoxy, a new dogma. Then differences become viewed, not as positions to be examined and debated, but as heresy. At that point, laws, regulation, social pressure, and policy institutionalize and enforce the dogma and place harsh penalties for deviation. In the case of nursing, these penalties take the form of declaring that graduates from schools who do not conform are ineligible to take the licensing examination and of denying the schools the blessing of accreditation. Most probably the difficulty lies not in the theories, the positions, and in the ideas themselves, but in the very human inclination to translate these ideas into dogma and prescriptive orthodoxy.

In nursing, Tylerian behaviorism, the currently prescribed orthodoxy, is not bad in and of itself. It is excellent for those aspects of curriculum that are oriented toward memorization and skills. Its misuse has come in trying to make it uniformly applicable to all nursing curriculum matters and in limiting curriculum exploration to behaviorist theory.

A national effort to loosen these bonds will be ineffective unless there are workable alternatives. It is the goal of this book to offer such an alternative in the expectation that it will engage the minds and imaginations of nursing educators and thereby promote freedom to choose among possible models.

There are several problems inherent in using behaviorist theory in the form of the Tyler rationale to guide all of nursing education. However, there are three assumptions that are most problematic and that probably influence all other difficulties that nursing has with the model. They are described in the following paragraphs.

1. There is one type of learning, and one coherent group of compatible theories sufficient to support and explain learning.

2. Educated, mature learners can be graduated using behaviorist theory and the teaching methods that are consistent with it.

3. The schooling system based on behaviorism is capable of liberating, educating, and helping people to be integrated.

This paradigm must help educators take another look at these assumptions, challenge them, and offer another possibility. Therefore, throughout the book there is criticism of the behaviorist model.

AN EXPLANATION: BEHAVIORIST CRITICISM

It seems somewhat disloyal to suggest that nursing alter the premier place of behaviorist learning theory in nursing curriculum development. Behaviorism in the form of the Tyler rationale has been the tried and true keystone of nursing curriculum for 35 years. In fact, there has been a question raised, justly so, about the necessity of being so critical of a model that has done so much for nursing education, a theory of learning that is supported by so much excellent research and has so many reputable adherents and such a large body of literature sustaining it. Throughout the book, behaviorist doctrine is continually examined for what it can and cannot do for nursing education. These criticisms seem necessary for the reasons that follow.

1. The model is so widely accepted and commands such uncritical loyalty that if its limitations are not highlighted and exposed, nurse educators may not be attentive to the need for change. This requires challenging its assumptions and consequences.

2. We find behaviorism flawed in that its acceptance and validity are confirmed by its own hypotheses. By suggesting that all learning is evidenced in some form of empirically observable behavior, the necessary sequitur is without empirical validation the existence of that behavior is called into question. A better position to confirm oneself could not be found. With that as a premise, all research findings are empirically validated; when they are not, it is attributed to no learning having taken place. So the design for research verification is circular in that it admits no indicators except empirical ones. This position requires that if one is to offer an alternative, then one must confront this self-fulfilling confirmation head-on, because it is responsible for some of the problems inherent in behaviorist education.

3. Behaviorism is a masculine theory. It is materialistic, instrumentalist, reductionistic, and empirical. It consists of deductive logic and supports procedural knowledge. As masculine theory, it lacks the elements necessary to the feminine needs of both teaching and nursing.

4. Nursing and education are caring social services and feminine fields. As feminine fields, they are based on human science, not traditional science, and require as a base theories that are flexible, open, and whole and that allow multiple realities and intuitive and constructed knowledge as well as procedural knowledge. The areas where the conflict occurs must be consistently illuminated in order to justify the investigation of alternatives. Additionally, workable alternatives must be generated and tested.

5. There has been a shift in paradigm for nursing philosophy and research. For many years, and until the mid-1950s, nursing was based on the medical model: dualistic, reductionistic, objective, logico-deductive, quantitative, and diagnosis and treatment oriented. Slowly it began to change to be humanistic-existentialistic, holistic, subjective, intuitive, phenomenological, and human experience oriented. Its research paradigms were slower to change. It has only been in the last 10 years that qualitative research was sanctioned and valued, but it has become viewed as such now. Since it too has shifted its base toward research more befitting a human science, nursing education is out of step with its philosophy and its research. Such a dissonance within the structure of the field cries out for remedy . . . for as it currently exists, schools write out a philosophy that is human-science human-experience valuing, holistic, quantitative, and caring oriented, yet plan a curriculum that is based on behavioral objectives and oppressive. This inconsistency is a handicap to nursing.

The needs of modern health care—increased technology, chronicity, and acuity—require a well-educated—not just a well-trained—nurse. Both are needed in today's world. To do justice to our mission we must alter our paradigm.

Throughout the book, therefore, interwoven with suggestions for alternatives, there are criticisms of the objectives-behaviorist models. These are offered not only on the basis of my belief in the validity of these criticisms but in the belief that without very good reasons, nursing educators will not support the change in paradigm that is needed.

THE CENTRAL THESES OF THE PARADIGM

Several converging lines of thought are used to establish a new curriculum-development paradigm for nursing. The first involves defining curriculum as interaction. The central thesis of this book—all else being commentary—is that *curriculum is the interactions and transactions that occur between and among students and teachers with the intent that learning occur.* All other aspects of curriculum, programs of study, written plans, and extracurricular activities are adjuncts to teacher–student and student–student interactions. The interactions and transactions are conceived as occurring between collegial participants—co-learners— in ways that are egalitarian and sororal/fraternal.

The second position maintains that active learning—learning that engages the intellectual efforts of both students and teachers—is necessary to the development of the creative thinking that is the mark of the educated person. Frontal lecture, as with other passive teaching strategies, has limited usefulness in the educational scene and little place in the lexicon of strategies used for educative teaching.

A third position is that the maturity of the learner is intimately tied to the modalities of teaching and that behaviorist methods reinforce students in the immature position of anticipatory compliance with the faculty's agenda. To move students into mature positions requires teaching strategies that compel students to take the leadership and responsibility for their own learning agenda.

A fourth position is that no one theory can explain the complex and multifaceted thing called learning, and, therefore, there is not one type of learning but six different types. These types fall into two categories, training and education.

A fifth position is that all curriculum development commences with faculty development. Faculty are ill prepared by higher educational programs for anything but behaviorist curricula. Faculty need guidance, help, and support to grow and to develop for themselves a *repertoire* of teaching tools and skills that supports active, educative, egalitarian learning.

These central positions converge into a total picture, a paradigm, that gives substance to and a direction for curriculum-development change that is educative in nature.

The significance of the curriculum-development paradigm espoused in this book is that it highlights the fundamental relationship between how the teacher teaches and the attainment of the educational qualities that lead to and aid in the achievement of critical thinking. Critical thinking, not training, is perceived of as an outcome of education and as necessary to the roles and functions currently required of nurses. This highlighted relationship places primary emphasis upon the *teacher's pedagogic skills in educating learners* rather than upon training them as the key element in a new direction for nursing education. Furthermore, it accentuates the training nature of the Tylerian models and underscores the necessity of educative models.

In that vein, there were road signs that saturated U.S. highways a few years ago in solicitation of contributions to colleges, saying, "The mind is a terrible thing to waste." Nowhere do we have a better example of the accidental waste of the mind by people who wish with all their hearts to harness its potential than in classrooms from elementary schools through doctoral programs. To stop this waste, we must first acknowledge the need to alter the teacher's role radically and to make that alteration the primary commitment of curriculum development. If this position is not accepted—that the teacher's role must be reconceived—then curriculum changes are sabotaged by the continued use of passive learning modes. Therefore, until we reconceptualize and restructure the nursing teacher's common and usual way of both perceiving and enacting the teaching role, no other curriculum changes will effect substantive changes in nursing graduates and consequently in nursing practice. Furthermore, any mode of conceptualizing the nursing teacher's role in an authoritarian, frontal teaching, information-giving, control-laden way (ultimately politically oppressive) is inimical to the caring paradigm that is nursing's moral imperative and nursing education's moral activity (which must be ultimately politically liberating). Consequently, we must change the politics of the classroom and the clinical area. If we fail to do this, the effect will be that the desired substantive changes will not occur because they are politically impossible.

To change the fundamental relationships between and among teachers and students requires a reconceptualization of the ideas that influence relationships. Among these ideas are such matters as the nature of curriculum, what it is, and how such perceptions influence curriculum development; student maturity as learners and the teacher's influence on such maturity levels; the way learning is conceived and how those perceptions influence teaching and learning; the nature of learning activities and what criteria are used for their selection; and how one goes about teaching in ways that engage students in the whole process, for example, making colleagues of them, not dependents. These problems are dealt with throughout this book in ways that provide a series of theoretical models based upon a succession of assumptions, documented assertions, real-life experiences, intuition, insights, and hypotheses.

THE NEED FOR RESEARCH

The models presented in this work need to be researched; most have been successfully field-tested, but few have been researched. It is hoped that as they are researched, they will be improved and changed so that never will there ever be another model that freezes in form and is institutionalized as nursing educational dogma. The tendency of nursing education to institutionalize theoretical positions that are attractive and of timely use is well documented (nursing diagnosis and nursing process are two examples in addition to behaviorist learning theory). The structure of this paradigm is deliberately loose in an attempt to discourage such doctrinaire proceedings, but the possibility remains.

ORGANIZATION

This book consists of three parts. Part I makes a case for a new paradigm of curriculum development. It consists of Chapter 1, which looks at the development of nursing education and how we came to this historical intersection. It is also an attempt to illuminate some of the issues. Chapter 2 examines the philosophical foundation of nursing as a caring, human-science, liberal-arts-based field. Chapter 3 more specifically discusses transformative thinking and the nature of a caring curriculum.

Part II lays out an educative-caring curriculum-development paradigm for professional nursing. It consists of six chapters. The first of these proposes a series of theoretical models that form the basis of the paradigm. The second describes those things that influence practical decisions about nursing curriculum in order to help faculty in their curriculum-development efforts. The next four chapters address teaching and learning as conceived in a paradigm that defines curriculum as teaching interactions and reality-based, active, learning episodes. The last chapter in this section offers ideas for a criticism model in lieu of behaviorist methods of evaluating learning.

Part III consists of three chapters. The first examines traditional behaviorist-curriculum development with the goal of determining what, if any, role the elements of Tylerian curriculum play in an educative curriculum. The second attempts to address when and under what circumstances this new paradigm will influence the course of nursing and the kind of care given to clients. In other words, so what? Why all this effort? The last takes a look at the future. What kind of nurse can we graduate and what roles will that nurse play in health care in the 21st century?

The paradigm is not a finished product that can remove all ambiguity, solve all dilemmas, and be reduced to prescriptive formula. It resists such formulations on the basis that dilemma, conundrums, and ambiguity are the progenitors of creativity and necessary to the ongoing vitality that must imbue a curriculum-development paradigm. To be true to its purpose, it must resist codification and dogmatization. It is structured to resist such formulations because of a belief that flexibility and freedom of choice give rise to the natural expression necessary to the educative curriculum and can only be found in a philosophy in which context dictates method and influences content choices. This means that curriculum is particular—a unique expression of each school's mission, faculty characteristics, student needs, and cultural influences.

Part I

Making a Case for a New Paradigm of Curriculum Development

We face the future fortified only with the lessons we have learned from the past. It is today that we must create the world of the future. . . . In a very real sense, tomorrow is now.

Eleanor Roosevelt

INTRODUCTION

How one defines curriculum and the paradigm used to develop it helps to influence the type and quality of graduates. It also influences the way nurses view their work, how nursing work is evaluated, and what types of research are sanctioned. No other nursing activity or enterprise has so affected nursing's historical course and its practice than the curriculum-development paradigm used for the last 40 years. A grandiose claim? Not so much as one might think.

The use of the Tylerian curriculum-development model cast nursing education into the behaviorist framework and entrenched nursing practice in a training modality, brought behavioral objectives and behaviorist-evaluation methods into primacy, and was responsible for the rise of competency-based education and evaluation as well as the dedication of nurses to nursing diagnosis and the stylized, rule-driven, problem-solving format called *nursing process*. It may be credited with much of the quality that nursing has achieved in the past. Its misuse through institutionalization has been partially responsible for the failure of nursing to move more swiftly into professionalism.

Nursing is encountering problems in moving further along the occupation-to-professional continuum. The well-educated, critical-thinking nursing professional emerges infrequently from colleges and universities. The origin of many of these problems rests in history. Yet when all is considered, it is clear that nursing is ready in all respects to

11

create, in Eleanor Roosevelt's words, "the world of the future"—a new now. Part I introduces the new wave of curriculum development.

It consists of 3 chapters. Chapter 1 examines the history of nursing educational paradigms. Chapter 2 provides a philosophical foundation for the new direction in curriculum development. Chapter 3 discusses transformative thinking and a caring curriculum.

The history of the evolution of nursing curriculum as institutionalized behaviorism is a long one and significant as background for this paradigm. Its length and relevance is such that a large part of Chapter 1 is designed to provide a historical perspective on the move from craftsmanship to professionalism and from training to education. The chapter proposes that there have been four significant turns in nursing and that a fifth turn is beginning. It provides a historical overview of the four curriculum-development models that have directed nursing education, and it explores the factors that supported institutionalizing behaviorist doctrine. Furthermore, it makes a case for changing the paradigm and suggests what must be done to move nursing education into a new era. In this new era—the fifth turn—the new models place emphasis upon teaching.

There are several new models being generated for curriculum development that are designed to educate nurses better. Curriculum, in most of these models, is the interactions, oral and written, that occur between students and faculty and among students. For this reason, this, an educative-caring paradigm, requires that curriculum development start with faculty development. Faculty are helped to make the transition from behaviorist training to educational practices: to the art of raising questions that provoke dialogue and facilitate insight, patterns, meanings, and all the other characteristics of education. Faculty development must concentrate on helping faculty alter their perception of their role.

Chapter 2 continues exploring why we need a new paradigm. Additionally, it describes the philosophical foundation for this new direction. It examines the rich tapestry of philosophical convictions that support nursing as a human science and liberal arts education as a natural basis for that human science. It provides the foundation for all the assumptions, postulates, posits, and theses found throughout all the rest of the chapters.

Chapter 3 proposes transformative thinking as liberation for students and teachers and as essential elements in a caring curriculum and new pedagogy for nursing.

1

Illuminating the Issues: Probing the Past, A History of Nursing Curriculum Development—The Past Shapes the Present

Em Olivia Bevis

The best thing about Herbart was himself; the worst that can be laid to his charge is the Herbartians.

Herbart taught the doctrine of interest in education. In the early part of the nineteenth century he startled the pedagogic world with a series of psychological experiments conducted at the university of Konigsberg-way-off-the-Rhine, Germany. He proved to the students who flocked to his lectures, by actual and repeated demonstrations, that, in teaching a puppy anything, say, to sit up on his hind legs, the quickest, most effective and lasting method is first to excite his interest by showing him a piece of meat. This basis dogmatically established, it may be proved in psychological terms, which the confines of this treatise will not allow us to reproduce, that the method of exciting interest is likewise best in the instruction of young human beings.

While to those who rely upon the uncertainties of common sense this idea may seem simple and one likely to have occurred to Adam when raising Cain, yet elaborated, as it is by the modern disciples of Herbart, in the terms of psychological pedagogy, it fills several hundred volumes.

Indeed, it is more than suspected that they have overdone the matter. So far as the Herbartians have succeeded in getting their ideas into the schools,—and that is not a little,—they have made the instruction and operations of the schoolroom a stupendous hippodromic exhibition; and they have turned the teacher into a vaudeville artist and professional entertainer. This in the language of Aesop's frog, may be fun for the children, but it's death to the high-pressure teacher.

Possibly it was not Madame de Stael who exclaimed, "O Herbart, what ineffable bosh has been perpetrated in thy name!"

Welland Hendrick,
A Joysome History of Education (1909)

INTRODUCTION

I think it significant that Hendrick, in his *A Joysome History of Education* poked fun not so much at Herbart as at the Herbartians. Herbart was, of course, the progenitor of behaviorism, and the schools, loving simple formulas, adopted and elaborated his work as they did later with Thorndike and Skinner. And, as Hendrick says of Herbart, it is probably not Tyler that is so much a problem as what nursing educators have done with him.

In contrast, I have a book by William James, published in 1912, 3 years after Hendrick's *A Joysome History.* Part of it is a collection of his talks to students on some of life's ideals. In it he talks about his own awakening to the "unidealized heroic life around me" (p. 276). Heroic life, he says, is simple, it has horny hands and often dirty skin; it is genuine, vital, unconscious, and it is unexpectant of decoration or recognition. His remarks reflect an innocent idea, yet one that brings things back to earth. Nursing is about caring for these people: ordinary, working people who live quietly heroic lives, sometimes the sheer boredom and drudgery of them, the toleration of burdens, the daily making do, living with pain, facing loss of health and continued vulnerability may not seem as heroic as they, in fact, are. These heroic lives and the ability to perceive them and appreciate them puts our theories, our ideas about teaching and learning, into perspective. No theory of learning that mechanically and reductionistically treats with the lives of humans can help to improve the quality of these heroics—hence this attempt to find additional options, additional ways of viewing the work of teaching nursing. This work is an attempt to bring nursing education into alignment with its philosophy, research, and practice paradigms. Nursing's philosophical base has shifted, its research paradigm has changed, and its practice modes are increasingly guided by human science. Only nursing's educational model remains to be altered to bring the whole into internal congruence. Additionally, there are demands now being placed upon nursing that cannot be met through its traditional educational system.

This chapter lays some groundwork (additional to the introduction) for and justifies the choice of creating a new curriculum-development paradigm designed to educate professional nurses. It briefly explores the problems and needs that give rise to a paradigm shift. It is designed to give the reader some sense of what the work is about, why, and where it is going. It also provides a history of how we got to be where we are.

BACKGROUND

The need for a change in the curriculum-development paradigm arises from at least three sources. The first is the ratio of nurses from associate of arts and diploma programs to those graduated with a baccalaureate degree and the indication for greater accessibility of baccalaureate programs. The second is the natural development of nursing as a human science and its need for congruence among its parts, philosophy, theory, research, practice, and education. The third is the social needs of the current age of health problems and modern technology.

The Need for Educational Accessibility

The present world of students nudges curriculum toward accessibility and flexibility, since most newly licensed nurses are not from baccalaureate programs. Based on first-time candidates for the July 1988 NCLEX (National Council Licensing Examination), associate degree programs now graduate 57 percent and diploma programs 10 percent of the total (National Council, 1988). This means that about 67 percent of new nurses lack the first professional degree. Increasing numbers of students are no longer immediate post-high school; increasing numbers are reentry persons with either second careers or second degrees, and more students than ever before work 20 or more hours per week. These realities force nurse educators to plan programs that allow associate of arts degree in nursing (ADN) graduates to seek baccalaureate degrees with the least redundancy and the fewest possible problems and roadblocks.

This situation forces educators to examine and reconstruct programs of study in such areas as the policies governing entry, part-time study, scheduling, articulation, and challenge exams or transfer of credit. Programs must be arranged so that they are flexible and accessible.

The Need for Congruence in Nursing

One origin of the needed change in educational paradigm arises from perceptions that nursing philosophy has moved from pragmatic empiricism to humanistic existentialism and that nursing theory and research have moved from a strict adherence to scientific empiricism to encompassing all investigative methods in creative combinations (inclusive of empiricism and such other methods as phenomenology, poetics, and hermeneutics). This leaves nursing's curriculum paradigm in a position of incongruence with its philosophy and research (Munhall, 1981; Watson, 1988). Watson points this up in making a case for restructuring nursing as a human science rather than considering it among the traditional natural sciences:

> There is greater acknowledgment and public recognition that continued adherence to a medical model for nursing practice and adherence to a traditional natural science model for nursing science is not adequate for addressing the phenomena of human care in nursing and human responses to actual or potential health problems.
> For perhaps the first time in its scientific development, nursing has recently had the opportunity to explore its own heritage, become recommitted to nursing values, goals and philosophies, and explore research methods and options consistent with prevailing views about the nature of nursing. In so doing, nursing scholars and clinicians have begun to admit openly that an inconsistency or anomaly has existed and continues to exist between the medical tradition and/or natural science paradigm and the nature of nursing. . . . In addition, nursing is investigating alternative methods for researching nursing phenomena. (pp. 18–19)

Watson further maintains that the medical tradition arises from a quantitative-rationalistic inquiry model, that nursing as a human science derives from a qualitative-phenomenological or naturalistic form of inquiry, and that these two perspectives derive from disparate assumptions about the nature of reality, the nature of the relationships between inquirer and subject/object, and the nature of truth (p. 20). Munhall (1981) points out the basic incongruence between nursing's philosophy and its sanctioned research methodologies. She concludes that the reductionism, the dependence upon observable or measurable indicators, and realities and objectification necessary to empiricism or scientific methods are out of step with the basic tenets of nursing philosophy. Such observations, coupled with the acknowledgment of the value of the contributions of phenomenological and grounded-theory researchers in nursing, have moved nursing from strict conformity to traditional quantitative research paradigms to paradigms more in keeping with nursing's philosophical underpinnings.

This growth has left nursing education as the last bastion of behaviorist/empiricism in nursing. The incongruity of nursing's sanctioned educational paradigm and nursing's philosophy and research paradigm has begun to damage its capacity to be socially responsive, for one consequence is that nursing graduates are caught in a bind between the commitment to caring for persons as unique, perfect wholes, and behaviorism's reductionistic objectification of person.

Today's health care system has reached a point in which the nature of providers and the kind of care they give must radically alter. Social health-related problems require this.

THE SOCIAL MANDATE

Based on events in the current health care system and predictions for future health care problems, the position is taken that the empiricist/behaviorist curriculum-development paradigm used in nursing is antithetical to the graduation of the kinds of nurses needed in today's health care system. To support this assertion requires an examination of the health problems facing the world: increases in the numbers of eldest elderly, prolonged survival of the chronically ill and disabled, and the global epidemic of acquired immune deficiency syndrome (AIDS). All three of these are problems for which nursing care is *the* major health industry provider (Diamond, 1988; Smith, 1988). Therefore, it can be assumed that the need for nursing care will rise logarithmically and that nursing personnel shortages will continue to be an industry problem. Nursing care for persons with these health problems requires nurses who are compassionate, well educated, creative, capable of independent judgment and action, and morally astute and courageous. Our very technology mandates this.

Advances in medical science have brought us to impossible choices that disturb our deepest sense of ethics and our moral commitments as nurses. Our ability to enable more people to live out the full extent of human life expectancy has had a major effect on the strains now placed upon the ability of society and nursing to cope with the numbers of persons needing health and nursing care. As a result, we can make the following assumptions:

1. Practicing nurses must be ethically grounded and must be perspicacious, wise, and compassionate in order to shoulder their share of responsibility for the morality of health care.

2. Medical science will continue to place emphasis upon high levels of technology. Nurses must not only be able to work effectively in these technically complex environments, but they must also be able to humanize these environments with caring and concern so that clients are persons, not objects of health care.

3. The increasing numbers of persons with health problems brought about by aging, chronicity, and AIDS will stress the health care system to the point that the fiscal balance of the country will be placed in jeopardy.

4. The United States is the only developed country in the world except South Africa that allows 37 million of its population to be without any form of health care coverage. Most of these are nonwhite, women, or children. This cannot endure for long in a "civilized" nation.

5. These problems require a total shift in the health care paradigm. Nursing will need to assume a major role in the restructuring process both in policy setting and in care delivery.

These health problems and issues are the ones that will be faced by current and future graduates. It is posited that the current nursing educational paradigm does not support the graduation of persons capable of fulfilling these roles. The proposition is offered that only by being educated as scholar-clinicians can nurses be professionals who are responsive to the needs of society for compassionate, skilled nursing care.

THE FOUR SIGNIFICANT CURRICULUM-DEVELOPMENT MODELS

Every present requires an understanding and appreciation of the past. Without that perspective, we grow intolerant of the pace of change, and our progress would be more often circular than it is already. Each new generation would repeat the errors and forget the successes of the preceding generation. Progress requires memory. Memory enables us to analyze where we have been, where we are going, and to generate new approaches for bettering our efforts. Therefore, it makes sense to examine the history of how we got from there to here, and then to explore some of the issues that influence the next step—a step forward.

When examining the past of nursing education, one can see that there have been four significant changes, or turns, in direction and substance of curriculum models. Each turn took us further along the way to more humanistic, society-responsive, caring, intelligent nursing care by improving the way nurses were taught to nurse.

The First Turn

"The first hopeful step toward reform," said Stewart (1947), in speaking of nursing education in the Western world, came in the 17th century from the French Sisters of Charity. Until that time, untrained helpers, mostly servants, were nurses. The older system of ascetic religious orders still persisted to some extent in Catholic holy orders, but basic nursing care was given by untrained, often illiterate, persons or by those in the servant classes. When the order was formed in 1633, the prescribed course of study was a 2-month probationary period followed by 7–8 months of instruction and supervision. The instruction consisted of lectures, quizzes, and religious exercises. It was successful during the life of its founders, St. Vincent De Paul and St. Louise de Marillac, but deteriorated after their deaths. It had a resurgence in modern times and is still a force in the nursing world today. It is an interesting coincidence of history to observe the Mlle. le Gras and Florence Nightingale had many parallels. Mlle. le Gras (née Louise de Marillac), belonged to a family popular in the court circles of late-16th and early-17th century France. The daughter of Marie de Medici's male secretary, she was well educated in Latin, Greek, literature, philosophy, the sciences, and the arts (Pennock, 1940). She was as much an educational anomaly for her time as was Nightingale.

Part of this same turn in nursing curriculum was composed of the Lutheran Deaconesses at Kaiserwerth. The Fliedners, in founding the Lutheran Deaconesses, followed the general guidelines of the Sisters of Charity, except that they prescribed that study be concurrent with practice in the field (*Encyclopaedia Britannica*, 1968; Stewart, 1947).

Protestant motherhouses spread, and the Sisters of Charity experienced a resurgence. The curriculum pattern consisted of three parts: the practical (skills and procedures); the theoretical, made up of rules and precepts regarding practice; and the code of conduct containing the ideals and general philosophy, loyalties, and obligations of nurses (Stewart, 1947).

The Second Turn and the Beginning of Modern Nursing

The second turn in curriculum development occurred in 1860, due, of course, to the efforts of the founder of modern nursing. Enough has been written about Florence Nightingale and the school at St. Thomas that it need only be briefly mentioned here.

The school had two types of nurses, lady probationers and ordinary probationers. Note that "probationer" is the term used for the full year of training, not the first few months, as became common in the 20th century. There was a year of training (probationary) and 3 years of hospital service as part of the obligation. The curriculum was based upon required characteristics and functions. There were 12 character-istics, according to the "Duties of Probationers under the Nightingale Fund," written by Florence Nightingale (1867). Probationers were re-quired to be "sober, honest, truthful, trustworthy, punctual, quiet, and orderly, cleanly and neat, patient, cheerful, and kindly" (p. 304). (It can be presumed that at the successful end of their obligation, they were sainted rather than graduated.)

The functions were a list of what we would now call "competencies." It is interesting to note that the content of these 13 functions and skills may have changed, and certainly the equipment with which the work is done has changed, but the basics (except for leeching and applying fomentations and poultices) are familiar to any nurse. Florence Nightin-gale, in providing the "Duties of Probationer under the 'Nightingale Fund'" (1867), wrote:

You are expected to become skillful:

1. In the dressing of blisters, burns, sores, wounds, and in apply-ing fomentations, poultices, and minor dressings.
2. In the application of leeches, externally and internally.
3. In the administration of enemas for men and women.
4. In the management of trusses, and appliances in uterine com-plaints.
5. In the best method of friction to the body and extremities.
6. In the management of helpless patients, *i.e.*, moving, changing, personal cleanliness of, feeding, keeping warm, (or cool,) pre-venting and dressing bed sores, managing position of.

7. In bandaging, making bandages, and rollers, lining of splints, etc.

8. In making beds of patients, and removal of sheets whilst patient is in bed.

9. You are required to attend at operations.

10. To be competent to cook gruel, arrowroot, egg flip, puddings, drinks, for the sick.

11. To understand ventilation, or keeping the ward fresh by night as well as by day; you are to be careful that great cleanliness is observed in all the utensils; those used for the secretions as well as those required for cooking.

12. To make strict observation of the sick in the following particulars:—

    The state of secretions, expectoration, pulse, skin, appetite; intelligence, as delirium or stupor; breathing, sleep, state of wounds, eruptions, formation of matter, effect of diet, or of stimulants, and of medicines.

13. And to learn the management of convalescents. (pp. 304–305)

It was a well-organized curriculum, highly structured and exported all over the world. It was an idea whose time was right. But, shortly after it was imported to the United States, the Nightingale model started to deteriorate, and the expansion of nursing schools without controls or standards led to the exploitation of students and to poor nursing care.

The Third Turn: The Age of the Curriculum Guides

Improvements were being made here and there, including some movement into higher education, but there was no real third "turn" in curriculum until the publication of the *Standard Curriculum,* prepared by the Education Committee of the League of Nursing Education in 1917. Described as an "optimum" curriculum so that schools could voluntarily improve their programs, it came about at a time when state requirements were minimal and not at all uniform. The League's book provided objectives, content, and methods for each course and listed materials, equipment, and bibliographies. It even provided a schedule for operating a school on an 8-hour plan (a new concept for that time). The objectives were not the prescriptive behavioral objectives to which we have grown accustomed today but instead were more in the line of general and specific goals. It was revised in 1927 with the word "Standard" dropped from the title. A third revision was published in 1937 under the title of *A Curriculum Guide for Schools of Nursing.* World

War II came along and so changed nursing that the book was never again revised. It left a vacuum.

From the postwar 1940s until the mid-1950s, there was a hiatus in curriculum-development paradigms. The old *Curriculum Guide* was not republished and nothing else existed.

The Fourth Turn: Tyler and Behaviorist Theory

Into this vacuum came the fourth turn in curriculum development, the adoption of the Tyler model (1949) and its institutionalization by the approval and accrediting bodies at state and national levels.

In 1955, Ole Sand published the report of 3 years of action research in curriculum revision, conducted at the University of Washington School of Nursing with Ralph Tyler as consultant. That publication substantiated the practicality of using the Tyler Rationale to develop nursing curriculum, and the methodology of curriculum development used and recommended to American nursing educators was, of course, the Tyler model.

THE MOVE TO COLLEGES AND UNIVERSITIES

The context in which the Tyler model was institutionalized is significant and merits consideration here. Unrelated to curriculum-development models, a great deal of progress in nursing education was being made, especially in the movement of nursing education from hospital-based training programs to academic settings. As early as 1893; a university program for nursing was established at Howard University in Washington, D.C. It was, however, short lived. In 1898, university courses for graduate nurses were developed in New York in Teachers College at Columbia University, although a real university school of nursing that endured was not founded until 1909. In that year, the University of Minnesota "put the whole school of nursing connected with its university hospital on a dignified standing as a professional school of the university" (Dock & Stewart, 1925). Nursing needed to be in control of its own practice, its education, and its research. To do this required movement into settings of higher education. During the 50 years that followed, more than 350 college and university schools of nursing opened.

A second educational factor that greatly influenced nursing practice was the experiment by Mildred Montag (1951), who, like Nightingale, structured two levels of nursing. This was also the advice of nursing educational experts (Brown, 1948; Chayer, 1947; Wolf, 1947). Montag designed a 2-year course of study for "technical nurses" and tried them out in a funded project with selected 2-year community colleges.

Following Montag's successful experiment (1951), hundreds of 2-year colleges developed associate of arts degree nursing programs, gradually filling the slot in the health care scene held by hospital diploma schools. So it was that the midcentury found baccalaureate programs emerging to herald a new era: real higher education for nursing.

Higher education for nurses was designed to move nursing toward professionalism, a shift that placed professional nursing education (baccalaureate programs) on a base of 2 years of prerequisite courses and liberal arts. However, unlike the traditional professions such as theology, law, and medicine, nursing has attempted to include both the cognates (prerequisites and liberal arts) and the professional courses in a 4-year baccalaureate program. The truncation of the professional curriculum into only 4 years left nursing with many unsolved problems, the most obvious being that 4 years is inadequate time to provide the liberal arts necessary to the humanities-based professional nurse. The generic master's and generic doctorate in nursing are approaches to solving this problem.

During the 1950s and throughout the 1960s and 1970s, there was a geometric explosion of college-based programs and a corresponding decrease in hospital schools. One interesting aspect of this explosion was the exclusive use of the Tyler model to develop curriculum in both types of programs. In those years of progress using the Tyler model, few questioned the assumption that the same model was valid for both technical and professional programs. A second problem, perhaps unrelated to truncation but equally enigmatic, developed. It was during this time of tremendous growth in collegiate nursing education that the fourth turn in nursing curriculum development occurred. The usefulness and practicality of the Tyler model for training caused it to become the only model acceptable to approval and accrediting bodies for use in developing nursing curriculum in all levels of nursing education, hospital, community college, and baccalaureate programs despite its limitations for professional education.

THE TYLER RATIONALE

First published as *Syllabus for Education 360* at the University of Chicago in 1949 and then reprinted in 1950 as *Basic Principles of Curriculum and*

Instruction, Tyler's book of 128 pages has had a massive impact on education around the world and has become mandatory practice for schools of nursing. His paradigm states that a curriculum developer needs to ask four questions:

1. What educational purposes should the school establish?
2. What learning experiences should be selected which will likely be useful in attaining these objectives?
3. How can learning experiences be organized for effective instruction?
4. How can the school ascertain whether or not the purposes are being attained?

When Tyler raises questions about purposes, he is in fact (if one reads his discussion on pp. 3–43) writing about behavioral objectives. He says they are derived from three sources: the students, the society, and the subject matter. These tentative objectives are then "screened" through the accepted faculty philosophy and a psychology of learning. When the screening process is finished, what is left is a refined list of objectives that are to be stated in a form helpful in guiding teaching and selecting learning experiences and are couched in terms that reflect the changes required in the student's behavior.

Next, the learning episodes are selected that will promote attaining the objectives and are then organized for instruction into a program of study, courses, and units. Last, procedures for evaluation are examined. Since it is a behaviorist model, Tyler goes straight to the heart of the matter by stating:

> The process of evaluation begins with the objectives of the educational program. Since the purpose is to see how far these objectives are actually being realized, it is necessary to have evaluation procedures that will give evidence about each of the kinds of behavior implied by each of the major educational objectives. (p. 110)

This model makes a neat, circular package that begins with identifying behaviors and ends with evaluating to see whether those behaviors that have been identified have been met. Since it is behaviorist, it holds that all learning is manifested in changes in behavior. If behavior has not changed, learning has not taken place (see Fig. 1).

Figure 1
The Tyler Curriculum-Development Paradigm

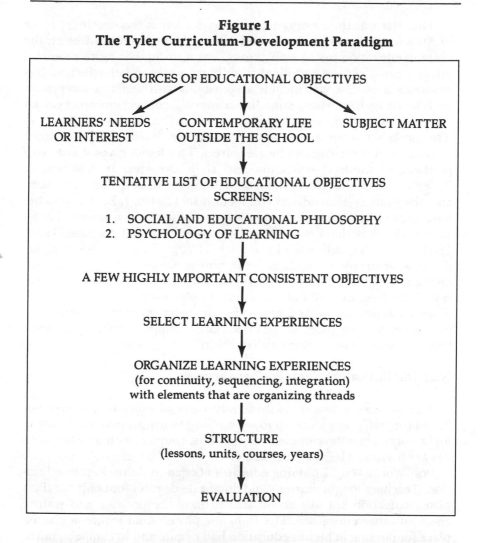

SOURCES OF EDUCATIONAL OBJECTIVES

LEARNERS' NEEDS   CONTEMPORARY LIFE   SUBJECT MATTER
OR INTEREST   OUTSIDE THE SCHOOL

TENTATIVE LIST OF EDUCATIONAL OBJECTIVES
SCREENS:
1. SOCIAL AND EDUCATIONAL PHILOSOPHY
2. PSYCHOLOGY OF LEARNING

A FEW HIGHLY IMPORTANT CONSISTENT OBJECTIVES

SELECT LEARNING EXPERIENCES

ORGANIZE LEARNING EXPERIENCES
(for continuity, sequencing, integration)
with elements that are organizing threads

STRUCTURE
(lessons, units, courses, years)

EVALUATION

INSTITUTIONALIZATION OF THE TYLER PARADIGM IN NURSING EDUCATION

The Emergence of Behaviorism

A great many forces merged to make it inevitable that nursing would institutionalize the Tyler paradigm through its accrediting and approval bodies.

The first was the emergence of behaviorism as the dominant force in American education. By the mid-1940s, the influence of Dewey, the giant in education for so many years, was waning. His more powerful but less easily researched ideas rapidly gave way to behaviorism. (*Behaviorism* is used here to include all positions with similar assumptions, such as neobehaviorism, stimulus–response, connectionism, associationism, and operant conditioning.) Behaviorism, in short, adheres to Thorndike's famous assertion that "whatever exists, exists in some amount" and therefore can be measured. This belief gives shelter to a plethora of kindred educators and their theories. In addition to Tyler's ends-means curriculum-development model, there are such contributions as Thorndike's connectionism (1949), J. B. Watson's behaviorism (1924), Skinner's stimulus–response-associationism (1953), Bloom's work both on mastery and on the educational domains (1956, 1968), Gagne's conditions of learning (1970), and Taba's learning activity or inverted curriculum-development model (1962). These are only a few of the writers who formed and influenced modern education. The sheer quantity of the work of behaviorists is overpowering. They are articulate spokespersons for the behaviorist movement. Furthermore, all—or most all—curriculum-evaluation paradigms arise from the empiricist-behaviorist tradition.

Nursing Educators Seek Higher Degrees

The persuasive power of these advocates of behaviorism may not have been sufficient alone to move nursing to institutionalize a behaviorist curriculum-development model, but, coupled with another accident of history, it became inevitable.

Post-World War II nursing educators began to desire higher education. Teachers sought master's and doctorate degrees, not only for their own satisfaction but also to be able to have the prestige and stature awarded other educators. The fight for professional legitimacy and a place for nursing in higher education had begun, and to compete, nurse educators had to seek higher degrees. Because of the dearth of master's programs in nursing (and the complete absence of doctoral programs in the late 1940s and 1950s), nursing teachers seeking higher education majored in fields that promised some relationship to nursing. Most popular were subjects such as education, sociology, anthropology, microbiology, business, anatomy, and physiology. For teachers and nursing educational administrators, degrees in education were by far the most popular. Even today, with fairly easy access to doctoral programs in nursing, the doctorate in education remains a popular degree for nurse educators.

The progression of events is obvious. Nursing educators seeking higher degrees received them in schools of education. Schools of education were being swept by a tidal wave of behaviorist literature. The Tyler curriculum-development paradigm was the outstanding model, and all other models studied were those that prescribed the same or similar products as the Tyler model or had variations on it. (These were philosophy, conceptual framework, behavioral objectives for program, level, course, unit, and learning activity, and a program of studies and criteria for evaluating student progress that were built on the behavioral objectives.) Teachers, earning degrees in schools of education, came back into nursing schools armed with the logic of behaviorism and backed by Sand's work at the University of Washington School of Nursing.

Improving the Accrediting and Approval Processes and the Institutionalization of Behaviorism

Concurrently with the increasing influence of behaviorism on nursing curriculum, state boards of nursing were seeking ways to change from the traditional quantitative method of approving programs to a more qualitative one. Most state boards of nursing, empowered by state laws to govern and regulate the quality of nursing schools, did little beyond counting the "experiences" of students. Programs were approved if they provided the required number of days in each of the designated services, for example, the specified numbers of deliveries, scrubs, and circulation nurse experiences in the operating room and so many days in the supply room, the linen room, the nursery, pediatrics, post partal, general medicine, general surgery, and other places deemed necessary. It was an improvement to examine schools to determine that they had the correct curriculum-development products according to the Tyler-type paradigm and that there was consistency among the parts.

Accreditation by the National League of Nursing Education avoided the mistakes of the state approval agencies. Requiring "numbers" of experience tended to stereotype programs and to decrease freedom and initiative by virtue of the counting of days or experiences. The first National League of Nursing Education accreditation visits were completed in 1939, and the first list of 70 schools was issued in 1941. When the Tyler curriculum paradigm came along in 1950, it furnished some fresh ideas to the membership. By the late 1950s and early 1960s, the criteria for the appraisal of all three types of programs reflected the

Tyler Rationale. Gradually state boards of nursing adopted this more reasonable method. Thus, the Tyler curriculum-development paradigm became institutionalized by state boards of nursing and the NLN. Through the use of regulations, criteria, and the way visitors were oriented, these powerful agencies made it mandatory to use a philosophy, concepts or strands, and all levels of behavioral objectives for every one of the wide variety of types of nondoctoral programs in nursing: diploma, associate of arts, baccalaureate, and master's.

One consequence of this forced "sameness" in curriculum-development model was some degree of similarity in the graduates. It was, and is, very difficult to differentiate among graduates of the three most popular types of generic programs: diploma, associate of arts, and baccalaureate. The mandated sameness in the curriculum-development model has not been the single cause; nothing is that simple. While many factors have had an influence, certainly the utilization of the same curriculum-development model—and that one a technical or training model—is a major factor.

Among the forces that affirmed the Tyler-type, curriculum-development products as nursing curriculum dogma were two more that should be mentioned. The first and most obvious is Bevis' book on curriculum-development (Bevis, 1972). This book, the first to translate primary and secondary school curriculum-development behaviorist theory into a useful handbook for the practice field of nursing, became a standard text for students in curriculum courses and faculty working to develop curriculum. The second force was Mager. Soon after the publication of his book, *Preparing Instructional Objectives* (1962), workshops were held throughout the United States to ensure that every nurse educator had an opportunity to attend sessions to learn to write and use "measurable, behavioral objectives" correctly. The reverence for behavioral objectives reached such a peak (and remains there) that even their development has become formula driven and rigid.

At present the Tyler-type, curriculum-development products have been translated into essential components. Without evidence of these components, there cannot be approval by the state board of nursing. Therefore, if a school does not follow the technical models and cannot show the products of these models, its graduates are not allowed to take licensure examinations. Until recently, a school also could not be accredited.[1] That is institutionalization at its most powerful. Beginning in 1988

---

[1]The present posture of the NLN Council of Baccalaureate and Higher Degree Programs is to support paradigms transcending self-study criteria, thereby permitting a wide choice of curriculum-development paradigms.

with the National Nurse Educator Conference in Philadelphia, and the sixth edition of the *Criteria for the Appraisal of Baccalaureate and Higher Degree Programs in Nursing* (1988), the NLN Council of Baccalaureate and Higher Degree Programs began the long and difficult task of deinstitutionalization of the Tyler model. It took about 10 years for it to be institutionalized and to consolidate its mastery over nursing curriculum. In all, it enjoyed a 35-year reign without competition. One can hope that it can be deinstitutionalized without loss of quality and that paradigm transcending criteria will be devised.

BENEFITS OF THE TYLER MODEL FOR NURSING

This model has done much for nursing. The strict insistence of measurable behavioral objectives backed by the force of law, custom, and accreditation has focused the training and instructional aspects of nursing in such a way as to lift it to a highly organized, evaluation-oriented, and regulated group that provides services of reliable quality. Along with improved state rules and regulations governing schools, licensure, and excellent accreditation procedures, schools of nursing have attained a quality seen in few other service fields. They have an ability to monitor and police themselves that is unusual and a sense of responsibility and commitment to the public trust that is not found in any like group such as medical, legal, or clerical. This, of course, is not due exclusively to Tyler's curriculum model. However, Tyler's curriculum-development products became tools to be used in the search for quality and then, sadly, ends in themselves.

THE LIMITATIONS OF THE BEHAVIORIST, TYLER PARADIGM AND THE NEED FOR A NEW DIRECTION FOR NURSING CURRICULUM DEVELOPMENT

What was, and in some ways still is, a blessing to excellence in nursing care in an earlier phase of the profession's development has become a liability and danger in achieving its current developmental task, that of graduating educated, caring scholar-clinicians capable of meeting the complex needs of today's society. Since Tyler-type models are all that are known in nursing, these models are used for all curriculum development without ascertaining whether or not other models exist that might be better for some levels of nursing education. Perhaps, what was good for nursing education in its developmental phase, and still has qualities that are helpful to some of the training aspects of nursing, promises to be a liability when used for developing the professional level of curriculum. In other words, all generic nursing education, which is the initial nursing education leading to licensure, has some content that lends itself to behaviorism regardless of level. But for certain aspects of baccalaureate education and most of master's and doctoral education, it is too limiting. One of the main problems of the model is the requirement that behavioral objectives be devised for all planned learning. Another is the rigidity and narrowness of the model's conceptualization of behavioral objectives.

As conceived, behavioral objectives as the sole arbiters of learning are too narrow and lack the creative energy necessary to guide the awakening discovery that must earmark true education. Behavioral objectives represent minimal achievement levels, are useful primarily for skill training and instruction, and leave no room for the student's individual interest pursuits, enculturation into the profession, and introduction to the ways of identifying, classifying, and solving the problems of the discipline. They stifle creativity and provide rigid and restrictive guides for evaluations. When one remembers that evaluations and the feedback thereby derived, including grades, are the essence of reinforcement (a behaviorist concept) in learning, one can see how restrictive behavioral objectives can be. If used exclusively—and the Tyler-type, technical curriculum-development models currently are the only sanctioned models—they become inhibitors of achievement of the very purposes of professional education, both undergraduate and graduate.

Essentially, behavioral objectives spell out what the faculty perceives as important (and those only if they are concrete, i.e., measurable behaviors) and ignore the student's values, interest, and natural bent. Because of their nature, they cannot facilitate the achievement of goals that are not empirically verifiable. Behavioral objectives are congruent with empiricism and training but are out of step with transformative education and nursing as a human science.

Watson (1988) offers the following criticism:

> In nursing it is easy to fall prey to current trends and fads of education and practice. Nursing is becoming established as an academic discipline that requires a liberal arts education. It is therefore incumbent on the profession and the academic community to adhere to the purpose of a university education—to gain knowledge and understanding. More energy is now expended in the acquisition of scientific knowledge than of understanding. Nursing tries to understand people and how they cope with health and illness.

. . . It [nursing] tries to understand how health and illness and human behavior are interrelated. Nursing education rarely concentrates on that level of understanding. In some ways nursing schools are still technical, professional schools. Many teachers and schools state attempts to develop self-actualization. However, they end up hidden, primarily teaching specialized terminology, procedures, scientific principles, the basic content of behavior, pathophysiology, and the disease processes.

Teaching mostly the rules and procedures—the "trim"—of nursing does not lead to understanding people and how they cope with health and illness. Even if all the rules and procedures could be taught (they cannot), many things taught today are outdated in a few years. (pp. 2–3)

This is a commentary on some of the problems professional programs face *because* of the behaviorist orientation of curriculum and the resulting measurable objectives that determine curriculum. Understanding cannot be and should not be measured. Other characteristics necessary to nursing as a human science exceed our measurement skills, and attempts to measure them place them in the reductionistic-mechanistic-materialistic sphere. Compassion, caring, loving, pain, hope, suffering, wonder, and excitement are human experiences that occur daily to the vulnerable persons who are our clients and to nurses giving care to those vulnerable persons. Criticism may be given to nurses learning to use themselves as instruments of healing, but measurement is out of place.

Kliebard (1968) puts it even more strongly than Watson:

From a moral point of view, the emphasis on behavioral goals, despite all of the protestations to the contrary, still borders on brainwashing or at least indoctrination rather than education. We begin with some notion of how we want a person to behave and then we try to manipulate him and his environment so as to get him to behave as we want him to. (p. 246)

Nursing uses the Tyler Rationale in a way never intended by Tyler: as a "guide" to a code—laws so immutable as to make the Ten Commandments easier to break without bringing down organized condemnation and punitive consequences. Currently, regardless of the deviations, reorganization, or alterations in approach conceived by curriculum experts, the products of curriculum-development remain Tyler-type products: philosophy, screens that evolved into a conceptual framework, measurable (behavioral) objectives, and a plan for evaluating learning based

upon the objectives. These products and codified processes have constituted nursing educational dogma and created a single-track educational
prescription that has ignored all aspects of education not covered by
behaviors and *finite* preconceived measurable outcomes. This has as
consequence a curriculum that for the professional level is inadequate
and limited in its conception and its implementation. It leaves as irrele-
vant the unmeasurable mass of individually conceived, individually discovered, creative body of things learned by experiences both directed
and not directed by teachers—learning possibilities that sometimes,
most times, are not even imagined by teachers and curriculum developers. It discounts insights, analysis, and detail—formed and unformed
into patterns.

It discards any and all joy taken by the student in the private world of
discovery, in walks alone through the peaks and valleys of the student's
own mind. It ignores what Watson calls "soul." Watson uses the concept
of soul to refer to the

> geist, spirit, inner self, or essence of the person, which is tied to a
> greater sense of self-awareness, a higher degree of consciousness,
> an inner strength, and a power that can expand human capacities
> and allow a person to transcend his or her usual self. The higher
> sense of consciousness and valuing of inner self can cultivate a fuller
> access to the intuitive and even sometimes allow uncanny, mystical,
> or miraculous experiences, modes of thought, feelings, and action
> that we have all experienced at some points in our life, but from
> which our rational, scientific cultures bar us. (Watson, 1988, p. 46)

To ignore this idea places in peril the professionalism all nurses strive
for. That is because that "soul" is the unique human science orientation,
the human caring-human experience component, of the developing
field of nursing.

Educative learning is, after all, a private journey that nourishes the
student's selfhood. The public, prescribed journey is not so much educative as instructive learning and leads only to smartness, whereas the
private journey leads to wisdom.

Behaviorism can produce efficient nurses on a technical level. The
long, successful use of behavioral objectives has proven this beyond any
doubt. What it cannot do is to support the changes necessary to keep pace
with society's changing demands and the natural evolution of nursing as a
profession. What is sought for nursing education is a legitimization of
the practical elements and aspects of curriculum; an endorsement of the

dynamic, creative whole of education; a legitimization of what many educators are doing "under the table": the teaching of inquiry, reflection, criticism, independence, creativity, and caring, inclusive of all aspects of nursing education—planned, prescribed, accidental, individual, public, and private. A methodology for curriculum development is needed that will provide a new graduate, a substantively different graduate, because the curriculum-development process has different outcomes. It emphasizes the selection of experiences and the character and quality of teacher–student interactions rather than the closely held, highly structured prescribed outcomes. The graduate must be different because the values are different, the emphasis placed is different, and the roles of teachers and students are different. The consequence must be a substantively different graduate.

Therefore, it is essential that nursing educators and curriculum experts seek a new model for curriculum development that offers a means for developing curriculum that will facilitate students in cultivating creative, dynamic modes of approaching nursing care. This can be achieved only with different products of curriculum development— ones that provide a wider range of options, a greater scope of ideas, a valuing of process-teaching strategies, teacher development as primary goal and curriculum development as its by-product, a deliberate placement of student creative thought as the essence of education, and an underlying assumption that nursing is a human science.

REFERENCES

Bevis, E. O. (1972). *Curriculum building in nursing: A process.* St. Louis: C. V. Mosby.

Bloom, B. S., Englehart, M. D., Furst, E. J., Hill, W. H., & Drathwohl, D. R. (Eds.), (1956). *Taxonomy of educational objectives.* New York: Longmans, Green.

Bloom, B. (1968, May). Learning for mastery. *Evaluation Comment,* 1–11.

Brown, E. L. (1948). *Nursing for the future.* New York: Russell Sage Foundation.

Chayer, M. (1947). *Nursing in modern society.* New York: G. P. Putnam's Sons.

Dock, L., & Stewart, I. (1920). *A short history of nursing.* New York: G. P. Putnam's Sons.

Diamond, M. (1988). *Nursing and the aging chronically ill.* Paper presented at the 16th Annual Meeting and Scientific Session of the American Academy of Nursing.

Encyclopaedia Britannica (Vol. 17). (1968). Chicago: William Benton.

Gagne, R. (1970). *The conditions of learning* (2nd ed.). New York: Holt, Rinehart and Winston.

James, W. (1912). *Talks to teachers on psychology: And to students on some of life's ideals.* New York: Henry Holt and Company.

Kliebard, H. (1968). Curricular objectives and evaluation: A reassessment. *The High School Journal,* 241–247.

Mager, R. (1962). *Preparing instructional objectives.* Belmont, CA: Feron Publishers.

Montag, M. (1951). *The education of nursing technicians.* New York: Putnam.

Munhall, P. (1981). Nursing philosophy and nursing research: In apposition or opposition? *Nursing Research, 31*(3), 176–181.

National Council of State Boards of Nursing. Telephone conversation with staff regarding data for NCLEX, July, 1988.

National League for Nursing. (1988). *Criteria for the appraisal of baccalaureate and higher degree programs in nursing* (6th ed.). New York: National League for Nursing.

National League of Nursing Education, Committee on Curriculum. (1917, 1927, 1937). *A curriculum guide for schools of nursing.* New York: National League of Nursing Education.

Nightingale, F. (1954). Suggestions on the subject of providing, training, and organizing nurses for the sick poor in workhouse infirmaries. In L. Seymer (Ed.), *Selected writings of Florence Nightingale.* New York: Macmillan. (Original work published 1867).

Pennock, M. (Ed.). (1940). *Makers of nursing history, portraits and pen sketches of one-hundred and nine prominent women.* New York: Lakeside Publishing Company.

Sand, O. (1955). *Curriculum study in basic nursing education.* New York: G. P. Putnam's Sons.

Skinner, B. F. (1953). *Science and human behavior.* New York: Macmillan.

Smith, G. (1988). *Influencing public policy: Rethinking the public health nursing practice dilemma.* Paper presented at the 16th Annual Meeting and Scientific Session of the American Academy of Nursing.

Stewart, I. (1947). *The education of nurses, historical foundations and modern trends.* New York: Macmillan.

Taba, H. (1962). *Curriculum development, theory and practice.* New York: Harcourt, Brace and World.

Thorndike, E. L. (1949). *Selected writings from a connectionist's psychology.* New York: Appleton-Century-Crofts.

Tyler, R. W. (1949). *Basic principles of curriculum and instruction.* Chicago: University of Chicago Press.

Watson, J. (1988). *Nursing: Human science and human care: A theory of nursing.* New York: National League for Nursing.

Watson, J. B. (1924). *Psychology from the standpoint of behaviorist* (2nd ed.). Philadelphia: Lippincott.

Wolf, L. K. (1947). *Nursing.* New York: Appleton-Century.

BIBLIOGRAPHY

Grove, P. (1971). *Webster's new international dictionary of the English language unabridged.* Springfield, MA: Merriam.

Watson, J. (1985). *Nursing: The philosophy and science of caring.* Boulder, CO: Colorado Associated University Press.

2

A New Paradigm of
Curriculum Development

Jean Watson

PHILOSOPHICAL FOUNDATION

The philosophical foundation for this curricular approach is based upon a belief in human freedom and what Maxine Greene (1978) calls a "Wide-Awakeness" in education—a wide-awakeness that she says is paradigm shattering and emancipatory. Such an approach calls for encouragement of self-reflection wherein the educators can come in touch with their own humanity and encourage the release of the human spirit in teaching–learning processes—caring processes that must be considered in nursing education as we seek to facilitate learning associated with human health and healing processes and expert human caring practices.

What we seek here is what Greene highlights in *Landscapes of Learning* (1978), that is, esthetic, moral, and intellectual encounters that disturb as well as confuse, because attention is paid to experiences and questions that have an emancipatory function. As she puts it, learning is a process of "'I' meeting the 'I'," which involves a futuring, a going beyond, what is not yet. In the current structure of education there is the tendency to deal with effectiveness and efficiency, often void of subjective human meanings. Such approaches become independent of moral propriety and have a bent toward equalizing the very condition of being human (Greene, 1978). The "Wide-Awakeness" of landscape

Greene proposes calls for an informed passion that frames the very perceptions and questions about knowledge and reality.

Nursing knowledge and learning processes for the future require much more thought, contemplation, and reflection upon the very concepts and phenomena associated with dramatically changing human conditions and life processes. In acknowledging a new philosophical starting point for nursing curriculum, we hope to stimulate critique and change. As we know, if we allow our teaching–learning approaches and knowledge to become "set" for too long, knowledge is used for domination and control. Furthermore, there is the danger of *fixing* the vision for the next generation on a reality that others have already defined.

This position of human freedom as a starting point for professional nursing education and practice is what distinguishes this work from the dominant curricular models of education generally and nursing education in particular. The officially sanctioned, dominant model of nursing education is based on control and conformity of the human mind and spirit—an ideology of dualism and a tendency to split emotional-rational-cognitive-personal-intuitive, and so on. Thus, the dominant approach separates fact from value and meaning, separates subject and object, focuses on value-free intellectual, factual, technical education and pedagogies to the exclusion of the intentional, the relational, the intersubjective, the contextual, the evolving, growing human consciousness, and the realization that all knowledge is constructed as a human endeavor, just as teacher–learning is a profoundly human and moral endeavor.

Nursing education and the medical care system parallel each other with their common emphasis on objectivist interventions, based upon a rationalist view of both science and education. Thus, nursing education has been handicapped by an oppressive model in both worlds of learning and practice; therefore, philosophical values and theory, and science and research, have become fragmented and often distinct from the nurse's internal human experiences associated with human care and caring in practice.

Until recently, nursing's dominant educational ideology was viewed as a neutral technical process, associated with biomedical science empiricism and a set of care tasks and functions (Moccia, 1988); imparting a form of technocratic rationality, void of human meaning and values (Greene, 1988); void of moral commitment, intentions, goals and moral ideals, or the covenantal relationship (Gadow, 1988) associated with human caring (healing and wholeness).

As Stevenson and Woods (1986) emphasized in their keynote address to the American Academy of Nursing, in the main to date, in spite of what we may profess, published nursing research has conformed to an empiricist view of science, and nursing theory, science, and philosophy have little relation to each other. Likewise, nursing education, in spite of what we may profess, teaches mostly the rules and procedures, rights and wrongs, specialized terminology, symptom and problem identification, basic disease processes, and technical interventions (Watson, 1985).

We all know that more is at stake in education than intellectual, technical growth and in health than treating disease and curing illness, to the exclusion of human caring–healing now called for in science and society. Self-understanding and connectedness is now deemed essential to human problem solving and even discovery of new knowledge. As Greene says, even committed rationality rests on . . . self-reflection.

In *Scientific Genius,* Simonton (1989) says that it is the intuitive, rather than analytical intellect, that is associated with subjective interconnections—interconnections that facilitate human's tendency toward self-organization of mental elements that underlie the creative processes of great science. The scientific learning discovery process appears to be more oriented toward discovery of order, harmony, and, in a word, beauty. Simonton points out that mental elements are both conscious and unconscious and must be free to enter into various combinations. He actually draws upon Keats' "Beauty is truth, truth beauty" in emphasizing the creative and esthetic aspects of value-based education and science.

Only recently have some of the moral processes and values of educational concerns captured national attention in nursing. The American Association of Colleges of Nursing (AACN) Report on Essential Values (1986), for an educated person and educated nurse, brought national focus to a values dimension as *essential* to nursing education. More recently, the National League for Nursing (NLN), an historically conservative body, sponsored a series of nurse educator conferences (1987, 1988, 1989) on a curriculum revolution, raising issues that mandate significant change in nursing education. The common theme of these conferences was a renewed emphasis of nursing's essential role, mission, commitment and function of *human* caring and a return to the human aspect of nursing and a moral-based educational perspective in our individual settings. The mandate is to shift from a focus on *training* to *education,* from *technique* to *understanding,* from *strict content* to *critical clinical decision making,* from *product line thinking* to *value-based human caring education for an educated person,* as well as an *educated values driven professional.*

The shifts proposed are now acknowledged as fundamental for human survival and the development of humankind (Peccei, 1984, p. xvi). The status quo training type of education has been referred to as maintenance-adaptation type learning versus anticipatory-innovative learning (Botkin, Elmandjra, & Malitza, 1984). Maintenance learning is the acquisition of fixed outlooks, methods, and rules for dealing with known and recurring situations. It works for solving problems that are given, in order to maintain an existing system or an established way; however, maintenance learning is ineffective during times of turbulence, change, or discontinuity, so evident in society today and most dramatically experienced in the changing world of nursing and the broader fields of health and medical care. For example, maintenance learning does not prepare the learner with the capacity to reconcile value conflicts under crisis conditions. Another feature of traditional teaching–learning approaches that perpetuate maintenance learning is the idea that they sustain a mode of unconscious adaptation, the neglect of contexts, the circulation of information with the pretension of being understood (Botkin et al., 1984). However, we are now cognizant of the reality that "as contexts widen and multiply, and as the values that these contexts encompass grow more varied, the process of understanding becomes more difficult" (Botkin et al., 1984, p. 19). The characteristic of maintenance learning is to fall back on reliance of old formulas in the midst of uncertainty, crisis, or change.

The alternative approach to education proposed in this text is more consistent with anticipatory-innovative learning. Such learning is linked to the reality that humanity must not be subjected to the whims of crisis and uncertain destiny, but must be an active participant in guiding its own destiny and not lagging behind events that will determine human conditions (professional nursing practice). Rather, innovative learning is a necessary means of preparing individuals and societies to act in concert in new situations. Anticipatory learning is contrasted with adaptation. As Botkin et al. (1984) point out in the book *No Limits to Learning,* adaptation suggests reactive adjustment to external pressure, and anticipation implies an orientation that prepares for possible contingencies and considers long-range future alternatives. For example, anticipatory learning uses techniques such as forecasting, simulations, scenarios, and models. It encourages teacher and student to consider trends, to make plans, to evaluate future consequences and possible injurious side effects of present decisions, and to recognize the global implications of local, national, and regional actions. Furthermore, it employs imagination, but is based on hard fact as well as values context (pp. 12, 13).

A primary feature of anticipatory-innovative learning is participation. As the book points out, participation is more than the formal sharing of decisions: It is an attitude characterized by cooperation, dialogue, and empathy. It means not only keeping communications open but also constantly testing one's operating rules and values. Anticipatory learning and participation must be tied together in order to be effective. These characteristics need to be combined with values. The context is that one must be willing to question the most fundamental values, purposes, and objectives of any system, and not just reinforce values inherent in the status quo. Furthermore, the "no limits to learning approach" adopts a normative value position as the survival of humanity—however, not "just survival" but also preservation of human dignity and the inherent concept of freedom of the human mind and spirit, consistent with caring and reverence for humanity as a whole, and also the mutual caring and respect for individuals in culturally diverse societies, including self-respect and self-care. All of these features are consistent with the views of Greene, Noddings, and others frequently referenced in this work.

Thus, the notion of medical and nursing science and technocure (Quinn, 1989) knowledge that is given antecedently as maintenance, adaptation learning, independently of knowers and doers and ways-of-being in caring-based education and practice, is rejected. That is, the knower and the known, the one-caring and the one-being-cared-for are both present, each modifying and shaping the other. Therefore, it is now openly acknowledged that knowledge development and the teaching–learning process are distinctly alive anticipatory human processes and participative activities, as opposed to merely cognitive, rational, and technical status quo adaptation.

This work is concerned with release of human creativity, freedom, development of a new consciousness, and morality for nursing education and expert human caring practices. Release of the human imagination and appeal to human freedom, creative critical thinking, and an expanded educational, teaching–learning order is necessary in nursing to create and imagine what *might* be, rather than conform to what is, an educational and medical care system that is in turmoil and chaos; a system that is unable to cope with the changing nature of health and illness, a system that is increasingly unable to respond to the values and ideals of professional nursing. These ideals aspire toward wholeness of mind, body, and spirit within a context of human caring-healing and health.

In the broadest sense, an anticipatory caring approach to nursing education and nursing curriculum is consistent with Maxine Greene's work on the dialectic of freedom (1988). Both caring in education and freedom are concerned with a critical awakening of the evolving human consciousness; the human spirit or life spirit; a consciousness of wholeness, health, and healing; a consciousness of possibility; a release of creative, artistic, and scientific imagination; and a recognition of alternative realities for science and society.

Such a framework for nursing education offers nursing an opportunity to become its full professional self. Moreover, such thinking offers each nursing educator and each nursing student and practitioner the opportunity to more fully actualize and utilize self as the ultimate therapeutic process in a caring–healing relationship, be it in teaching or in clinical practice. Such an orientation to nursing education and practice helps nursing collectively to redefine itself for new health, caring–healing roles demanded for a new century.

As Greene (1986) says, "Such changes can be learned as persons begin to move toward one another, appearing to one another, articulating different perspectives, becoming concerned." She goes on to say, "It is only in our intersubjectivity, our coming together that we create social space for caring, for values literacy, where transformation can occur" (p. 243). Noddings (1988) and Benner and Wrubel (1989) help us to understand the relational aspects of caring in education and nursing care reminding us of the need to refocus on the human beings involved in the ethics and praxis of caring, including concern for relation, responsibility, mutuality, reciprocity, intersubjectivity and informed passion; returning us to the power, if not reverence and regard for the sacred space which each caring occasion potentially contains, be it between educator and student, or between nurse and patient (Watson, 1985).

The Brazilian author of *Pedagogy of the Oppressed* (Freire, 1988) said that our advanced technological society is rapidly making objects of most of us and subtly programming us into conformity. Such processes are linked to human freedom and moral actions. In an anticipatory teaching–learning, curriculum-building sense, caring is informed moral action (Schultz, 1989) that adamantly resists reducing persons (students or patients) to the moral status of object (Gadow, 1985, 1988; Watson, 1985). As such, human caring curricular approaches require a personal, social, moral, scientific, and spiritual engagement of the nurse educator and a commitment to self and other. Thus, anticipatory moral concerns and moral actions associated with preservation of humanity, human dignity, and caring help to inform our knowledge and teaching practices.

Palmer (1987) puts it this way, "I believe that it is here—at the epistemological core of knowledge (our processes of learning and knowing, and our views of person, being, and what it means to be caring)—that our power for forming or deforming human consciousness is to be found. I believe that it is here, in our modes of knowing, (and being in teaching–learning) that we shape souls by the shape of our knowledge" (p. 22, my parenthesis).

It is here in the way we think about human caring that a difference from other disciplines appears; the way we think about human caring as one of the central missions for the profession—not just adaptation to the status quo, but the generation and transmission of anticipatory caring knowledge and practice. It is here in our views of knowing and being that the idea of human caring must take root and have impact if it is to reshape higher education and the larger health care system.

However, to date, our current educational and practice worlds have not had the open context, public space, or what Freire (1988) calls the critical consciousness, the *conscientizacao,* to acknowledge the void, to liberate and free the mind to reflect and imagine how things might be (see Chapters 5 and 6). We have lacked the *conscientizacao* to identify the trouble and sufferings generated by the dominant adaptation-maintenance educational and practice model that has labeled and framed the existential questions (Greene, 1988) about human learning and human caring and healing (in relation to birth, death, wholeness, reverence, sacred covenant, health, pain, anxiety, fear, dread, vulnerability, and "sickness unto death"). It is through the exercise of anticipatory *conscientizacao* that it is "possible for humans to enter the historical educational process as responsible subjects in the search for self-affirmation" (Freire, 1988, p. 20). As Jean-Paul Sartre put it, "It is on the day that we can conceive of a different state of affairs that a new light falls on our troubles and our suffering and that we decide that these are unbearable" (1956, p. 435; in Greene, 1986, p. 237).

In an existential sense, nursing's awareness and commitment to human caring and its responsibilities help us to awaken to our own knowledge and our own unique service to society. Therefore, the development of anticipatory teaching and practice of expert human caring knowledge, knowledge that is values driven and placed within a philosophical and moral context, calls for alternative educational curricular pathways.

Pedagogy for the nonoppressed is required for the new social and professional order emerging in this postmodern era and set forth in this text.

Pedagogy of the sort fundamental to this curriculum approach offers the most fundamental liberation of all—freedom from oppressive thoughts and actions. Because nursing is considered a profession of the oppressed, the issue of human freedom and release of human spirit is foundational for nursing education and practice in a changing and turbulent world. Before moving to the heart of this text, it seems necessary to give some more specific attention to the issue of oppression, however. In light of women and nursing being so intertwined with common sociohistorical influences, a feminist context of nursing's oppression seems warranted.

PEDAGOGY OF THE OPPRESSED AND
A FEMINIST CONTEXT

We are already painfully aware that nursing education, being primarily an education for women has suffered from the sociohistorical political forces of women in society (see Chapter 6). Oppressed groups are controlled by outside forces that have greater prestige, power, and status and therefore can exploit the less powerful group (Lynaugh & Fagin, 1988). While radical feminists insist that women's oppression is the most fundamental form of oppression, enlightened nurses now acknowledge that nursing is a clear paradigm case of women's oppression in society. Not to belabor the connections between female oppression and nursing as an oppressed group, some key points need to be recognized still.

Tong (1989) summarized some of the claims about women's oppression that carry over, directly or indirectly, into nursing as a predominant women's profession, striving for equality in education, practice, and even personhood. These claims are:

1. That women were historically the first oppressed group.
2. That women's oppression is the most widespread, existing in virtually every known society.
3. That women's oppression is the deepest in that it is the hardest form of oppression to eradicate and cannot be removed by other social changes, such as the abolition of class society.
4. That women's oppression causes the most suffering to its victims, qualitatively and quantitatively, although the suffering may often go

unrecognized because of the sexist practices of both the oppressors and the victims.

There is a relationship between women's oppression generally and nursing's oppression specifically, in both education and the medical systems and technocure institutions. After all, hospitals and physicians controlled nursing education and practice until recent times and, to a great extent, still exercise control and barriers to nursing education and practice. Moreover, since we are all subjected to such an ingrained sociohistorical perspective on women, our perspective becomes a world view that is too powerful to ignore but rather needs to be unveiled as outdated myths that perpetuate oppression and directly impact our educational systems. Also, there is a tendency for oppressed groups to oppress others. Darlene Clark Hine, in a recent essay, "They Shall Mount Up with Wings as Eagles: Historical Images of Black Nurses, 1890–1950," reminds us of the treatment given black nurses by fellow nurses, and how black nurses had to overcome racial injustices that were perpetuated and internalized by the nursing profession (in Watson, 1988, p. 61). Nursing has a continuing history of oppressing its young, thereby socializing a new generation into a system of oppression and control that often perpetuates adaptation to the status quo. Thus, oppressive acts of socialization are transmitted from one generation to another.

A major feminist critique tenet of oppression that has hindered women and nursing is the dominant order of patriarchal thinking that invokes duality; a duality that sets humans in opposition to each other; a duality that sets humans in opposition to nature and the larger universe. Thus, traditional linear, oppressive thinking has conceived of a view of humans and what it means to be human; that is, to be separate, independent, distant from and in control over others, with a desire to manipulate others as well as the universe. Likewise, a world view is created wherein what it means to be a physician and what it means to be a nurse is based on a system of control, manipulation, and domination of one (the male subject) over the other (the female object); a system wherein disease is separate from health and something to be controlled, something disconnected from the person and separate from nature, separate from one's relation with a higher order of meaning or the broader universe. Therefore, medical science and curing has been positioned as the highest order of power and control over patients and health–illness, rendering nurses' (and women's) work of caring as a means to the physicians' goal of cure. Nursing, of course, as a subset of medicine, is to be similarly directed, dominated, and controlled.

Kathryn Montgomery Hunter defines the identity crisis of the nursing profession as part of the larger predicament shared by all women—including the experience of social repression and the lack of social value ascribed to caring. She highlights the key point: "Nursing is a metaphor for all women and the problems posed by women for men" (in Watson, 1988, p. 61). Hunter uncovers the surprising fact that the idealized view of nursing and caring in both classic and contemporary literature is portrayed by men not women. For example, she references the literature of Dickens, Kesey, Irving, Tolstoy, and Whitman as presenting *man* to deliver a "translocated ideal of nursing and caring."

Leslie Fiedler has emphasized that "in the popular mind, the deep psyche of the mass audience, not merely . . . does Nurse equal Woman, but on an even profounder mythological level, Woman equals Nurse" (in Watson, 1988, p. 61). The implication, of course, is that not only are stereotypes of woman transferred automatically to the specific category of *nurse,* but it becomes a vicious, entrapping metaphorical circle of almost doubling the stereotype of woman-equal-nurse-equal-woman. Is it any wonder that nursing is considered an oppressed profession, stifled in its educational and practice worth, value, and human and professional goals? Is it any wonder that nursing is the health profession with unmet expectation? Is it any wonder that women nurses oppress other women nurses?

Education and socialization has therefore suffered the plight of maintenance-adaptation education for women generally. More specifically, nursing education has been oppressed, because of the double burden of nurse-equal-woman-equal-nurse phenomenon. On the other side of the issue, however, Wollstonecraft's (1759–1799) early feminist work advocated that women be treated as, and to act as, autonomous decisionmakers. Furthermore, her "cure" for women was to let them be provided with a real education, one that would sharpen and focus the mind and give women a chance to develop rational and moral capacities, and full human potential. These issues are still alive today, 200 years later, with nursing educational patterns and practices a clear example. Wollstonecraft's view was consistent with Kant's perspective on human nature, that unless a person acts autonomously, he or she is acting as less than a fully human person. Thus, society owes females (and nurses) the same education as males (and physicians) because all persons deserve an equal chance to develop their rational and moral capacities so that they can achieve personhood. The connection between this view and feminist thinking is the shared goal of "a just and compassionate society in which freedom flourishes" (Tong, 1989, p. 13).

The educational and practice challenges for nurses is anticipatory-innovative learning that calls for us to rework the world of health care so that the work of both sexes is respected. As Muff says, "nurses for the first time are being asked to define or perhaps redefine their competencies and delineate the boundaries of their profession. Acknowledging that the work of women and nurses is powerful and worthy of reverence will require a reworking of the profession that will challenge the core of traditional patriarchal beliefs" (in Watson, 1988, p. 62).

With this challenge, what is now called for is an approach to education and practice that appeals to freeing human potential, an approach that allows one to develop not only rational and moral capacities, but emotional, expressive, intuitive, esthetic, personal capacities and bring one's full self to bear with one's life work—in this instance, work of human caring. Changes in nursing education and practice can anticipate the highest development of person as one engaged and committed to human caring as a way of being—as a person and as professional; a person and professional with equal privileges and opportunities to study and practice one's life work.

While Wollstonecraft called for a new order for women and education in the 1700s, Annie Goodrich reported in 1917, "A nurse should have a liberal and broad education, languages, history, and the social and physical sciences, and she, like the physician . . . should keep up with the development in her own profession" (p. 48). However, in spite of early advocates for education for women and nurses to be equal with men and physicians, nursing has yet to come of age, even as we enter the next century. Even today we are still having to make a case for education of nurses as women. Nevertheless, times are changing and Annie Goodrich's wisdom prevails and predicts our yet to be, but realizable future. Her 1921 message lingers, "When the public grasps the fact that we are not seeking to elevate nursing into an aristocracy of learning, but to apply all available knowledge, there will no longer be this effort to cramp and stultify her education. And when the doors of knowledge are freely opened, students will awaken to the import of the nurses' task and will flock to our schools of nursing in far greater numbers than ever before" (p. 26). As nursing becomes liberated, the range of possibilities for a new social order are anticipated and thus created.

REFERENCES

American Association of Colleges of Nursing (AACN). (1986). *Essentials of college and university education for professional nursing: Final report.* Washington, DC: Author.

Benner, P., & Wrubel, J. (1989). *The primacy of caring, stress and coping in health and illness.* Menlo Park, CA: Addison-Wesley.

Botkin, J. W., Elmandjra, M., & Malitza, M. (1984). *No limits to learning.* New York: Pergamon Press.

Freire, P. (1988). *Pedagogy of the oppressed.* New York: Continuum Publishing Co.

Gadow, S. (1985). Nurse and patient: The caring relationship. In Bishop & Scudder (Eds.), *Caring, curing, coping* (pp. 31–43). Tuscaloosa, AL: University of Alabama Press.

Gadow, S. (1988). Covenant without cure: Letting go and holding on in chronic illness. In J. Watson & M. A. Ray (Eds.), *The Ethics of care and the ethics of cure: Synthesis in chronicity* (pp. 5–14). New York: National League for Nursing.

Goodrich, A. (1917). The trained nurse. In A. Goodrich. (1973), *The social and ethical significance of nursing. A series of addresses.* New Haven: Yale University School of Nursing.

Goodrich, A. (1921). Education versus training. In A. Goodrich (1973), *The social and ethical significance of nursing: A series of addresses.* New Haven: Yale University School of Nursing.

Greene, M. (1978). *Landscapes of learning.* New York: Teacher's College Press, Columbia University.

Greene, M. (1986). Toward possibility: Expanding the range of literacy. *English Education*, pp. 231–243.

Greene, M. (1988). *The dialectic of freedom.* New York: Teacher's College Press, Columbia University.

Lynaugh, J., & Fagin, C. (1988). Nursing comes of age. *Image, 20*(4), 184–190.

Moccia, P. (1988). A critique of compromise: Beyond the methods debate. *Advances in Nursing Science, 10*(4), 1–9.

Noddings, N. (1988, February). An ethic of caring and its implications for instructional arrangements. *American Journal of Education.*

Palmer, P. (1987). Community, conflict, and ways of knowing. *The Magazine of Higher Learning, 19*(5), 20–25.

Peccei, A. (1984). Foreword. In Botkin et al., *No limits to learning* (pp. xiii–xvi). New York: Pergamon Press.

Quinn, J. (1989). Personal communication. University of Colorado, Center for Human Caring.

Schultz, P. (1989). Personal communication. University of Colorado, School of Nursing.

Simonton, D.K. (1989). *Scientific genius.* New York: Cambridge University Press.

Stevenson, J., & Woods, N. (1986). Nursing science and contemporary science: Emerging paradigms. In *Setting the agenda for year 2000: Knowledge development in nursing.* Kansas City, MO: American Academy of Nursing.

Tong, R. (1989). *Feminist thought. A comprehensive introduction.* Boulder, CO: Westview Press.

Watson, J. (1985). *Nursing: Human science and human care.* New York: Appleton-Century-Crofts.

Watson, J. (1988). Of nurses, women and the devaluation of caring. *Medical Humanities Review, 2*(2), 60–62.

Wollstonecraft, M. (1975). (C.H. Poster, Ed.). *A vindication of the rights of woman.* New York: W.W. Norton.

BIBLIOGRAPHY

Belenky, M., Clinchy, B., Goldberger, N., & Tarule, J. (1986). *Women's ways of knowing, the development of self, voice, and mind.* New York: Basic Books.

3

Transformative Thinking and a Caring Curriculum

Jean Watson

Although transformative thinking can begin to liberate us, it also presents an extraordinary challenge for education and practice. Transformative thinking requires that we move away from oppressive status quo educational and practice structures. In this sense, the transformative thinking of Simone de Beauvoir (1952) has relevance for nursing. She posited the following (in Tong, 1989, p. 210, author's parentheses):

> Woman (nurse) need not continue to be what man (male-
> dominated medical institution) has made her be;
> –woman (nurse) can be a subject, can engage in positive action
> in society, and can redefine or abolish her roles . . . ;
> –woman (nurse) can create her own self.

She goes on to point out that what is holding woman back from self-creation in society is patriarchal thinking—a patriarchy that, however, is breaking down and nearing its end. To paraphrase her, what is certain is that while hitherto women's (nursing's) possibilities have been suppressed and lost to humanity (and the health care system), it is high time that she be permitted to take her chances in her own interest and in the interest of all. Woman, like man, is a subject, rather than an object—and it is high time for man (medical system) to recognize this fact (Tong, 1989). Such reflective awareness provoked by de Beauvoir may arouse our felt deficiency to date, our sense of what is not yet, but perhaps ought to be. In fact, such an experience of possibility depends a great deal on the awareness of incompleteness—on the awareness that there is more to see, to grasp, to know as we expand our consciousness and envision new possibilities (Greene, 1986, p. 237).

De Beauvoir made it clear that if we want to be all that we can possibly be as individuals (nurses), we must first clear the social space for the project. For our purposes, therefore, that social space can begin with what this work proposes: education for freedom. The social space that a new model for nursing curriculum can create is intimately related to a transformative world view that contains some of the following beliefs:

- A belief in power and primacy of person and power of human consciousness, human imagination, and human spirit as inner resources and key components in teaching and learning and in health–illness outcomes.
- A belief in wholeness, harmony, and beauty.
- A belief in the wholeness of human and environment and the larger universe.
- A belief in ways of knowing and teaching–learning that incorporate not only rational, cognitive, technical, empirical, but call upon esthetics, ethical values, moral ideals, intuition, personal knowing, process discovery, and spiritual-metaphysical dimensions.
- A belief in the context of intersubjective, interhuman events, processes, relationships, and human-environment energy fields.
- A belief in an ontology of evolving consciousness, human freedom, release of human spirit, while adhering to caring as an absolute value and special way of being in education and practice.
- A belief in world view for human destiny that is open.

Therefore, through transformative thinking it is now openly acknowledged that knowledge development and the teaching–learning process is a distinctively human process and activity, as opposed to merely cognitive, rational, and technical; all knowledge is created; all knowledge is constructed; therefore, it is contextual, emotional, subjective, intersubjective, rational, passionate, controlled, evolving, and so forth (Belenky,

Clinchy, Goldberger, & Tarule, 1986; Kidd & Morrison, 1988; Moccia, 1988; Schultz & Meleis, 1988; Stevenson, 1988; Watson, 1985).

In this expanded transformative educational framework, knowledgeable human caring teaching–learning and clinical practices become the ethical principle and human science *pedagogical* standard by which nursing education, teaching–learning, and curricular approaches are evaluated (Gadow, 1988; Watson, 1988a, b, c, 1989). This framework accommodates an evolving professional consciousness and allows for methods that attend to the moral ideals and values that are relational, subjective inner experiences, while honoring intuition, personal, spiritual, cognitive, and physical senses alike.

An approach to curriculum development and teaching within a human caring–human science perspective combines and integrates the cognitive with the beauty, art, ethics, intuition, esthetics, and spiritual awareness of the intersubjective human-to-human caring processes and moral ideals embedded in the curriculum and intrinsic to the teaching–learning process in nursing. As a result, a model of curriculum development that is philosophically and morally consistent with phenomena and practices of human caring in nursing's clinical world is now called for in nursing education and professional curricula.

Within a transformative perspective for nursing education, an ethic of caring as a moral ideal must be considered. An ethic of caring provides an expanded context for nursing education by calling upon the highest ethical self in the process of an evolving consciousness. Caring is concerned with the human center of self and other. In this sense, caring is linked to healing; thus, as caring educators, we are all healers as we provide alternative pathways and enable others to find their own voice.

Just as nurses enable others to find their own voice and meaning during life's most vulnerable moments, likewise the discipline and profession of nursing is now seeking its own voice as it constructs and transmits its caring knowledge and advanced practices. An ethic and curricular model for human caring, healing, health, and wholeness is values-based, relational, intentional, intersubjective, contextual, and evolving (Noddings, 1984, 1988; Benner, 1984; Benner & Wrubel, 1988; Gaut, 1983; Leininger, 1981; Gadow, 1985, 1988; Watson, 1985, 1988 a,b).

Caring, like teaching–learning, is a human process, not a product or commodity to be bought and sold as human capital, or a substance to be manipulated and controlled by an oppressive system of education or practice. Thus, a framework for a caring curriculum is a transformative paradigm that is philosophically and morally consistent with phenomena and practices of human caring in both educational and clinical worlds.

RECREATING THE IDEAL

The Paideia Proposal (in Adler, 1982) reminds us of common traits we share as we move toward a values-based anticipatory caring curriculum, yet traits we often abandon in our current adaptation-maintenance system of education. For example we share:

- Common humanity.
- Personal dignity.
- Human rights and aspirations.
- Common future destiny.

It is significant that *paideia* is a Greek word which incorporates the Latin concept of humanities, signifying that *general learning* should be the possession of all human beings. The educational manifestos recommended are still waiting to be implemented, especially in nursing education. It must be remembered, as well, that nursing education largely means education for professional women. Perhaps if nursing responds to the educational challenges of early and contemporary feminist writers, as well as nursing leaders such as Annie Goodrich, the new generation of young men and women will not have to enter traditionally dominant men's professions to receive a general and liberal and liberating education for a professional career of their choice, be it in medicine, law, business, dentistry, pharmacy, or be it nursing with its "soft" human science focus and commitment to health and caring–healing. After all, it has been predicted that the so-called soft sciences of today will be the hard sciences of tomorrow.

Ernest Boyer (1989) points out that it is connectedness through liberal education that can help nursing fulfill its worthy goals and essential values. He emphasizes the critical role of language in helping connect us through the exquisite use of symbol and capturing feelings and ideas. He also points out that in teaching and using language we should also teach the value of silence, being able to listen to each other and to ourselves. Indeed, listening is the heart of healing professions and establishes the quality of patient–professional interaction and trust.

A second feature highlighted by Boyer in relation to nursing education is the empowerment and connectedness that a liberal education brings in putting the work of nursing into a larger context. As the human agenda becomes more global, often our education becomes increasingly parochial (adaptation-maintenance level). Indeed, Boyer points out that current educational practices indicated a "frightening almost 'anti-connectedness' to much of the world" (p. 104). At the same time, he reminds us that we must become increasingly sensitive to the interdependent nature of our physical world and our responsibility to live according to the laws of nature, both as a global community and in our personal lives.

A third point raised by Boyer is the critical need for the nursing profession to be placed within a social and ethical perspective. Otherwise we run the risk of having so-called professional people who do not make their decisions within the context of moral judgment, people whose confidence is not guided by conscience. Indeed, according to the Carnegie report, every professional field should be asked to place its own work in historical, social, and ethical perspective (p. 105).

HUMAN CARING THEORY APPLIED

Noddings (1988) points out that moral education for caring involves *modeling, dialogue, practice,* and *confirmation*. As a result, our methods of curriculum and instruction about caring must include the human dimensions. Thus, our technocratic cognitive knowledge and skills are not the same as our lived human learning experiences and needs as part of a caring context for nursing education.

Modeling

Educators model caring when they encourage self-affirmation and self-discovery in students. When educators are interested in development of fully moral persons, they are modeling. Again, as Boyer (1989) points out, "connectedness is established in the classroom by teachers who serve as models and mentors" (p. 105). In applying human caring theory to educational practices, the nurse educator uses teaching moments as "caring occasions"—recognizing that in every human encounter there arises the possibility of a caring occasion (Noddings, 1988; Watson, 1985). In every caring occasion, those involved must decide how they will respond to each other. Teaching and learning are filled with caring occasions, or quite often, with attempts to avoid such occasions (Noddings, 1988, p. 13). For example, as Noddings points out, overuse of lecture, without discussion, impersonal grading in written quantitative form, or modes of punitive decision making that respond only to the behavior and refuse to encounter the subjective meaning, or broader understanding of the person, all risk losing opportunities for moral education, mutual growth, and modeling of caring in action.

Dialogue

To consider dialogue as an integral part of a caring-based curriculum, opportunities need to be created wherein the faculty and student can engage in genuine dialogue, and genuine caring can be expressed (see Chapters 5 and 7). Noddings (1988) reminds us again that dialogue is essential to a caring, moral education. "True dialogue is open; that is, conclusions are not held by one or more of the parties at the outset. The search for enlightenment, or responsible choice, or perspective, or means to problem solving is *mutual* and marked by appropriate signs of reciprocity" (p. 140). There is attention to the individual and contextual human meaning that arises from the interhuman, intersubjective events. To quote Moustakas, "The opportunity to engage in genuine caring is a process of intuitive awareness, sensing and knowing, a recognition of the mystery, the awe, the capriciousness, the unpredictability of life, the possibility of the power of silence and of real dialogue with others in the deep moments of life; . . . and indeed spiritual qualities of our energy interchange via the caring relationship" (in Newman, 1986, p. 134).

Practice

In a clinical field such as nursing the praxis of caring occurs; theory and practice live together, each informing the other. The educational setting is where caring theory can be first applied and later translated from pedagogical practices into the clinical world of nursing practice. Thus, it is critical that modeling and dialogue emerge into practice opportunities, wherein students and faculty can demonstrate caring. This can occur as students are encouraged to help and support each other; opportunities for peer interaction are co-created; the quality of the interaction is attended to. Use of small groups that contain "caring occasions" can be created even if the class sizes are large and less desirable than one would choose. Furthermore, recent attempts to pay attention to the contextual wholes of human learning are generating class exercises that seek to integrate personal learning and prepare an informed passion and moral ideal in the class setting. For example, progressive faculty are reporting approaches such as deep breathing, stretching, touching, centering exercises, quiet preparatory moments with affirmations of what each hopes to give and receive during the class, use of music, color, and other esthetic modes to deal with whole person learning and teaching. While these approaches may sound tangential for this moment in time, the future will demonstrate the effectiveness of such approaches, especially if we are to model and practice caring for self and others, and if we are to integrate all ways of knowing and learning into our curricula.

Confirmation

Of all of the above dimensions that are essential in a caring, values-based moral curriculum, Noddings (1988) again especially emphasizes the process and importance of confirmation. The goal here, as she puts it, is to assist in the shaping and construction of one's ethical ideal.

> When we attribute the best possible motive consonant with reality to the cared-for, we confirm the other; that is, we reveal to the other an attainable image of self that is lovelier than that manifested in the present acts. In an important sense, we embrace the other as one with us in devotion to caring. In education, what we reveal to a student about self as an ethical and intellectual being has the power to nurture the ethical ideal or to destroy it. (p. 16)

Such a perspective is consistent with Palmer's earlier advice, in that it is here, perhaps at the very core of our teaching–learning caring occasions, that we have the power for forming or *deforming* human consciousness; it is here in our modes of modeling, dialogue, practice, and confirmation that we shape souls. And it is here in our educational caring occasions where we lay the very foundation for human caring in health care; we lay the very foundation for creating a context of community for, and of, caring, that affirms the relational, the mutual, the communal, the interhuman moral response and responsibility, and reciprocity. Thus, it is that an ethic of caring curriculum builds its now, its future humanity, and forms or deforms its practitioners of human caring in society.

All of these dimensions of caring in education need transpersonal caring contact between students and faculty. Such caring occasions celebrate the relational, reciprocal human quest for the best ethical self, and a "yearning for the good" (Noddings, 1984). The one-caring educator in this instance thus creates an ideal wherein another human should be able to request, with expectation of positive response, an educator's help, advice, and assistance, and a promotion of caring as a moral ideal that is mutually affirming. However, the process depends upon the will and intention of the one-caring to remain in a caring relation to the other. Knowing and being in a teaching–learning caring process are communally connected relational acts. They require a continual cycle of modeling, dialogue, practice, and confirmation; . . . "a continual cycle of discussion, disagreement and consensus over what has been and what it all means" (Palmer, 1987, p. 24). Thus, the broader system is impacted. However, again as Noddings (1984) reminds us, caring takes place at the individual, human level as we make up and influence our systems of education and practice. She puts it this way:

> The duty to enhance the ethical ideal, the commitment to caring, invokes a duty to promote skepticism and noninstitutional affiliation. In a deep sense, no institution or nation can be ethical. It cannot meet the other as one-caring or as one trying to care. It can only capture in general terms what particular ones-caring would like to have done in well-described situations. Laws, manifestos, and proclamations, (Patient's Bill of Rights) . . . . are limited, and they may support immoral as well as moral actions. Only the individual can be truly called to ethical (caring) behavior, and the individual can never give way to encapsulated moral guides, although she may safely accept them in ordinary, untroubled times. (p. 103, author's parentheses)

Such thinking again returns us to the call for anticipatory and participatory teaching–learning and contextual connectedness in all of nursing education:

> Nursing education requires a rare combination of knowledge, skills, and values. And at its core, it would call for an understanding of the connectedness of things. Connectedness through a careful, sacred use of language. Connectedness through the interdependent world in which we live. Connectedness through a vision of great teachers. Connectedness between theory and the values of our lives. And finally, connectedness between the classroom and the imperative of service. (Boyer, 1989, p. 107)

Finally, the caring curriculum and emancipatory, liberating education we are proposing for nursing is a call for a decision to care, to choose to care, to dare to care, in the worlds of education and health care—two worlds where caring is not valued (Moccia, 1989). The decision to care is a political, philosophical, and moral act, and involves risk. It is the risk of "Saying Yes" (Moccia, 1989) to releasing the power of human caring in the act of educating in an all too often care*less* system.

REFERENCES

Adler, M. J. (1982). *The Paideia proposal: An education manifesto.* New York: Macmillan.

Belenky, M., Clinchy, B., Goldberger, N., & Tarule, J. (1986). *Women's ways of knowing, the development of self, voice, and mind.* New York: Basic Books.

Benner, P. (1984). *From novice to expert: Excellence and power in clinical nursing practice.* Menlo Park, CA: Addison-Wesley.

Benner, P., & Wrubel, J. (1989). *The primacy of caring, stress and coping in health and illness.* Menlo Park, CA: Addison-Wesley.

Boyer, E. (1989). Connectedness through liberal education. *Journal of Professional Nursing, 5*(2), 102–107.

Gadow, S. (1985). Nurse and patient: The caring relationship. In Bishop & Scudder (Eds.), *Caring, curing, coping* (pp. 31–43). Tuscaloosa, AL: University of Alabama Press.

Gadow, S. (1988). Covenant without cure: Letting go and holding on in chronic illness. In J. Watson & M. A. Ray (Eds.), *The ethics of care and the ethics of cure: Synthesis in chronicity* (pp. 5–14). New York: National League for Nursing.

Gaut, D. (1983). Development of a theoretically adequate description of caring. *Western Journal of Nursing Research, 5*(4), 315.

Greene, M. (1988). Toward possibility: Expanding the range of literacy. *English Education,* 231–243.

Kidd, P., & Morrison, E. (1988). The progress of knowledge in nursing: A search for meaning. *Image, 20*(4), 222–224.

Leininger, M. (Ed.). (1981). *Caring: An essential human need.* New Jersey: Charles B. Slack.

Moccia, P. (1988). A critique of compromise: Beyond the methods debate. *Advances in Nursing Science, 10*(4), 1–9.

Moccia, P. (1989, May). *Deciding to care.* Keynote address presented at 11th International Caring Conference, Denver, CO.

Newman, M. (1986). *Health as expanding consciousness.* St. Louis, MO: C.V. Mosby.

Noddings, N. (1984). *Caring: A feminine approach to ethics and moral development.* Berkeley, CA: University of California Press.

Noddings, N. (1988, February). An ethic of caring and its implications for instructional arrangements. *American Journal of Education.*

Palmer, P. (1987). Community, conflict, and ways of knowing. *The Magazine of Higher Learning, 19*(5), 20–25.

Schultz, P., & Meleis, A. (1988). Nursing epistemology: Traditions, insights, questions. *Image, 20*(4), 217–221.

Stevenson, J. (1988). Nursing knowledge development: Into era II. *Journal of Professional Nursing, 4*(3), 152–162.

Tong, R. (1989). *Feminist thought. A comprehensive introduction.* Boulder, CO: Westview Press.

Watson, J. (1985). *Nursing: Human science and human care.* New York: Appleton-Century-Crofts.

Watson, J. (1988a). New dimensions in human caring theory. *Nursing Science Quarterly, 1*(4), 175–181.

Watson, J. (1988b). Human caring as moral context for nursing education. *Nursing & Health Care, 9*(8), 422–425.

Watson, J. (1988c). Of nurses, women, and the devaluation of caring. *Medical Humanities Review, 2*(2), 60–62.

Watson, J. (in press). Human caring: A public agenda. In *Monograph of the wingspread conference: Knowledge about care and curing.* Kansas City, MO: American Nurses' Association.

Wollstonecraft, M. (1975). (C. H. Poster, Ed.). *A vindication of the rights of woman.* New York: W.W. Norton.

Part II

A New Age Exemplar Curriculum Paradigm

After the First World War our historians abandoned the vision of the Enlightenment that had evoked the dream of unlimited moral progress. Even before the war some academic movements of thought were leading in this direction. Positivism had set out to eliminate all metaphysical claims of knowledge. Behaviorism had started on the course that was to lead on to cybernetics, which claims to represent all human thought as the working of a machine. Sigmund Freud's revolution had started too, reducing man's moral principles to mere rationalizations of desires. Sociology had developed a program for explaining human affairs without making distinctions between good and evil. Our true convictions were being left without theoretical foundation.

Michael Polanyi, *Meaning*

INTRODUCTION

Although the age Michael Polanyi (1975, p. 22) speaks of had a long run, it is the end of an era, the end of an epoch—one in which humans were perceived as machines; in which flesh and blood were assumed to be mere atoms explicable by biological and physical laws and principles; where imagination, creative thought, ambitions, the highest goals and ideal thought, the tender or pain-filled memories, complex motives, frailty, fallacy, fantasy, wishful thinking, and intuitive inspiration were all labeled "mind" and believed to be revealed and investigated by cybernetics and computer science. It was an age well described by Polanyi in the extract above—an age that started after World War I and is just beginning to end. We have finally arrived at the conclusion, probably because some have discovered that Elizabeth Barrett Browning's "ends of Being and ideal Grace" are not so easily explained by empiricism, logical positivism, behaviorism, and Freudian psychology.

63

And truly, the "ends of Being and ideal Grace" is the ultimate goal of education.

Since this is an end, so too there must now be a beginning—on a new age. It is an age that, unlike so many other ages, does not turn its back on our past for having been laced with errors and mistakes among its many successes. This age must and will create a future that takes our past with us. For it is in the past, in its successes and failures, that we learn. Our past serves as our beacon, an electric torch lighting our way toward a better world, a better education, a truly professional nurse providing a kind and quality nursing care not yet dreamed of, only glimpsed in our peripheral vision.

So here we are with a dream to build, hopes to fulfill, visions to realize, and a future to construct. To do this, we must not turn our backs on the past but work with it. Positivism, behaviorism, cybernetics, analytical psychology, scientific sociology, and anthropology have been productive. In nursing they have simply been lifted from possible theoretical positions and options to the dogma of incontrovertible truth. Such dogmas results in a perversion of the possibilities of human intellect. Such dogmas result in suppressing doubts and punishing doubters while accepting none but the scientifically detached who use methods of scientific rationalism and empiricism. Establishment scientists for three generations have had little regard or respect for those who dared conduct inquiry in ways that discredited or rejected the position that there could be any researchable phenomenon not verifiable by measurement. These investigators were given the worst of all possible labels: metaphysical.

Now that that phase of history is closing, we must not create the same problems as our forbears. Rather, we must take their successes with us. We must do this for the good they did us, for the infusion of wonders, discoveries, inventions, theories, truths, and half-truths they revealed. We must find a balance, a truce, a truly liberated climate of teaching, of inquiry, so that we fuse the "scientific" with the metaphysical, and infuse a new respect for those things uniquely human: morality, judgment, intuition, reflection, imagination, creativity, values, meaning, and spiritual sensitivity.[1] This paradigm is offered in the spirit of building on the past,

---

[1] Spiritual here used is not a religious reference. It has more to do with "geist" than with soul. Spiritual is used to mean that part of human beings that is responsive to beauty, searches after truth, appeciates kindness and compassion, accepts the obligations to care for fellow beings, motivates our efforts, energizes our lives, and opens the gates to laughter and tears. Spirit has as little to do with religion, or as much, as he or she who has it, wishes.

of using what we have learned and of providing an option, not another dogma. What is needed for the professional level of nursing education is teaching, delivered from the dogmatism of the Tyler Rationale, from the tyranny of lectures, and recast as teaching that, by its nature, demands that students bring their enthusiasm, energy, and best efforts to the task of creative, investigative, and liberating learning. It is within this context that Part II is written.

The first part of the book provided a brief history of nursing education and the four major curriculum development turns to date. It also provided a brief critique of the behaviorist movement, a discussion of what it has helped nursing education accomplish and its limitations for nursing's new professional dimensions. The implication in this is that a new turn, a fifth turn, has arrived.

These criticisms of the behaviorist influence on nursing education raise several issues: (1) If not the Tyler models—not the behaviorist-empiricist-quantitative paradigm—what then? (2) What kinds of theoretical constructs could support a paradigm that is nonbehaviorist? (3) What kinds of guidelines for curriculum development are appropriate to graduate an educated professional nurse? The first and second issues are the topic of concern here.

An early task of any ethical iconoclast is to offer alternatives. Criticism of an existing model without some proposals for new pathways would leave nursing education directionless at a time when it is very vulnerable to political and health industry pressures on nursing's very right to exist as a profession. Therefore, Part II examines one possible curriculum-development paradigm in two chapters. Chapter 4 offers an exploration of the theoretical formulations and models that make up the professional curriculum model and shows how these ideas are linked to serve the whole. Chapter 5 addresses the practical issues of how to identify and select content, how to structure learning episodes, and, in general, how to write curriculum plans using the new paradigm. Chapters 6–8 focus on teaching, for teaching is the crux, the essence, of a humanistic-educative curriculum. Chapter 9 addresses evaluation as interpretive criticism.

4

Nursing Curriculum as Professional Education: Some Underlying Theoretical Models

Em Olivia Bevis

The health care scene has changed and is still rapidly changing. Not a little of this is due to the changing attitude and needs of the client of the system. An increasingly sophisticated professional is demanded to deal not only with the technological explosion in health care but also with the more sophisticated needs of the client who increasingly is involved in self-care and in the care of his or her family. These clients therefore need more sensitive caring, teaching, prevention, guidance, and advice from a professional who communicates well, has insight and foresight, and can quickly and reliably gather appropriate data for use in working with clients in helpful ways. This new professional needs to be wise and mature, two things education cannot provide. But education can provide the tools with which one can become wise and mature (or unfortunately, merely clever at being foolish). Dr. Hanna Gray, the president of the University of Chicago, said in the president's annual address to incoming freshmen (1987) that

> They [the Renaissance humanists] believed that the kind of knowl-
> edge worth having resided in those studies which looked to the

enduring questions of meaning related to the nature of the human community, its dilemmas and possibilities, and which taught men not only how to think, but to act, not only how to appreciate, but to emulate, not only to know, but to carry on a creative dialogue with the past which would continue on beyond their own time.

Alas, the Renaissance humanists had not solved the problem of education either, but they certainly had some rich ideas about it. And what we seek today for nursing education is the kind of nurse that can accept the ambiguities of the modern medical and health care world—a complex world—in which there are no certainties or any easy and clear solutions, and everyday judgments are fraught with ethical and moral dilemmas that require daily reevaluation of our most basic ideas about human life. The nurse we seek is one who can act and reflect and who has the nature of compassionate scholar with a mind that never ceases to inquire, quest, and expand.

To accomplish this for society and for nursing, our whole approach to the education of professional nurses must be reexamined and new directions established with new strategies that are devised to realize these new directions.

TOWARD A DEFINITION OF CURRICULUM

The traditional first task, even that of developing a new future, is that of defining that which is to be constructed. Definitions are necessary so that there is some agreement regarding what is meant in a discussion. Beyond that, words are quite powerful and invoke ideas and meanings beyond their surface implications. Since this book is about curriculum, it seems important to pause a moment and examine what the word means to those who write about the subject, how it will be defined for use in this book and why it will be defined that way.

Those who write about curriculum define it in a variety of differing ways. To simplify matters, they are placed in four categories below:

1. Curriculum as the program of studies.
2. Curriculum as planned learning experiences or as a plan for learning.
3. Curriculum as all the experiences that students have under the auspices of the school.
4. Curriculum as a structured series of intended learning outcomes.

There has been more written about defining the word *curriculum* than could interest any educator or would be useful to discuss. Therefore, only a few brief and important points will be made here.

Curriculum as a Program of Studies

The first definitional grouping, curriculum as the program of studies, is the definition most often used by lay persons. When a copy of the curriculum is requested, what is really sought is the program of studies that lists the course offerings and the academic credit attached to each course. Sometimes course descriptions, prerequisite sequencing, and other accouterments are also intended to be part of this definition of curriculum. Beauchamp (1981, p. 206) comes close to this meaning when he defines curriculum as "a written plan depicting the scope and arrangement of the projected educational program for a school." However, his "scope and arrangement" might be intended to be more inclusive than this limited interpretation. In this book, a program of studies is always a list of the courses, the academic credit they carry, and the suggested sequencing.

Curriculum as a Plan for Learning

Curriculum as planned learning experiences or as a "plan for learning" was popularized by Taba (1962). Bevis (1973) used Taba's definition in her book on curriculum development in nursing and so made it a popular definition for nurse educators.

Beauchamp's definition, cited above, also spoke of curriculum as a plan, although a written one was designated. Macdonald and Leeper (1965, p. 3) also refers to it as a written plan for action. However, they distinguish, as does Taba (1962) and Johnson (1967), between the plan and the implementation. These authors believe that implementation becomes the domain of instruction, not curriculum. This distinction between the plan and carrying it out is consistent with behaviorist curriculum models that separate the ends and means (objectives and teaching strategies). Popham and Baker (1970, p. 48) make the same popular distinction and designate curriculum as a plan, although they define curriculum differently as can be seen below.

Oliva (1982, p. 10), in defining curriculum as a "plan or program for all the experiences under the direction of the school," is somewhat similar to Saylor and Alexander (1974, p. 6), who define the curriculum as "the plan for providing sets of learning opportunities to achieve

broad goals and related specific objectives for an identifiable population served by a single school center." Eisner (1985, p. 45) is not too far
from this when he says, "The curriculum of a school, or a course, or a
classroom can be conceived of as a series of planned events that are
intended to have educational consequences for one or more students."
These definitions are certainly broader than the more simplistic Taba
definition but still relegate it to paper or merely plans.

Curriculum as All Experiences in School

The curriculum as experiences "had" under the auspices of the
school is the prototype of curriculum writers such as Caswell and Campbell (1935) and the earlier work of Saylor and Alexander (1954).
Caswell and Campbell (1935, p. 66) defined curriculum as "all the
experiences children have under the guidance of teachers," and Saylor
and Alexander (1954, pp. 4–5) elaborated that classical definition with
". . . the total effort of the school to bring about desired outcomes in
school and in out-of-school situations." Further along they add, "The
curriculum is the sum total of the school's efforts to influence learning,
whether in the classroom, on the playground or out of school." Doll
(1978, p. 6) defines curriculum as ". . . the formal and informal content and process by which learners gain knowledge and understanding,
develop skills, and alter attitudes, appreciations and values under the
auspices of that school." Oliva's definition, quoted above, is consistent
with these definitions. Huebner (1968) has an interesting twist. He
objects to any definition of curriculum that addresses "learning opportunities" and instead suggests "opportunities for engagement." This
phrase certainly fits the interactive nature of the paradigm under discussion in this book.

These are broad definitions that do not separate curriculum and
instruction or teaching. They are appealing to those who believe
ends–means separation is meaningless unless the curriculum
paradigm is behaviorist, where the ends are spelled out specifically as
behavioral objectives, and these objectives and the materials developed around them are the curriculum. However, it is interesting to
note that some of the definitions in this category are written by persons who advocate some form of the Tylerian model. Usually, authors
in the behaviorist paradigms see curriculum as the plan or the objectives, and all else is naturally seen as something other than curriculum,
for example, teaching or instruction. This leads naturally into the last
category.

Curriculum as Intended Learning Outcomes

This is the ultimate position of the behaviorists. If one believes that all teaching is guided by preconceived, specific, behaviorally defined objectives, and all evaluation of teaching is how well those objectives were addressed, and all evaluation of learning is whether or not and how well the students achieved those objectives, then in order to be consistent, curriculum must be defined in terms of the intended outcomes or the objectives.

Gagne (1967), a behaviorist, defined curriculum as "a sequence of content units arranged in such a way that learning of each unit may be accomplished as a single act, provided the capabilities described by specified prior units (in the sequence) have already been mastered by the learner" (p. 23).

He goes on to say that by a specified curriculum, he means (and here he addresses the behaviorist paradigm clearly), "when (1) the terminal objectives are stated; (2) the sequence of prerequisite capabilities is described; and (3) the initial capabilities assumed to be possessed by the student are identified" (p. 23). This definition was chosen to illustrate the constraints of curriculum when it is behavioral objective-driven and sequentially arranged. Popham and Baker (1970) are less detailed but within the same framework when they define curriculum as "all the planned learning *outcomes* for which the school is responsible" (p. 48).

Tyler (1949) did not define curriculum as such in his book *Basic Principles of Curriculum and Instruction,* but his intent cannot be mistaken. He writes, "These educational objectives become the criteria by which materials are selected, content is outlined, instructional procedures are developed and tests and examinations are prepared" (p. 3). From that statement, one can deduct that to Tyler, especially for the purposes of his rationale, curriculum is (1) a plan, (2) objectives, and (3) objective-driven selection of materials, content, instructional procedures, and examinations.

Johnson (1967) is brief and to the point, clearly supporting this position. His "a structured series of intended learning outcomes" (p. 129) encompasses curriculum both as *intended,* that is, plans, and as *outcomes,* that is, objectives.

Definition of Curriculum for Use in This Book

The definitions of curriculum that come closest to expressing the position of this book are those in group three, "curriculum as all the experiences that students have under the auspices of the school." As pointed out earlier, there is too much covered under this definition. *For this book, curriculum is defined as those transactions and interactions that take place between students and teachers and among students with the intent that learning take place.* As such, it includes Huebner's (1968) "opportunities for engagement"—for such opportunities are the material from which curriculum is made. Lest this definition be too succinct, several of the key definitional issues necessary to setting the stage for a new curriculum paradigm designed to establish a new direction need to be explored.

ISSUES

The First Issue: A Plan Is a Plan

The first issue to be addressed is that the curriculum is not a plan. A plan may or may not be part of the curriculum, but the plan is just that, a plan. It is by no means the curriculum. The curriculum is what happens, what actually takes place among teachers and students, students and students, so that learning occurs. The *plan* may or may not have included what actually took place. What occurs can be quite spontaneous, or it can happen to a student alone when pursuing some meaningful idea triggered by something read, discussed, or investigated that is quite different from where the train of thought was supposed to lead. In fact, a good curriculum should be full of such gates of stimulation and inspiration. It cannot and should not be entirely preplanned and prescribed. Freire (1970) postulates that one of the basic elements of educational oppression is prescription. He says, ". . . the behavior of the oppressed is a prescribed behavior, following as it does the guidelines of the oppressor" (p. 31). A curriculum that is planned in too much detail must be oppressive to both teachers and students by its very nature. The problem faced by faculties in practice disciplines such as nursing is that to a certain extent, by nature of students being required to pass a state licensing examination, certain content is prescribed. If the students do not learn this content, often by rote, they may not pass the board examination and may not be able to practice nursing. Such penalties pose a grave threat to the existence of a school of nursing. Thereby training, under a rigidly defined preplanned curriculum, is perceived as the safe way to proceed. Since educative learning for professional nursing practice demands more than the prescribed training of such structured curricula, faculty must achieve some balance between prescriptive and goal-directed curricula. The unresolved question remains, can the incompatible opposites oppression and liberation coexist within the same curriculum?

The Second Issue: Curriculum Wholeness

A second but equally important issue is the separation of ends and means. Even if one rejects the idea of behavioral objectives and their tyranny over the curriculum, and even if one substitutes ends-in-view or goals and continues to separate those goals from the means of achieving them, the result is an artificial fragmentation of something that is an irreducible whole. If curriculum is the interactions among and between students and teachers, then it is basically teaching, and all else is commentary, including the plans, the goals, the philosophy, the course content, and the evaluation strategies. These items may be a part of the curriculum, but they are not essential to it, since the curriculum is what actually occurs.

The Third Issue: Curriculum Has Education or Training Value

A third issue is whether or not one can legitimately capture all the experiences students have under the auspices of the school and call that curriculum. According to Webster (1971), "auspices" means protection, patronage, and kindly guidance. Students certainly learn much in school that in a more innocent era they would not have learned, but even in the most innocent of times one would hesitate to label as curriculum *all they learn under the auspices of the school.* In the schools of today, students learn about drugs, rape and other violence, dancing, courtship, deportment, and how to "beat the system." These are not within the purview of the curriculum. Curriculum must have an educational or training value attached to it. Therefore, if it is not of training or educational value, it is not curriculum. All things that might at some time have value to the life of the student are not necessarily training or education. What is training and what is educational is addressed in more detail later in this chapter. Briefly, education is that which enriches the learner in the syntactical, contextual, and inquiry categories of learning (see pp. 91–94) and/or helps the learner grow in maturity (see pp. 83–87).

The Fourth Issue: Four Types of Curriculum

A fourth issue is whether a curriculum must be overt to be a curriculum. When one defines curriculum as those transactions among faculty and students so that learning occurs, it encompasses much that is not evident. Eisner (1985, pp. 87–125) speaks of three curricula that schools teach and calls them the explicit, the implicit, and the null, respectively. This nomenclature ignores the fact that the explicit curriculum has two aspects: one that is legitimate, or sanctioned by the faculty or those in authority to approve curricula, and one that is not sanctioned. In nursing this is due to educational content and processes that do not fit into the behaviorist paradigm of explicit, measurable behavioral objectives. Eisner's implicit curriculum is called by others the "hidden curriculum" (Vallance, 1973–1974).

His null curriculum has the same quality of truth of the White Knight in *Through the Looking Glass:*

> But I was thinking of a plan
>   To dye one's whiskers green,
> And always use so large a fan
>   That they could not be seen.

It is, in fact, not only that although often in the plan it is seldom seen, but that, as in another whimsical story, "The Emperor's New Clothes," everyone thinks it is there when it is not.

Rather than ignore the dichotomy of the two curricula encompassed by Eisner's explicit curriculum, I shall propose that every school has four curricula. These are:

1. *The legitimate curriculum:* the one agreed on by the faculty either implicitly or explicitly. Sometimes it is written into plans, sometimes not. But, regardless, it is recognized and acknowledged by faculty and students as the "real" curriculum. It is sanctioned by the approval and accreditation bodies and is the one that generates the learning tasks, episodes, papers, and tests with which both students and teachers contend. Currently in nursing this curriculum is generally behavioral-objectives driven. In other words, only those items describable in behavioral terms, explicitly chosen by faculty as worthy, and correctly formulated into prescriptive objectives, fuel the curriculum by dictating the learning episodes to be chosen and the evaluations to be made. This is the curriculum that is aboveboard and generally acknowledged

or owned by the faculty. The normal discourse regarding curriculum refers to this curriculum.

2. *The illegitimate curriculum:* the one kept in the closet, that all professional nursing teachers of worth not only know is there but actively teach. It is a curriculum that values and teaches, among many other things, caring, compassion, power and its use, ethics, politics in health care settings, and being accountable and responsible. This is the curriculum that, because of the constraints of the behavioral-objective driven curriculum prevalent in nursing, cannot be graded or officially acknowledged or sanctioned because it does not lend itself to descriptors that are behavioral. This curriculum exists in the behaviorist curriculum and is often taught quite openly because teachers feel a moral obligation to their students to recognize things beyond the explicit.

In many of these curricula, there is much activity around trying to structure behavioral objectives in such a way as to cover these phenomena (King, 1984; Krathwohl, Bloom, & Masia, 1964). They seem to work only if one is a behaviorist; otherwise they seem artificial, strained, and unnecessary. In fact, the illegitimate curriculum seldom exist in curricula that do not have to conform to strictly sanctioned plans or meet specified, behavioral objectives.

This is the curriculum of insights, patterns, creativity, strategies, inquiry, and understanding: a curriculum that is seldom expressed in easily manifested behaviors and lies softly within the learner influencing life choices, taste, approaches, values, and style.

3. *The hidden curriculum:* the one very appropriately called the "implicit" by Eisner (1985) and "hidden" by Vallance (Vallance, 1973–1974). It is the curriculum in which we are unaware of the messages given by the way we teach, the priorities we set, the type of methods we use, and the way we interact with students. This is the curriculum of subtle socialization, of teaching initiates how to think and feel like nurses. It is the curriculum that covertly communicates priorities, relationships, and values. It colors perceptions, independence, initiative, caring, colleagueship, and the mores and folkways of being a nurse. It is taught by subtle, out-of-awareness things that pervade the whole educational environment: when classes are scheduled, how much time is given a subject in relationship to other subjects, how many test items are assigned a topic or whether or not a term paper is given to the area, who addresses whom in what way, how the teacher responds to students who openly differ in opinion from the teacher, how students are or are not encouraged to work together, and how teachers interact with students.

All of these give the value messages to students that shape their learning in this curriculum.

4. *The null curriculum:* the curriculum that does not exist (Eisner, 1985, pp. 97–99). It is the one talked about with colorful rhetoric, believed in by all teachers in higher education, as popular as Mom, apple pie, and the flag. The curriculum of humanities, liberal arts, critical thinking, inquiry, creativity, and the full range of human intellectual capacity. Most curricula plans and materials, especially philosophies, speak highly of these things, and faculty mouth the right words in faculty meetings and over coffee, and believe in it in their heart of hearts—*but.* These conversations almost always are ended with a "but": "But where would we put courses in the arts, in the humanities, in philosophy? We only have 4 years to cover all we cover, and the student must have all these other *very essential courses.*" We speak of critical thinking, inquiry and intellectual development, and would like to teach it, but seldom do we raise the questions with students that would require any response beyond the "rationale" for a nursing decision. This is the curriculum that exists only in the hearts and minds of educators but, outside the doctoral level, seldom exists in reality. This may be because teachers are not taught the art of provoking cognitive dissonance and raising issues and questions that support these general aims of education.

It is the goal of all good professional programs to be educative, to have no null curriculum and no illegitimate curriculum, and to reduce the hidden (implicit) curriculum to the barest minimum.

However, in the schools of today we have four curricula (see Table 1): the legitimate, the illegitimate, the hidden, and the null. These curricula, although they may differ in content, are also different in reality because of the primacy of their agreed-upon acceptability by the faculty and their fit within the approved curricular philosophy regarding learning and the perceived importance of sciences to nursing. In other words, it is not the content that makes them legitimate, illegitimate, or hidden, but the degree of value placed upon the content, how overtly that value is spelled out, or the implicit messages in the environment

Table 1
The Four Types of Curriculum

1. The legitimate curriculum—sanctioned by the faculty
2. The illegitimate curriculum—not sanctioned
3. The hidden curriculum—socialization; mostly contextual
4. The null curriculum—thought there but not there

and climate of the school. The material in the hidden curriculum is often very powerful and is never acknowledged, because to acknowledge it is to raise it into awareness, and it then becomes no longer hidden. If it is retained, it usually moves either into the legitimate or the illegitimate curriculum.

One example of such material is assertiveness. In the mid-1960s, as the women's movement was beginning to help people become aware of the effects of institutionalization of women's traditional roles and behaviors on nursing, the Edwards Personal Preference Inventory was given to incoming nursing majors at San Jose State University in California. The study showed that the new nursing majors were very high in deference (low in assertiveness). The faculty agreed that deference in graduate (registered) nurses was in part responsible for the subservient role of nurses in the health care system and that subservience was probably part of the hidden messages given to students in the clinical courses by exposure to the autocratic bureaucracy of hospitals and schools of nursing. Based on these studies and a goal of having assertive graduates, assertiveness training was added to the legitimate curriculum. The Edwards Personal Preference Inventory tests were again completed by the same students the week of graduation and showed a marked decrease in deference scores (Bevis & Bower, 1972). This is typical of what happens when part of the hidden curriculum surfaces into awareness and faculty deliberately plan and execute curriculum to alter the results.

Currently in nursing the legitimate curriculum is behaviorist. Being training-oriented and technical, it cannot support professionalism and is best used for the technical aspects of nursing.

There are many more issues that could be discussed here. However, most issues will surface in subsequent chapters of the book. It is sufficient that one is clear about what is meant in this book when one speaks of curriculum.

PROFESSIONAL EDUCATION: A THEORETICAL POSITION

There are four mini-models that, taken together, make up the theoretical position of this paradigm: the learner maturity continuum, the typology of learning, criteria for teacher–student interactions, and criteria for selecting and devising learning activities. All of the models rest upon interlocked assumptions and propositions. These assumptions and propositions provide direction not only to the mini-models offered here, but also to how these models will be used to develop curriculum. They give the shift in paradigm a value system.

Assumptions

These theoretical constructs are based on several assumptions that are basic to the curriculum development paradigm. Some of these are:

1. The classroom and practica are political arenas.
2. The behaviorist curriculum paradigm is politically oppressive in that it is authoritarian and highly controlled, primarily contains teacher-selected content, and thereby discourages discourse that is not objectives relevant.
3. The educative/professional curriculum is best supported by models that are politically liberating in that the learning activities require the active participation of the learner and teacher–student interactions that are egalitarian.
4. Learning is the responsibility of the student.
5. Course and learning episode structure is on a progressive continuum from high to low structure by the teacher and low to high by the student.
6. As the teacher's structure decreases, the student's self-structure increases, playing an important part in learner maturity.
7. For best results in facilitating students' maturity level, teachers devise/select/support learning episodes that facilitate the movement of the student progressively from high to low teacher structure and from low to high student self-structure.
8. Structure can be oppressive or liberating. Some kinds of structure are necessary to liberation.
9. When working with students who are high on the learner maturity continuum, at the liberated (low structure) end of the teacher structure continuum, the student self-structures and requires little to no external motivation.
10. The liberated, self-structuring student who matures to the fifth level of the learner maturity continuum will be a substantively different graduate from those graduating from behaviorist curricula and will be the true professional nurse.
11. There is not one type of learning but several. Therefore, different learning theories support different types.

12. Different learning types require different teaching modalities.

13. Training can be differentiated from education by the types of learning involved.

14. The cognitive processes one teaches are as important as the content, and because of the utility and durability of cognitive processes, most are more important than the content.

15. The teacher–student interactions are inseparably linked to the kinds of learning episodes engaged in, and both are linked to the types of learning to be attained.

16. No one part of the four theoretical constructs can be altered without altering some aspects of the other three constructs.

17. Caring is the moral imperative of nursing and is an integral part of teacher–teacher, teacher–student, student–student and teacher–student–patient–staff interactions as well as a deliberate component in the curriculum.

Propositions

These theoretical constructs generate the following propositions that are basic to the educative curriculum development paradigm:

1. Oppressive classroom environments (climates) support only immature/low-level student positions; higher level positions may occur but do so in spite of climate.

2. Conversely, liberating classroom environments support high-level student positions. However, some students may not be willing to risk more than positions 1, 2, or 3 (see pg. 83).

3. The more oppressive the teacher–student climate, the lower the student's place on the learner maturity continuum will be. Conversely, the more liberating the student–teacher climate, the higher the student's place on the learner maturity continuum will be.

4. Cultural conditioning, life history, schooling conditioning, and personality characteristics are factors that influence the student's ability to move up the continuum.

5. The greater the number of criteria for educative teacher–student interactions met by the teacher and the greater the number of criteria for educative learning activities that are met, the higher the probability that students will move into maturity levels 4 and 5 and the greater the speed with which they will so move.

6. The more accepting the teacher is of the grief process precipitated in the student by the loss of passive learning roles, the more likely the grief will come to resolution and enable the student to move up the continuum toward learning maturity.

7. The behaviorist paradigm supports positions 1–3 but is antithetical to positions 4 and 5 on the learner maturity continuum. In other words, positions 1–3 are supported by behavioral objective-driven content and by evaluating and grading and take the position that knowledge is received. By contrast, positions 4 and 5 are supported by humanistic existentialism, thrive on criticism, and take the position that knowledge is constructed.

8. Differences in technical and professional nursing programs can be determined by evaluating the relative proportion of training and educative types of learning in each curriculum. Professional programs will contain more content that is educative, while technical programs will contain more content that is training.

9. The higher the nursing educational program is on the educational ladder, the greater the percentage of educational learning will be in the curriculum. Conversely, the lower the nursing educational program is on the educational ladder, the greater the percent of training types of learning will be in the curriculum.

10. Among generic nursing educational programs, the generic doctorate will have the greater percentage of educational types of learning in the curriculum.

11. Liberating teacher–student interactions are necessary to support educative learning.

What becomes clear is that in order to achieve what Botkin (1979) refers to as "innovative" learning and what the American Association of Colleges of Nursing (1986) calls "professional nursing," one must alter the curriculum in ways that promote teaching that educates instead of trains. To do this the nature and amount of the syntactical, contextual, and inquiry learning must alter throughout the curriculum. All generic programs, including the generic master's and doctorate, contain some training. Some nursing content must be memorized, and rules for the use of skills and their underlying rationales must be learned. However, the focus of professional nursing must shift toward educative learning for nursing to graduate the scholar-clinician that will mark the future.

THE MODELS

The goal for the use of these theoretical models is to provide a basis for educating for the human possibility—an education that will teach persons to think as well as act; to know, to continually seek a better knowing, and to discourse about knowing; both to seek and doubt truth while developing a splendid sensitivity and devotion to it; to appreciate the enduring values that make nursing a moral activity; and to shape faculty's wills and focus their energies on this meritorious endeavor called teaching so that nursing may evolve into a service guided by a commitment to enlightened compassion and vigorous scholarship making the 21st century a renaissance for nursing.

The first mini-model is a learner maturity continuum in which degrees of learner maturity are defined. The major assumption is that the characteristics that distinguish maximum learner maturity is the aim of all higher education. The second is a typology of learning in which content categories have been used as a framework for grouping learning into six types: three types designated as training and three as education. The basic assumption here is that in order to progress to truly professional status, baccalaureate and higher degree nursing must provide significantly more emphasis upon the educative types of learning. The third is that certain kinds of teacher–student interactions support educative learning and are useful in moving students forward on the learner maturity continuum and some kinds are counterproductive for that goal. The last is that learning episodes or experiences that meet specified criteria support educative learning and concomitantly are useful in moving students forward on the learner maturity continuum. For these last two mini-models, criteria must be developed that will be useful for faculty in choosing those teacher–student interactions and those learning episodes that are appropriate to their goals.

As mentioned earlier, the theoretical basis for this book begins with the position that all education (as opposed to training) has the goal of graduating students who are independent, self-directed and self-motivated, and life-long learners with questing minds and a familiarity with inquiry approaches to learning. In this paradigm, learners with these characteristics are called mature learners. It is a basic thesis of this book that learner maturity is supported by teachers who choose teacher–student interactions that promote educative types of learning and who structure or choose learning episodes that fall into syntactical, contextual, and inquiry learning types.

Graphically, Figure 1 portrays the way these factors interact.

Figure 1
Educative Factor Interaction

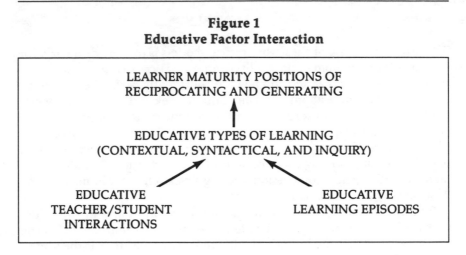

The corollary of this is that using teacher–student interactions and choosing or devising learning episodes that promote types of learning that are training are by nature oppressive and inhibit learner maturity. Such a model is illustrated in Figure 2.

Each of these four ingredients will be discussed individually and reference made to their unique synergistic influence on each other.

Figure 2
Training Factor Interaction

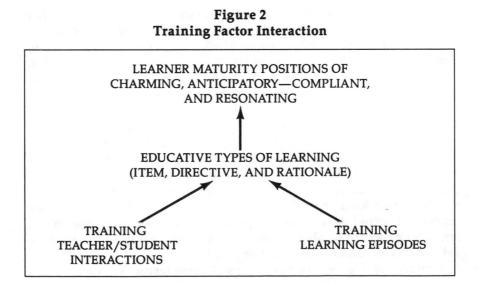

Figure 3
Five Basic Positions on the Learner Maturity Continuum

CHARMING   ANTICIPATORY   RESONATING   RECIPROCATING   GENERATING
COMPLIANT

LEARNER MATURITY CONTINUUM

There are five basic positions on the learner maturity continuum. From lowest to highest level, these are (1) charming, (2) anticipatory-compliant, (3) resonating, (4) reciprocating, and (5) generating. Each of these positions is represented by the relationship the student and teacher have with each other. The positions are student positions and are described in terms of learner attitudes, attributes, characteristics, and/or goals. Some mention may be made of teaching modes, but the emphasis is on the learner. The first three positions represent oppressed positions; the last two represent liberated positions (see Fig. 3).

Immature Positions

There are three immature positions. Each position of student immaturity is supported by oppressive teacher behaviors. Oppression breeds immaturity because it rewards it and it punishes behavior that is not adaptive to the system in place. Therefore, if the teacher structures the course around preconceived behavioral objectives, teaches to those behaviors, and tests those behaviors, students must, in order to survive and make acceptable grades, be charming, adaptive, or resonating.

1. *Charming* is the most immature place on the continuum. When the student is in this position, the student's goal is to please the teacher. It represents a seductive and manipulative stance on the part of the student, and in it students vie for teacher attention and the teacher "liking" them. In elementary school it is represented by the "teacher's pet" idea. Students wish to dupe the teacher into seeing them as special, being more forgiving, and liking them. Sometimes this "manipulation" is out of awareness, to be sure. In this position students bring gifts, apples, and cartoons; they pay compliments and have other forms of seductive behaviors in lieu of serious scholarly activity. The student's message to

the teacher is, "I'm cute and you are wonderful." It is a parent–adaptive child relationship. This is not to say that every time a student pays a compliment, brings a cartoon, or enjoys a nonscholarly time-out moment with the teacher, this constitutes a regression to this position. In this position these activities are the focus of the student's energy and the ultimate goal.

2. *Anticipatory-compliant* is the second-most immature student position. The student's goal is to preguess the teacher. Energy is spent in trying to figure out what the teacher wants so that the student can give the teacher what he or she wants and thereby get a good grade. As in position 1, the focus is on getting a good grade, not on learning. From this position, one hears such statements as, "I always make a low grade on the first test; it takes me at least mid-term to psych out the teacher and learn what he or she wants." Obviously in this position, students do not accept responsibility for success or failure personally but place it on their ability to second-guess the teacher. It too, is the adaptive-child position. The teacher is again authority-parent, and the student is anticipatory (through "psyching out") and compliant (by studying only what it is anticipated that the teacher wants learned).

3. *Resonating* is the center position on the continuum. One can liken it to the student being a crystal goblet and the teacher's lecturing or modeling eliciting in the student an exciting, vibrating resonance. The student finds the teacher attractive in some ways, usually perceiving the teacher as charismatic, stimulating, admirable, and enjoyable. Students in this position find themselves highly motivated. They read and prepare for class, not wanting to miss any part of the experience, and they are eager recipients of the teacher's wit, information, and wisdom. There tends to be great respect and admiration for the teacher. The student position is still primarily passive, with the teacher in control doing frontal teaching and conducting discussions that are alternating teacher to student, student to teacher. It is the most productive of the oppressed positions.

Stenhouse (1967) discusses the role of the teacher in the classroom and the history of that role. He maintains the tradition of authority based on force was a legal position, and reward and punishment were used to direct the child's learning. In this light, he speaks of the teacher making "war on misunderstandings with chalk and talk," and that these teacher modalities teach more than content. They also teach attitudes and approaches to learning. He maintains that force has disappeared in the classroom and other modes of authority have evolved. Among them is charismatic leadership, which depends upon the force of personality.

These teachers "cast a spell rather than wield a cane" (p. 66). He warns that

> charisma dominates the pupils in a way that can become oppressive. Charismatic leadership shades over into propaganda rather easily, and it may well be that teachers who use this power tend from time to time to imprison the minds of their pupils rather than liberate them. (p. 66)

One cannot afford to take his warning lightly.

It is evident that this position is the biggest trap for both students and teachers, for it is rewarding and enjoyable for both. Teachers feel especially good about themselves and are reluctant to relinquish the perks associated with their frontal lectures. Students are not bored and are excited about the subject. However, they are often more excited about the excellence of the teacher and want to take other courses from this teacher, regardless of the content being offered. Nevertheless, it is a good position from which to move into the liberated positions, because students often get the windows of their minds opened to the fresh air of curiosity, inquiry, and love of learning that sweeps through with an intoxication that precludes a subsequent mental shutdown. Also, the students may use this position to develop confidence in the teacher's ability to guide learning (even if it is a traditionally oppressed manner). This confidence provides a platform for liberation and independence.

One must not interpret this as meaning that it is necessary to begin on the continuum only in an oppressed position. One can begin in a liberated position. Teachers can structure courses and teacher–student interactions so that positions 4 and 5 are required from the beginning.

Flip Sides

Each immature position has its flip side. The flip side of *charming* is *hostile*. This opposite behavior is seen in the student who seems to bristle. Hostility radiates from this student even though he or she may be silent, not saying much to either other students or to the teacher. This student shows little interest in the course or its activities and usually gives the teacher a poor evaluation. This student does the work assigned and often does it well. This student may even challenge you with "you can't teach me anything" and sit there hostilely not learning anything just to prove him or herself right.

The flip side of *anticipatory-compliant* is passive-aggressive. The passive-aggressive student is resistant to suggestions regarding what the teacher thinks is adequate scholarship. Ways are found by the student to resist in indirect modes, such as misunderstanding directions, forgetting homework assignments, procrastination, being slow, or becoming stubborn. This person can be more difficult to work with than the overtly hostile person. Working with the passive-aggressive person can be like working with steam: You can see it and feel it, but it's hard to hold.

The flip side of *resonating* is critical. The critical student can't be pleased and is a master of the double bind. If you give thorough directions about a paper or an activity, you are too rigid; if you give much leeway and few instructions, you are too unstructured and disorganized. If you make jokes, you are not serious enough; if you don't, you are too serious and need to loosen up. The tests are too hard or too easy; the room is too cold or too hot; the subject is never interesting and the teacher is always dull. The critical part of this student is in gear all of the time.

Mature Positions

4. *Reciprocating* is the next-to-most mature position for the learner. It is characterized by a course environment that requires students to take responsibility for their learning. It is an environment that frees students to exchange ideas, to challenge each other and the teacher and to take the dialogue in directions that will meet their needs. In it the students have reciprocal relationships with each other and with the teacher. It is a position in which students actively look for patterns, express insights and puzzlement, find meanings and have egalitarian/ collegial relationships both with peers and with teachers. In this position, as in position 5, the teacher–student relationship is one of adult to adult: mutual respect and exciting exchanges. Teachers supply information, cues, models, and paradigms only when asked and when the student is stymied in working with a problem, issue, or client. The student–teacher relationship revolves around transactions that meet the criteria for educative teacher–student relationships and are involved in learning episodes that meet the criteria for educative learning activities. The course climate is liberating.

5. *Generating* is a creative position. Student initiative is high, passivity low to nonexistent. In this position students initiate problems and introduce topics, content, and issues. They move in new directions and

explore ideas relevant to their goals and directions and are searching and inquiring. Teachers are used as true consultants and as expert learners,[1] as content experts, as strategy or methodological experts, or as respected colleagues with whom students bounce ideas around. In this position ideally teachers relinquish their agenda and support the agenda of the student. It is legitimate to have a dialogue or debate about the agenda but not legitimate for the teacher to insist on an agenda. Evaluation for grades is replaced by criticism. Trust is the hallmark, and creativity and inquiry the motif. The position is best illustrated by the doctoral student, especially in the dissertation phase, but it can exist on any level. Teacher–student interactions are those that meet the criteria as discussed later in this chapter.

Uses of the Learner Maturity Continuum

The learner maturity continuum helps teachers establish where their students are on the scale, what their goals are for learner maturity, and what types of learning to select that will best move students to the desired position. It is not the goal of all teachers to have students at position 5. Some teachers, particularly those involved in training programs, might be thwarted by the very fact that students at this position have a low tolerance for frontal lecture, demonstration, return demonstration, memorization, and recitation—all of which are demanded by training. Students at position 2 or 3 might be ideally suited for this type of instruction. If teachers wish to facilitate movement of students into positions 4 and 5, they must involve themselves in three things:

1. Teachers must focus their teaching away from training content and upon educational content as described in the types of learning models (see next section). In typing learning, there is a distinction made

---

[1] The appellation "expert learner" is derived from Stenhouse (1975, p. 91). He proposes that a teacher should be a learner along with students but must accept the responsibility for guiding the learning of students. He suggests that the teacher is a "senior learner" capable of offering something of worth to the junior learners (students). These matters of worth are skills in finding things out, refining skills and knowledge, understanding the subject, and understanding deep structures and rationale in the field of study. I propose that the teacher, because of experience, knowledge, and skill, is the "expert learner" working with and tutoring junior or novice learners. The teacher must also be an expert in content, with knowledge of the literature, clinical skills, and a grasp of the issues, problems of nursing, and methods of inquiry.

between instruction, which relates to training, and teaching, which relates to education.

Furthermore, the three types of learning designated as educative require that teachers interact with students from a position of fellow learner, albeit an expert learner. The whole focus of the teacher–student relationship becomes egalitarian and liberating. The political climates of oppression and liberation as a curriculum phenomenon are discussed in Chapter 6. Teaching students to be egalitarian learners requires the teacher to move from the high structure students to those who are accustomed to low structure and simultaneously teach students to self-structure, so that while the teacher is decreasing teacher structure, the student is increasing self-structure (see Fig. 4).

2. Since the educative types of learning require teacher–student relationships of a kind and nature that support education and movement toward learner maturity, there must be some intelligent way to choose those interactions that are facilitative. Building on the work of Raths (1971), Murray and Merrefield (1989) have developed criteria for selecting teacher–student interactions designed to facilitate educative learning. In a curriculum fashioned to move students toward maturity, the teacher–student interaction is a key ingredient.

3. If one truly wishes to educate rather than train, focusing learning on educative questions is essential. Learning activities are sometimes spontaneous, sometimes preplanned, sometimes teacher designed, sometimes student designed. Regardless of any of these factors, it is the expert teacher's responsibility to pattern the learning episodes (activities, experiences) or to help students learn to pattern them so that they are educative. Again, criteria must be developed so that wise choices

Figure 4
Teacher and Student Structures

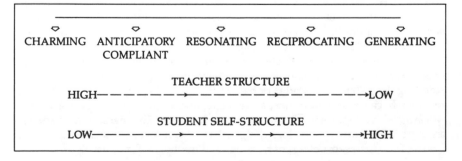

can be made by teachers and/or students when fashioning learning episodes that are educative. In all probability, faculties need to develop their own criteria so that they "own" them and use them. It becomes, in the educative model, one of the key products of a faculty's efforts in curriculum development.

Four entities are irrevocably intertwined: (1) The learner maturity model enables teachers to develop curriculum that supports learner maturity (for without learner maturity, education reaps few lasting benefits to students); (2) clarity regarding the types of learning enables teachers to select types that are educative and thereby facilitate learner maturity; (3) the criteria for student–teacher interactions enables teachers to modify their relationships with students in ways that support educative learning (and therefore maturity); and (4) the criteria for selecting learning episodes that provide the platform, the content, and the focus for educative learning. Since these four aspects of education act as an irreducible whole and since they are postulated to be essential to educative learning, the *most curricular energy must be given to faculty development so that these ways of being a teacher can become natural and normal and thereby shape the curriculum.*

TYPES OF LEARNING

If one accepts the position that maximum learner maturity is the ultimate desired position on the learner maturity continuum, then the query naturally follows, what will foster learner maturity? The answer to that question lies in part in a typology of learning.

The development of learning theory seems to have been undertaken with the assumption that one theory could be devised that would serve for every learning situation. Learning theorists advocate one theory over another, but those who struggle to teach find, that in practice, all theories seem to work to some extent, depending upon the subject matter, the environment and the teacher's abilities.

The assumptions behind the assumption that one "pan-theory" of learning applies to all learning could be one or more of the following: (1) There is only one type of learning; (2) there are "types," but these are in reality "conditions" for learning and exist sequentially on a learning continuum (Gagne, 1970); or (3) there are types of learning, but differences among them are so insignificant that one theory is sufficiently broad to guide the teaching of students.

The problem arises when teachers, in dealing with reality, find that for some learning situations and problems, one theory works better than another. This suggests that there are distinct types of learning, and these types are substantively different.

If one took a different assumption, for instance, that there are different varieties of learning, then it would follow that various theories of learning may be more appropriate or relevant to one variety than to another. It would also follow that, for different purposes, a teacher would choose teaching modalities that employ theories supportive of the kinds of learning desired.

In this sense, a typology of learning could be approached in several ways. For example, when one looks at Bloom's categories of behavioral objectives, one sees immediately that it could become a classification system for learning: cognitive, psycho-motor, and affective (Bloom, 1956). Of course, that would assume that learning follows the dualistic model, which is, of course, the companion of behaviorist theory. Such a typology would be incompatible with this curriculum paradigm. Furthermore, those who teach know from experience that much of human learning is organismic and affects all domains simultaneously. It is not surprising that this "experience" is not easily validated by research, since empirical research methods are the ones most often used, and these methods lend themselves to researching behaviorist theory much better than other types of theory. A second way one could approach a typology would be from the neurological framework, for example, right brain, left brain (Hampden-Turner, 1981). This would use the kinds of brain or intelligence function assigned to the respective hemispheres and the necessary neurological pathways to create a typology. Again, I suspect that, like the senses, the best learning occurs when both hemispheres are used.

Neurolinquistics offers another possible framework (Bandler & Grinder, 1975) which addresses such categories as visual, auditory, and kinesthetic. It might be possible to use these as touchstones for learning categories. However, experienced teachers know that, as suggested before, the more of these categories one reaches, the better the learning, so the same criticism applies, that is, the fact that the best learning is organismic and affects all categories simultaneously holds here as it does for Bloom. However, it should be noted that Bandler and Grinder propose neurolinquistics as useful for improving communications. Therefore, if teachers can perceive which avenue (visual, auditory, or kinesthetic) is the primary perceptual route of a student, communications can be improved, and better teaching should follow.

From this discussion, one can see that the way one types learning depends upon the framework used to generate categories. Since the category system offered here is designed to be helpful to teachers of a practice field, specifically nursing, the type of content to be learned is the influencing factor. Therefore, the typology suggested here assumes that the type of content is directly related to learning types, that is, that people learn different types of content differently. One does not go about memorizing a list of medical vocabulary and abbreviations in the same way one goes about learning to innovate nursing care strategies for a patient with difficult problems. Carried to another level, it seems appropriate to define learning differently according to the various types.

Another factor supporting a typology of learning is this: perhaps training can be differentiated from education by the types of learning involved. How one goes about training a person differs from how one goes about educating a person. Perhaps the reason for these differences is that there are entirely different types of learning involved. If several types of learning do exist, then it would follow that such a typology of learning could be used as a means (1) of sorting content, (2) of differentiating between technical and professional education, (3) of sorting among levels within professional education, (4) for devising or choosing educative or training teacher–student interactions and learning episodes, and (5) for choosing the types of learning most likely to move the student further along the learner maturity continuum. It certainly would be useful as a research framework for any or all of the above.

Assuming the typology is useful for the five purposes mentioned above, it would follow that such a typology would be exceedingly useful to curriculum developers in selecting and sorting content that is educational (as compared to training) and that moves students forward on the learner maturity continuum. In this spirit, types of learning are categorized and offered here (see Table 2).

Suggested Typology[2]

1. *Item Learning* is a category that deals with learning separate pieces of information, individual factors, and simple relationships, such as lists, procedures, and the use of tools and materials. It deals with acquiring the ability to complete a task mechanically and ritualistically, for example, how to take a temperature and appropriate sites for taking it.

---

[2]This material was developed in collaboration with Tamar Bermann, Chief Researcher, Work Research Institutes, Oslo, Norway.

Table 2
Learning Typology

Item	Directive	Rationale	Contextual	Syntactical	Inquiry
Pieces of information	Rules	Underlying theory	Caring and concern	Grounded in practice	Creativity
Individual factors	Injunctions	Sequencing items and directives	Nursing culture, mores, and folkways	Wholes	Investigating
Lists	Do's and don'ts	Why's	Language-jargon	Broad relationships	Theorizing
Procedures	Expectations	Use of formal properties	Perceive world as a nurse	Setting aside rules	Strategizing
Using tools and materials	Instructions	Relationship of skills and interventions to items and directions	Politics	generating personal rules and guides	Researching
Simple relationships between items	Directions	Applying research to practice	Power	Individualized care	Idea generating
Task centered			Ethics	Using personal guides	Visualizing
Mechanical			Work-role relationships	Acknowledging personal paradigm	Determining assumptions and implications
Descriptions			Esthetics	experiences	Scholarly feelings, standards, activities
			Philosophy (nursing)	Consequential reasoning	Questioning
			Professional activities	Insights	Intuitive leaps
			Professional identification	Meanings	Analyzing
				Interpretations	Synthesizing
				Significance	Criticism
				Comparisons	
				Patterns	
				Using informal properties	
				Deeper structures of the field	
				Praxis	

2. *Directive Learning* is the learning of rules, injunctions, and the exceptions to the rules. It is similar to a set of instructions. This type of learning is concerned with the "do's" and "don'ts" regarding tasks and includes the assembling of items into a safe system of directions. By necessity, directive learning follows item learning or can be learned concurrently.

3. *Rationale Learning* uses theory to buttress practice. In other words, it provides the rationale for why one nursing intervention is better than another. Answers to questions such as "Why do you do that this way?" and "What is the rationale for this nursing intervention?" are placed in this category. Simply put, this category concerns learning theories and rationales, when they apply, and their use in practice. In part, it is characterized by arranging the items and directions in some logical order and finding theories to inform practice (or if one prefers, on which to base practice). It addresses the rational use of *formal* properties of activities and theories and enables one to relate information (data) and ideas to plan interventions and skills. It exerts influence on judgment and decision making and enables learners to apply research to practice. It permits grounding practice in realities that are classical and fit known patterns, and it facilitates the structuring of nursing work and knowledge in a manner consistent with common or expected consequences of nursing care or interventions.

4. *Contextual Learning* is the cultural framework in which the field of nursing and its practice exists. It is the essence of nursing, the things that characterize it and make it uniquely nursing and not medicine, physical therapy, or social work. This category pertains to learning the sociocultural context of the discipline and the mores, folkways, rites, rituals, and accepted ways of being of nursing. It is the aspects of learning nursing that help one become a person who thinks and feels like a nurse. It is the language of nursing and its symbolism. It is the development of political expertise in the profession and its use in health agencies, in education, and in government to shape policy and legislation. It is the acquisition of power and its use. This category deals with the relationships in the work role of coordination, collaboration, and colleagueship. It is learning the values, esthetics, ethics, and general philosophy of nursing. It is learning to perceive of nursing as a human science in ways that influence nurses' transactions with clients and with colleagues so that these transactions are caring, compassionate, and positive.

5. *Syntactical Learning* is characterized by the logical structure or arrangements of data into meaningful wholes. The qualities of the situation are used as data in ways that prompt the learner to depart from the

rules and from the usual or customary nursing interventions to provide care patterned specifically for the unique client in the unique situation of the moment. It enables the use of informal (feelings and intuition) as well as formal properties and helps one to relate experiences to modes of using information, skills, ideas, and plans in ways that allow for deviating from the normal. It influences how one uses all other types of learning.

This type of learning enables finding practice-grounded patterns, examples, and models that support formation of personal general guides and paradigms and provides help in knowing when and under what circumstances one departs from these. The extent of achievement in this category influences the degree of expertise as described by Benner (1984). Benner's work has greatly influenced the formation of this category.

Syntactical learning belongs to the real nature and essence of things as opposed to the classical, rule-driven models of practice. This may be because theories, by necessity, are based in the average, the common, or classical patterns, and usually do not allow for the individual uniqueness and differences among people, while nurses in practice find a wide variety of individuality. This category addresses the relationships that ideas, concepts, and theories have with each other in *practical* usage. It promotes consequential reasoning and a substantive view of relationships.

This type of learning is characterized by viewing wholes, having insights, finding meanings and significance, interpreting, evaluating and projecting, and predicting from knowns to unknowns using both data and intuition. This type of learning enables people to make intuitive leaps and to trust them. It is the welding together of theory and practice into praxis.

6. *Inquiry Learning* is the creative aspect of nursing. In this category is the art of investigation, the search for truth, the generation of theory, and the development of new ideas, dreams, and visions. It contains materials that help people learn how to identify, clarify, and categorize the problems of the discipline of nursing as it attempts to be responsive to the society it serves. It also contains the ways or approaches to solving these problems. It is more than research and research design. It is idea generating: fantasizing new ways of doing things, new configurations of old ideas, and alterations or adjustments that improve things and systems; generating creative leaps into new dimensions; posing questions; formulating positions; visualizing possibilities; and inventing ways to make them realities. In this category, one learns to derive assumptions that are behind positions and to question their validity, to see beyond words to their implications and applications, and to enjoy the quest.

USING THE TYPOLOGY

The following items are to be kept in mind when using this typology:

1. The typology represents "kinds" of learning, not levels. However, each type has within it various levels of expertise.

2. Type 1, item learning and type 2, directive learning, may be necessary precursors to all other types. However, the degree of focus and the amount of emphasis placed on them would be minimal when one is working in the inquiry and contextual types.

3. Except for types 1 and 2, the types are not tied into a sequential relationship. For instance, type 3 (rationale learning) must follow its two companions, types 1 (item learning) and 2 (directive), but may just as easily accompany types 6 (inquiry) and 4 (contextual learning).

4. These are "types" of learning, and the descriptions used to distinguish them are derived from content and scholarly processes. Not attempted here are the implications regarding the teaching methods to be used with each type. However, these might be derived if one attempts to match learning theories to each type of learning in the typology. That has not been attempted here.[3]

As mentioned before, this typology is useful in several ways. One way is to examine curricula to determine the degree of training or education addressed. The tables in this section illustrate a rough estimate of the types of learning included in the various curriculum development models in existence today.

Generic doctoral programs are projected to have a much larger emphasis upon educative types of learning than other generic programs. This is due to the increased amount of humanities and other liberal arts courses allowed by the pattern of the generic doctorate.

---

[3] It has been an interesting exercise for me to attempt to trace the authors who have influenced this typology. Since the work on it extended over several years and the ideas about it evolved slowly, several editions were tried and discarded as it formed. Consequently, much synthesis took place, and there is no way to be sure about the parentage of some categories, for none is pure. Item learning probably had its nucleus in Dickoff, James, and Wiedenbach (1968); directive, in Gagne (1970); rationale, just seemed right (intuition? a visit from the muses?); contextual had its origin in Stenhouse (1975); syntactical came from Benner (1985); and inquiry also had its origin in Stenhouse (1975). Considering the disparate nature of the various schools of psychology of learning and learning theory from whence these authors come, it seems certain that different learning theories could be found appropriate to each of the categories.

THE USE OF THE TYPOLOGY FOR
CURRICULUM DEVELOPMENT MODELS

The typology of learning can be used to determine curriculum content and to provide the teacher with help in structuring or selecting learning episodes so that learning is educative and learners move forward on the learner maturity continuum. Every level, except practical nursing, uses every type of learning to some extent. However, the probabilities are high that the percentages of learnings categorized within each type alters for each kind of program in nursing. Percentages are not the only things affected by alterations in programs. For instance, in contextual learning the very nature of the content included in the program may differ—so that both diploma and baccalaureate education may both have contextual (socialization) content, but the nature of the content chosen for the overt curriculum or existing in the hidden curriculum may vary considerably.

The American Association of Colleges of Nursing's final report on the *Essentials of College and University Education for Professional Nursing* (1986) states, "attitudes are inclinations or dispositions to respond positively or negatively to a person, object, or situation, while personal qualities are innate or learned attributes of an individual" (p. 5). (Is the implication here that attitudes are not learned?) They have obviously attempted to distinguish between an inclination or disposition (as in attitude) and an attribute (described as a personal quality) because Webster (1971) describes them both as qualities or characteristics but states that attributes are inherent; the distinction is not clear regarding the AACN's use of these terms. Be that as it may, and clarity of intent aside, the significance placed upon personal qualities and attitudes in this important report is refreshing. Attitudes arise from values, ethics, and morals, and research indicates that values are learned in schools at all levels (Felton & Parsons, 1984; Rest, 1979.) Furthermore, the AACN report takes the position that "Values are reflected in attitudes, personal qualities, and consistent patterns of behaviors," and it goes on to recommend seven values that are deemed essential for the professional nurse: altruism, equality, esthetics, freedom, human dignity, justice, and truth. All these fall into the category called contextual here and in the AACN report, "socialization."

The point here is that such values are probably inherent in nursing programs regardless of level—but the content chosen and the socialization aspects in the hidden curriculum would emphasize different aspects

Table 3
Categories of Learning

	Training			Education	
Item	Directive	Rationale	Contextual	Syntactical	Inquiry

of these values, place more or less stress upon them, choose different learning activities to teach them in the overt curriculum, and thereby make their differences evident. It would not be true that technical programs do not teach these values in either the overt or the hidden curricula. That so much value is placed upon a category of learning that can be so poorly evaluated under the behaviorist curriculum paradigm is indicative of the need for a paradigm shift. It also supports the position that most of the content in this learning type is truly professional and educative and, therefore, if it is used in conjunction with the appropriate learning episodes and teacher–student interactions, it moves students upward on the maturity continuum. Table 3 illustrates which categories of learning are generally conceived as educative and which as training. It is important to note, however, that to the expert, the items, directives, and rationales, usually perceived as "training," become "education." This probably occurs because the expert readily sees patterns and has a cognitive structure that provides order and meaning to new material.

TYPES OF LEARNING IN KINDS OF PROGRAMS

The key proposition here is that the more weight that is given the educative types of learning in a curriculum, the more professional is that curriculum. The corollary is that the more weight given to training types of learning, the more technical is the program. Figure 5 illustrates this. Another proposition is that the higher up the educational ladder a program is, the greater proportion of its curriculum is educational learning.

The diagonal line illustrates the relative proportion of types of learning in each of the levels of nursing education. It moves from PhD, which has the least item learning and the most inquiry, to ADN, which has the most item and the least inquiry.

Figure 5
Proportion of Types of Learning in Kinds of Programs

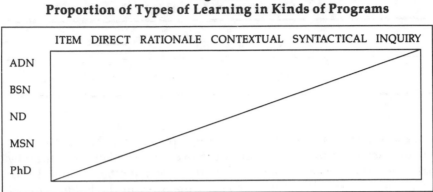

The basic assumption here is that in order to progress to truly professional status, baccalaureate and higher degree nursing must provide significantly more emphasis upon the educative types of learning. The question arises, can this be done in the traditional 4-year academic period allotted to "professional" education, or do we need to acknowledge the validity of the academic models of other professions and pursue the nursing doctorate?

Estimated Percentages of Types of Learning in Various Types of Nursing Programs

The following tables are a rough, unresearched estimate of kinds of learning that are the focus for each common type of program. These tables do not address the *nature* of the content selected for type of learning in each kind of program (see Tables 4 and 5).

Baccalaureate and master's programs are predicted to alter in the ways represented above because they are the programs that would be most affected by new ways of perceiving curriculum.

Doctoral programs are changing, not only because of curriculum development paradigms, but also because of an increasing awareness of the value of nonempiricist research methods and the world view that accompanies such shifts. It is expected that under a curriculum-development paradigm shift, baccalaureate programs would become more focused on the syntactical, an area that is inadequately emphasized by today's nursing educators, usually falling within the null curriculum in undergraduate programs.

Table 4
Estimated Percentage of Type of Learning Currently in
Nursing Curricula by Type of Program

	Item	Directive	Rationale	Contextual	Syntactical	Inquiry
Practical	60	27	10	3	0	0
Diploma	35	30	17	15	3	0
Associate	35	30	17	10	3	5
Baccalaureate	25	25	20	15	5	10
Master's	10	10	20	20	15	25
ND*	?	?	?	?	?	?
Doctorate	0	0	5	15	10	70

*ND, too few programs to estimate percentages.

Master's programs would also shift toward more syntactical content. One of the major purposes of master's programs is to prepare clinical specialists, and clinical expertise is the focus of syntactical learning. It may be that syntactical learning takes place best in the clinical area or in clinical simulation. Certainly, clinical experience is essential and central to it. Benner's work (1985) verifies this. This type of learning relies heavily on teacher–student interactions that help students search for and find meanings, view wholes, crystallize insights, evaluate, project, predict, and intuit. For these activities, human-to-human transactions

Table 5
Predicted Estimated Percentage of Type of Learning in
Nursing Curricula by Type of Program if Educative (Professional)
(Nonbehaviorist) Curriculum Development Models Were Used for
the Baccalaureate, Master's, and Doctorate Programs

	Item	Directive	Rationale	Contextual	Syntactical	Inquiry
Practical	60	27	10	3	0	0
Diploma	35	30	17	15	3	0
Associate	35	30	17	10	3	5
Baccalaureate*	15	20	25	15	15	10
Master's*	5	5	10	25	25	30
ND	10	15	15	20	20	20
Doctorate	0	0	5	15	10	70

*Programs that have percentages altered from Table 4.

may not be essential, but they are certainly facilitative. Generic doctoral programs assuredly will have a significant role in nursing's rise to professionalism, and, as mentioned earlier, the amount of educative learning predicted for these programs is possible because of their liberal arts base.

TEACHER–STUDENT INTERACTIONS

Raths (1971) argues that "activities may be justified for inclusion in the curriculum on grounds other than those based on the efficacy of the activity for specifically changing the behaviors of students" (p. 714). He goes on to suggest that schools, "while accepting a minimum number of training responsibilities, should take as their major purpose one of involving students in activities which have no preset objectives, but which meet other specified criteria" (p. 714). With these statements, he introduces a proposal that the major focus of schools should turn from learning episodes designed to bring about specific behavioral changes and that other mechanisms be devised to be used as a basis for justifying the selection of learning activities for the curriculum. He suggests that a list of value statements written as criteria be used as a guide for such selection. He calls these "criteria for worthwhile activities."

His idea was picked up by Stenhouse (1975) in his development of a "process model" of curriculum as an example of a possible way to select content according to principles that are not governed by behavioral objectives. He furnishes a critique in which he says, "The formulation of a schedule of behavioral objectives helps us little towards the means of attaining them. The analysis of the criteria for worthwhile activities and of the structure of the activities deemed to be worthwhile appears to point much more clearly to principles of procedure in teaching" (p. 87).

Stenhouse proceeds to discuss Peters' (1959) "principles of procedure" for teachers, as well as those of Metcalf (1963). Both authors advocate some principles of teaching (or, as Peters refers to it, "procedure").

Although all of these scholars stop short of recommending criteria for selecting appropriate teacher–student interactions for educative learning, the logical progression of their thought, taken to its conclusion, would embrace such criteria. This would seem true especially if one is searching for an alternative paradigm for curriculum that would provide some structure for both the processes and the content. If one devises a set of criteria for developing and selecting learning activities, it seems to follow that a similar set of criteria would be appropriate for guiding the teaching modalities.

Stenhouse's argument supporting emphasizing the responsibilities of individual teachers as a curriculum development tool (1975, p. 62) uses work done on a project with which he was involved called the "North West Development Project." He presents a list of items he calls objectives, which sound as if they could easily be translated into criteria for guiding teaching modalities. This list does not resemble the behavioral type of objectives we are accustomed to using. Among many others are these objectives: "Helping students develop interests, attitudes and esthetic awareness," "developing basic concepts and logical thinking," "posing questions and devising experiments or investigations to answer them," and "appreciating patterns and relationships and interpreting findings critically."

Stenhouse's Process Model has influenced Bevis' work considerably. Among the seminal features of his model are the elements committed to teacher development (1975, pp. 96–97). He advises using something similar to Raths' criteria for selecting and devising learning activities or episodes, suggests principles of procedure as guides for teaching (altered for this paradigm, to criteria for teacher–student interactions), and suggests using criticism rather than evaluation. It seems logical in a professional and educative curriculum that there must be a great deal of congruity among the criteria for selecting learning activities and those for guiding the way teachers relate to students. They both must come into play synergistically in order to support learning that is educative, liberating, and facilitates learner maturity.

Using Bevis' Educative Curriculum Development paradigm, Murray and Merrefield (1989) have developed, for research purposes, a list of criteria for teacher–student interactions and a list for selecting or devising learning experiences. (Murray and Merrefield use the term *experiences,* while I have chosen to call them *learning activities or episodes.*) In Chapter 7, Murray discusses the two aspects of the curriculum. The following are a few of their criteria as examples. Their criteria, however, can be found in Appendix I. As stated before, these criteria are necessary to devising curriculum-learning experiences and for selecting ways and modalities for teachers and students to interact, with the general educative goal of graduating mature learners who are educated for a profession.

CRITERIA FOR TEACHER–STUDENT INTERACTIONS

1. Teacher–student interactions provide teacher and student with intellectual stimulation that requires disciplined thinking about subject area.
2. Teacher and student select goals that are important and may not be behaviorally measured.
3. Teacher–student interactions occur in diverse situations calling for varied roles.
4. Teacher provides a positive milieu that is conducive to activities that promote learning, that is, discussion, small group work, confrontation, etc.
5. Teacher engages student in activities that develop cognitive structures and positive affective responses.
6. Teacher helps student to develop own meaningful ways of knowing and thinking processes.
7. Teacher–student interactions assist student in deriving meaning from the learning experiences.
8. Teacher–student interactions raise issues and questions about the subject matter that require the student to use a variety of heuristics.
9. Teacher's sharing the critique of student's work is more important than the concept of grading.
10. Teacher reacts in a constructively critical manner to the student's work, refining and developing standards and stressing a sense of scholarliness.
11. Teacher provides an atmosphere and climate that communicate valuing caring and concern as the moral imperative of nursing.

CRITERIA FOR LEARNING EXPERIENCES

1. Provides an environment that requires the student to be actively involved in learning.
2. Creates a cognitive dissonance that requires the student to engage in educative heuristics such as reflection, incubation, dialogue, debate, imagining, and hypothesizing to approach the resolution of the dissonance.

3. Requires the student to practice creative approaches to the subject matter.

4. Uses writing to encourage students to perceive, create, reflect, represent, and inquire.

5. Structures activities so that the student discovers solutions, alternatives, consequences, etc., for self.

6. Requires the student to use a variety of methods of inquiry in order to find or create information, raise questions, etc.

7. Requires the student to use a variety of theoretical frameworks from which to view issues/problems.

8. Engages the student in intellectual or higher thinking modes such as analyzing, critiquing, identifying and evaluating assumptions, inquiring into the nature of things, predicting, searching for patterns, engaging in praxis, viewing wholes, etc.

9. Requires student to support and defend formulated propositions, postulates, and hypotheses.

10. Allows for interaction between the teacher and student around the many possible outcomes of the experience.

11. Promotes encounters with the artistic aspects of nursing, such as meanings, relationships, context, patterns, and new insights.

12. Requires the student to use a variety of sources and rationales as evidence from which to draw conclusions.

13. Allows for dialogue around finding meanings in the experience, errors made, acknowledging paradigm experiences, differences, and diversity.

A last criterion must be added here that is not in the Murray–Merrefield list to ensure philosophical consistency with the paradigm:

14. Provides the structure and models so that students experience the productive compatibility of caring and concern with good scholarship.

USING THE CRITERIA FOR CURRICULUM

Since curriculum, as defined in this book, *is* composed of those interactions and transactions that occur between teachers and students and among students with the intent that learning take place, it follows that there must be some way to determine what transactions and interactions are to be used. Criteria such as these, devised by the faculty and used to guide their interactions and selection of learning activities, provide such a way. What of the subject matter called nursing? Whatever nursing content is chosen is done so with an eye to its compatibility with these criteria. Content has too long been the driver of curriculum and as consequence course outlines have bulged with content. Chapters 5–7 will address this problem and offer some guidelines for faculties attempting to use the mini-models to develop curriculum.

REFERENCES

American Association of Colleges of Nursing. (1986). *Essentials of college and university education for professional nursing, final report.* Washington, DC: American Association of Colleges of Nursing.

Bandler, R., & Grinder, J. (1975). *The structure of magic I: A book about language and therapy.* Palo Alto, CA: Science and Behavior Books.

Beauchamp, G. A. (1981). *Curriculum theory* (4th ed.). Itasca, IL: F. E. Peacock.

Benner, P. (1984). *From novice to expert: Excellence and power in clinical nursing practice.* Menlo Park, CA: Addison-Wesley.

Bevis, E. (1973). *Curriculum in nursing: A process.* St. Louis: C. V. Mosby.

Bevis, E. (1982, 1989). *Curriculum building in nursing: A process* (3rd ed.). New York: National League for Nursing.

Bevis, E., & Bower, F. (1972). *Comparisons of characteristics and preferences of students upon entering and exiting the nursing department curriculum.* Unpublished studies done as part of the evaluation of United States Department of Health, Education, and Welfare, Public Health Service, Division of Nursing Training Project Grant, identifying the core content of an advanced nursing curriculum. San Jose State University, San Jose, CA.

Bloom, B. S. (Ed.), Englehart, M. D., Furst, E. J., Hill, W. H., & Krathwohl, D. R. (1956). *Taxonomy of educational objectives.* New York: Longmans, Green.

Botkin, J. W., Elmandjra, M., & Malitza, M. (1979). *No limits to learning: Bridging the human gap.* New York: Pergamon.

Caswell, H., & Campbell, D. (1935). *Curriculum development.* New York: American Book Company.

Dickoff, J., James, P., & Weidenbach, E. (1968). Theory in a practice discipline. *Nursing Research, 17,* 415–435.

Doll, R. (1978). *Curriculum improvement: Decision making and process* (4th ed.). Boston: Allyn and Bacon.

Eisner, E. (1985). *The educational imagination* (2nd ed.). New York: Macmillan.

Felton, G. M., & Parsons, M. A. (1984). *The effect of education on the ability to resolve ethical / moral dilemmas.* Unpublished paper.

Freire, P. (1970). *Pedagogy of the oppressed.* New York: Herder and Herder.

Gagne, R. (1967). Curriculum research and the promotion of learning. In R. Tyler, R. Gagne, & M. Scriven (Eds.), *Perspectives of curriculum evaluation.* Chicago: Rand McNally.

Gagne, R. (1970). *The conditions of learning* (2nd ed.). New York: Holt, Rinehart and Winston.

Gray, H. (1988). The aims of education. *The University of Chicago Magazine, 80*(2), 2–8.

Grove, P. (1971). *Webster's third new international dictionary of the English language unabridged.* Springfield, MA: G. and C. Merriam.

Hampden-Turner, C. (1981). *Maps of the mind: Charts and concepts of the mind and its labyrinths.* New York: Collier.

Huebner, D. (1968). The task of the curriculum theorist. Teachers College, Columbia University. New York: Mimeographed.

Johnson, M., Jr. (1967). Definitions and models in curriculum theory. *Educational Theory, 17*(2), 127–140.

King, E. (1984). *Affective education in nursing: A guide to teaching and assessment.* Rockville, MD: Aspen.

Krathwohl, D. R., Bloom, B. S., & Masia, B. B. (1964). *Taxonomy of educational objectives, handbook II: The affective domain.* New York: Longman.

Macdonald, J., & Leeper, R. (1965). *Theories of instruction.* Alexandria, VA: Association for Supervision and Curriculum Development.

Metcalf, L. (1963). Research on teaching the social studies. In N. Gage (Ed.), *Handbook of research on teaching,* A Project of The American Educational Research Association, A Department of the National Education Association. Chicago: Rand McNally.

Murray, J., & Merrefield, S. (1989). Criteria for teacher–student interactions and learning experiences. In J. Murray, *Developing criteria to support new curriculum models for doctoral education in nursing.* Doctoral dissertation, University of Georgia.

Oliva, P. (1982). *Developing the curriculum.* Boston: Little, Brown.

Peters, R. (1959). *Authority, responsibility and education.* London: Allen and Unwin.

Polanyi, M., & Prosch, H. (1975). *Meaning.* Chicago: University of Chicago Press.

Popham, W., & Baker, E. (1970). *Systematic instruction.* Englewood Cliffs, NJ: Prentice-Hall.

Raths, J. D. (1971). Teaching without specific objectives. *Educational Leadership, 28,* 714–720.

Rest, J. (1979). *Manual for the defining issues test: An objective test of moral judgment* (rev. ed.). Minneapolis: University of Minnesota.

Saylor, J., & Alexander, W. (1954). *Curriculum planning for better teaching and learning.* New York: Holt, Rinehart and Winston.

Saylor, J., & Alexander, W. (1974). *Planning curriculum for schools.* New York: Holt, Rinehart and Winston.

Stenhouse, L. (1967). *Culture and education.* London: Nelson.

Stenhouse, L. (1975). *An introduction to curriculum research and development.* London: Heinemann.

Taba, H. (1962). *Curriculum development: Theory and practice.* New York: Harcourt, Brace, Jovanovich.

Tyler, R. (1949). *Basic principles of curriculum and instruction.* Chicago: University of Chicago Press.

Vallance, E. (1973–1974). Hiding the hidden curriculum. *Curriculum Theory Network, 4*(1).

BIBLIOGRAPHY

Huebner, D. (1966). Curriculum language and classroom meanings. In Association for Supervision and Curriculum Development, *Language and meaning.* Washington, DC: The Association.

Peters, R. (1973). Must an educator have an aim? In R. Peters (Ed.), *Authority, responsibility and education,* pp. 83–95. London: Allen and Unwin.

Scriven, M. (1967). The methodology of evaluation. *AERA Monograph Series on Curriculum Evaluation, No. 1. Perspectives of Curriculum Evaluation,* pp. 39–83. Chicago: Rand McNally.

5

Clusters of Influence for Practical Decision Making about Curriculum

Em Olivia Bevis

All formulas for meeting life—even many philosophies . . . are illusion.

Robertson Davies, The Manticore

INTRODUCTION

Davies is right. It is an illusion to think that things can be reduced to formulas. Yet we still hope for the formula and prefer the illusion to the more complex, but infinitely more interesting, reality. Methods and formulas often make mechanical the fluid, mercurial world of curriculum. Curriculum construction can never become a matter of routine or formula; it is too great a mixture of human elements. Good curriculum development relies on variety: variety in ideas, prejudices, imagination, knowledge, facts, theories, and creativity.

We search for formulas because of the complexity of the task and the interpersonal problems among faculty that these complexities often beget. Curriculum development is complicated because it involves people who have vested interests and private hopes and dreams. Although faculty have differing ideas about what nursing curriculum should be, they have a common desire to make the best possible education for students. Needless to say, there are widely differing ideas about what constitutes "best." Curriculum development is further complicated by the fact that faculty have various levels of curriculum expertise.

In curriculum development, faculty whose ideas differ often become so emotionally involved that dialogue breaks down and becomes polemics. Ambrose Bierce (1958) said that battle is "a method of untying with the teeth a political knot that would not yield to the tongue" (p. 11) and discussion is "a method of confirming others in their errors" (p. 18). Both, unfortunately, are reminiscent of what happens among faculty members embroiled in the business of trying to agree upon curriculum matters. It is no wonder that faculties seek formulas that will provide a route that avoids the pain, the emotional energy, and the trials of forbearance that often mark discussions about curriculum changes. What occurs too frequently are faculty curriculum meetings that are fraught with misplaced dreams and lost ideas. They are laden with ambiguity, laced with multiple, unpredictable variables, and characterized by clandestine conspiracies, secret hopes, closet anxieties, and mass confusion. These problems can be avoided. Avoiding them depends not so much on formulas for curriculum construction as on advice about how to have productive group meetings so that all agenda are legitimate, and people's needs are honored.

This chapter attempts to provide some advice regarding productive curriculum development meetings and some guidelines about the use of what I shall call "clusters of influence." These are groups of factors that influence practical curriculum decisions.

Any help offered here, however, must be taken as it is offered: as possible routes among many options, as steppingstones in a bog. There may be some light shed on the pathway but no overall illumination. Therefore, this chapter has the intent of providing discussion on the possibilities and the general directions that can be taken by faculties.

It is difficult to face curriculum development when one is attempting to move in a new direction that has only a group of mini-models as general paradigm. One can become so vague about the possible shape and form of the finished curriculum (outcome) that a vision can turn to nightmare. This chapter is an attempt to help educators avoid as many traps as possible, find their own parameters, plot their own directions, and stay as consistently as possible with educative-caring curriculum.

The goal is to help faculties develop a curriculum that by its nature emancipates both students and faculty, one that educates yet builds upon the base of skills necessary to expert care. One overall aspiration is to free students to cultivate their creativity and pursue their individual learning goals while helping them become professional nurses. In this way, schools would graduate a different kind of student, which in turn will enable the profession of nursing to attain a new level of excellence and to make new progress toward becoming a discipline.

Any curriculum paradigm can be expressed in a wide variety of curriculum structures. Some think of this ultimately as a program of study or courses that group content into manageable clumps. Other structures are such things as theories that are used as conceptual frameworks; the organization of the curriculum development products into such categories as philosophy, objectives, courses, and evaluation tools; the way clinical experiences are arranged; the decisions guiding the allocation of educational resources; the guidelines for setting up course outlines; the constraints within which faculty must teach; and, ultimately, the climate that establishes the patterns for teacher–student interactions. The ways in which these structures manifest themselves are largely dependent upon the framework used by the curriculum architects. These very frameworks that provide so much help can also be dangerously limiting by dictating the constraints that restrict exploration of new ideas about ways to approach teaching nursing. It can also restrict trials of liberating teaching methods, and it can restrict development of imaginative and creative new views of the world. Therefore, the disadvantage of any process guide is that it limits while enabling. The impossible intent of this guide is to enable without limiting. So, instead, it is offered as a loose structure that within the limits of the ultimate values inherent in the paradigm and expressed in the assumptions, propositions and mini-models can be invoked or omitted at will.

The best description of curriculum development I have ever encountered (Zukav, 1980) is one that is least formulalike and most appropriately fits the intent of the educative-caring curriculum:

> *When a child stands in awe and mystery of a falling rose petal, then it's time to teach the law of gravity.*

CURRICULUM DEVELOPMENT
AS INFLUENCE CLUSTERS

The idea that curriculum development can be viewed as, what I have named, "clusters of influence" needs explanation. Often, for instance in the Tyler (1949) rationale, the Taba (1962) inverted model, and the

Bevis (1973–1982; 1989) process model, there is a fairly clear process for curriculum development that is linear in nature. This works in those models because the parameters are established through fairly clear considerations and accepted traditions. One establishes a philosophy; looks at setting, students, and subject matter; derives some theories/concepts; and devises behavioral objectives at every level. From that, one selects the content that meets the objectives and sorts them into some order that seems to make sense to the faculty. And—voila!—you have a curriculum. It is then a simple matter to devise evaluation strategies that determine the merit of achievement of the specified behaviors (see Chapter 9). In a paradigm shift that frees us from the constraints of such clear parameters, the process of curriculum development is no longer linear. (It never was, it just seemed so.) It is not that curriculum development in an educative-caring model is more complex; it is only that each factor to be considered in curriculum development is acknowledged as having influence and the extent and manner of the influence is fluid.

The factors that do influence decisions about curriculum have a fairly natural pattern of classification. These groupings are the "clusters of influence" for practical decision making about curriculum. The factors cluster around four general topics or issues: (1) needs assessment, (2) faculty role development, (3) general goals/ends in view, and (4) program content (see Fig. 1). Of these, the cluster entitled "faculty role development" is the key to the substantive differences between this paradigm and a behaviorist one. This is true for contingency reasons. Without faculties developing new ways to perceive and carry out their roles, no real changes in curriculum will occur. And, without these changes, the general goals cluster (criteria for teacher/student interactions and criteria for selecting and devising learning activities) will never emerge as liberating and educating. Furthermore, the content will remain packed and laden with the details of a thousand

Figure 1
Clusters of Influence

ASSESSMENT	PROGRAM CONTENT
PRACTICAL DECISION MAKING	
FACULTY DEVELOPMENT	GENERAL GOALS

diseases and learning will remain defined as a change in behavior. Therefore, there seems a sequence and a power order of sorts, but for process purposes—for example, what comes first, second, or third—it is illusion, for none do and each can. Sometimes faculty development precedes needs assessment, although needs assessment seems the place to start. There just is no *one* place to start. A faculty may begin with the general goals cluster, the content, or the assessment cluster and from there enter the faculty development cluster after realizing that new teaching skills must emerge in order to realize the other aspects.

The idea of clusters of influence gives rise to this position: *No one factor is powerful enough to be singularly persuasive in shaping curriculum. It is the interplay of a whole group of factors that, acting synergistically, influence the character and direction curriculum development takes within a school.* These factors, although examined individually, in actual fact act as a cluster, as a whole. This whole gives impetus to the choices faculties make about curriculum.

DESCRIPTION OF THE CLUSTERS

The four clusters are so interwoven themselves that their influences are in all directions simultaneously. They are sensitive actors that complement, promote, inhibit, motivate, inspire, impel, arouse, alter, and modify each other. A good metaphor is a basketball team comprised of four instead of five players, in a game revolving around which of the players has the ball and what that player does with it. When running up the court toward the basket, the players fall into one pattern of interactions; when the ball is thrown at the basket they interact in a different way; when they are defending against another team, they arrange themselves in another distinctive mode. But to have a winning team, each player knows the other player's ways and moves smoothly to be responsive to the nuances of alterations in goal, patterns, style, and methods.

The same holds for the clusters. It is impossible to change a factor in one cluster without altering the whole paradigm in some way, even if it is a small alteration. By necessity, Figure 1, representing the four clusters, is static, and it would mislead one to think there is some significance in the way they are arranged. There is significance only to the extent that faculty development is, as explained earlier, a central factor. The explanation is simple. Neither undergraduate nor graduate education in nursing or in education has prepared faculty for any but the behaviorist curriculum model. This makes faculty development a necessary aspect of curriculum development at this stage of nursing history simply because most faculty, regardless of academic degrees, have not been prepared for the shift in thinking and interacting with students that this paradigm represents. Because of this, faculty development must revolve around each part of the process and become an integral part of all phases of curriculum development. Otherwise a curriculum will be developed that few can teach, although all may wish to do so. Failure will occur, not because the curriculum is poor, but because faculty changes in role perception and enactment have been insufficient to support an educative-caring liberating-transformative curriculum.

Figure 1 is an attempt to illustrate the clusters of influence. Each cluster will be discussed individually.

THE ASSESSMENT CLUSTER

Most faculties do not start with a formal assessment for curriculum revision. Only in situations in which new schools of nursing are under consideration does one think first in terms of an assessment. These assessments, in the form of feasibility studies, determine if a school is possible in that particular setting, at that time, and with the available resources. They look at student availability and costs, whether or not they can attract faculty, practice settings, and many other aspects of starting a program. Few people do a full feasibility study for curriculum revision. But some kind of assessment is necessary in order to determine present conditions and future directions and capabilities.

Usually change begins, not with a formal assessment per se, but with a sense in the faculty or in key members of the faculty that something could be done better. Often the spark is an approaching self-study. It might be a higher failure rate on board examinations than the faculty finds unacceptable—perhaps a workshop that ignites the imagination and affirms a subliminal dream of better things. The factors that can motivate faculties to begin to look at whether or not they wish to revise the curriculum are endless. Whatever the cause, there gradually grows a facultywide feeling that they would like to investigate the possibilities of curriculum change. This can either result in inviting a consultant or in some sort of study.

Most faculty have in place an ongoing assessment that helps them make the continuing adjustments necessary to the smooth conduct of every course and the curriculum. Otherwise schools have a built-in obsolescence factor so that doomsday curriculum changes must occur every 7–8 years. (Doomsday curriculum changes are those that occur because things get so bad that accreditation is threatened, state approval is jeopardized, students are unhappy, faculty turnover is high, community or state reputation is poor, health care agencies do not want the students/faculty to practice in them, and things must change or things will close down.) However, when changes, such as a major paradigm shift, are contemplated, yearly minor adjustments made in response to the ongoing assessments are inadequate.

Another phenomenon around curriculum change is the 7-year itch. This is a phenomenon concerning the cyclic degeneration of good curricula. About every 7 years in some fairly good schools, a major curriculum change is carried out. Everyone works hard as the faculty divide and debate issues such as integration, the use of nursing diagnosis, the kind of nursing care planning to use, where to put what content, what theories to choose, whether to have a conceptual framework and what it should consist of, how many class hours to allot to what, what to name the courses, and whether or not to teach intensive care in the undergraduate curriculum. The changes seem of some magnitude, and the energy and effort consumed would indicate that the changes are quite substantial. However, in reality it is merely shifting content around, renaming courses, and changing the emphasis here and there. The substance and character of the curriculum has not changed, and, as a result, some of the same problems exist. These might be things such as that the students are graduated worn out and burned out, the faculty have too many committees and too many student-contact hours, it is hard for associate degree students to matriculate into the program, it is difficult to accommodate part-time students, the students get obstetrics too early or too late, there is not enough clinical time, there is not enough gerontics or inpatient pediatrics, every faculty does not use nursing process the same way, there is no uniformity in the way faculty ask students to do nursing care plans, some faculty use nursing diagnosis and some do not, the audiovisual learning lab is underused, computer-assisted instruction is underused, the students do not know enough pathophysiology, and so on.

In the educative-caring paradigm, these questions do not become the energy-consuming issues they are under the content-oriented behaviorist paradigm. Instead, assessments examine the nature and direction of health care and the role of nurses in that care. They examine not only the role that nurses might play under present conditions but also what role they might play if they were prepared differently and what kinds of preparation would enable them to play those roles. The faculty examines in what ways nurses could influence the health care paradigm to be more health care oriented and less profit oriented, more preventive and less curative, more concerned with the whole citizenry and less concerned with only the insured majority, and more caring in a technological society that does not value caring.

Assessments examine who is "out there in the real world" of nursing or health care that has a vested interest in good nursing care and should be included in curriculum development. Where are the clinical experts (those clinicians who know and sometimes are unaware of the value of their knowing to students)? What are the major health problems now and in the foreseeable future? What are the characteristics of the population to be served? What nonnurses in the community have something of value to give the faculty and/or students? There are other questions that must be examined: What are the characteristics and abilities of the students currently entering and expected to enter nursing in the future, and how does this affect what and how we teach? In what future environments will graduates practice nursing, and what will be the nature of that practice? What is the cost of nursing education, and to what extent can we influence the costs of education without affecting quality? What is happening in society that affects the curriculum? In what direction is government moving, how do we shape policy, and how does it shape us? What are the graduates like now, what do they think and feel, where do they work, and what further education do they have? What are the faculty's hopes and dreams about nursing, about the curriculum, about their teaching and own lives? And, as desired changes evolve, how do they affect cost? These are only a few of the issues that cluster around the needs assessment (see Fig. 2).

Assessments need not all occur at once. They can, and usually do, go on and on. Assessment becomes part of the continuing efforts of the faculty to test their own ideas against reality. Our concept of that reality may rest on an elitist view that is somewhat insulated not only because of our education but also because of the environments in which we live and work. Our realities become skewed by our cultural conditioning, our familiarity with our daily world, our attention to our own immediacies, our preconceived notions of blame and responsibility, our wishful thinking, our authenticity, our materialism, and our notion of truth.

The assessments we make and the means we use to determine our directions must be those that help us to unveil our senses and capture a vision of what is and what can be, to diminish the power of our illusions, and to empower ourselves to shape a more healthful future.

Figure 2
Assessment Cluster

MAJOR HEALTH PROBLEMS

NATURE OF	CHARACTERISTICS OF
HEALTH CARE	THE POPULATION

CURRENT AND   DIRECTIONS AND TRENDS
FUTURE COSTS   IN NURSING

SOCIETAL NEEDS   **NEEDS**   STUDENT
AND TRENDS   **ASSESSMENT**   CHARACTERISTICS

NURSING AND   FACULTY HOPES
RELATED RESEARCH   AND DREAMS

CURRENT PROGRAM   REAL WORLD EXPERTS
STRENGTHS AND PROBLEMS   NURSING AND OTHERS

GRADUATES' THOUGHTS AND FEELINGS
WORK AND EDUCATION

THE FACULTY DEVELOPMENT CLUSTER

What currently characterizes the teaching of nursing is passive information getting (lecture, films, audiotapes, movies, television, reading),
demonstration and return demonstration, memorization, recitation,
repetition, and "discussions."

"Discussions" has quotation marks around it because most of the
so-called discussion consists of a teacher, standing in front of the room,
asking questions to which students are trying to guess what the teacher
wants them to respond. Instead of "discussion," it should be called
"guess what the teacher wants for an answer." Sometimes, much to our
surprise, a discussion breaks out in a room. At the end of such a discussion, the participants usually turn to the teacher (instructor) and ask for
an argument or point to be settled, turning by habit to an authority
figure for such arbitration. The teacher, feeling the press of time and
the responsibility for accuracy, provides truth as she or he knows it in
the form of an answer that settles the issue and curtails both discussion
and further explorative learning.

This mode of teaching is not bad. It follows the usual and accepted classroom procedures; it validates the traditional roles assigned to learners and teachers. It is not behaviorism that is particularly responsible for this—behaviorism lends itself to active teaching modes—it is habit, comfort, convention, and routine that consign us to these practices. Furthermore, teachers actually believe several untested assumptions that have assumed the power of axioms. These mythical axioms follow:

1. Course outlines should consist of content to be covered.
2. Content must be covered by teachers saying the content or assigning readings about it.
3. Lecture methods are the most effective and efficient ones for teaching.
4. Something is not learned until it is memorized and can be tested in an objective test or recited when questioned.
5. Objectives give direction to teaching and help us know where we are going and when we have arrived, and, conversely, without objectives we will wander off into the foggy, foggy swamps of lost time and lost opportunity.
6. The teacher's role is authority related both in content knowledge and in control of student behaviors and activities.
7. If the teacher does not maintain control, students will take advantage and not learn anything of value.
8. Everything the student may ever need to know must be covered in the curriculum.
9. Every student needs to have as nearly as possible the same experience as every other student.
10. Given the same assignments and environment, students will have much the same experiences and learn much the same things.
11. It is essential that every student have experiences in every major nursing specialty.
12. Classroom and clinical work need to be correlated as closely as possible for "good learning" to take place.

These myths persist in the face of expert opinion and evidence to the contrary.

The faculty development cluster (see Fig. 3) addresses not only teaching methods and styles but also role relationships with the experts in

Figure 3
Faculty Development Cluster

FACULTY DEVELOPMENT

VALUING AND COLLABORATING
WITH EXPERT CLINICIANS

DIFFERENT PERCEPTIONS
OF CURRICULUM

AS LEARNING ACTIVITIES
DELIBERATIVE APPROACHES   AND TEACHER/STUDENT
TO PRACTICAL DECISION   INTERACTIONS
MAKING   AS HAVING CARING
                                                  AS ITS ETHICAL IMPETUS
ROLE CHANGE   AS CLINICALLY BASED
                                                  AS INTENTIONALITY
NEW TEACHING APPROACHES

AS ACTIVE
   ENGAGING
   COLLABORATIVE   DIFFERENT TEACHING GOALS
   EXPERT LEARNER
   CO-LEARNING   MATURING
                                        EDUCATIVE
                                        PROFESSIONAL
   BASED ON EGALITARIAN   LIBERATING
   SORORAL/FRATERNAL, AND
   EDUCATIVE TYPES OF LEARNING

nursing practice, with students, and with colleagues. These relation-ships affect curriculum planning, teaching and, as Schwab (1978, pp. 288–291) calls it, "practical deliberation."

Faculty development is so closely tied to teaching and learning that much regarding it is covered in Chapters 6–8. Inevitably there may be some repetition, but only that necessary to make a few definitive statements about it as complement and introduction to the next three chapters.

To many, especially those employed in higher education, "faculty development" has a remedial ring to it. Faculty may perceive of the term as discounting their level of knowledge or expertise or as some commentary on the decisions they make about teaching, content, structure, or relationships. If, however, faculty development is viewed as postgraduate study, it shifts the connotation from one of discount to one of ambition to grow. Actually, it is *not* a commentary on the need for remedial work in education. In the first place, many educational programs in nursing have few if any education courses, and, in the second, those having education courses never intended them to be terminal or to cover all present and future possibilities in education. Therefore, the remedial aspect does not apply.

Neither is faculty development a commentary on the teaching/ curriculum decisions faculty have made. Those decisions were made under conditions and knowledge existing when the decisions were made, not on conditions as they were to exist in a future that was unreadable. No one can base decisions on ideas about teaching and learning that are yet to be developed.

Faculty development, if it is a commentary on anything, is a statement on the continually developing and evolving state of the human sciences of teaching and nursing and the constant struggle of faculty to keep abreast of ideas about education. Faculty development is also a dialogue among persons who have ideas about teaching that have often been submerged and suffocated in a system whose parameters did not allow them to become part of the legitimate curriculum. For that reason, they were forced into conformity and into participating in teaching a large illegitimate curriculum made of materials that were difficult or impossible to accommodate in a behaviorist model. In this way, faculty development is affirming of the best that is in us; it allows us to test ideas that have had to be concealed because there was no legitimate forum and no mode for creating one. Faculty development allows that which has been prohibited by sanction and tradition to be surfaced, examined, shared, developed, and validated. Every faculty departs from the behaviorist paradigm to teach those things that are educative and do not lend themselves to behavioral objectives: values, ethics, professional perspectives, inquiry, creativity, caring, educational heuristics and modes, significance, patterns, etc. Every faculty member thinks that the curriculum is too content laden and that some, if not all, of the mythical axioms listed earlier are illusions and not truths. Faculty development opens the opportunity for the individual and collective intelligence and creativity of faculty to take control of the curriculum instead of abdicating voicelessly to isolation and disappointment.

Faculty Development Leads to Role Change

Faculty development for an educative-caring curriculum has as primary goal that faculty change their traditional roles with students. There are powerful persuaders keeping both students and faculty in the traditional roles. The first and most powerful is the power of the teacher as grader. Some students can mature beyond the preoccupation with grades implicit in the present educational system. However, as long as the teacher must be "pleased" in order for students to "pass" or make good grades, there will be pressure to maintain the teacher-as-authority relationship. Therefore, one of the first problems faculty must examine is how to devise ways to monitor safety and excellence while sharing power. One suggestion that emerges is to separate training from education when possible so that faculty need not play two roles. This is not, of course, the only viable option, just the most obvious one for safety. It does not address the problems of excellence. The problem is not insoluble, and faculty working together can devise a solution that will work for them.

Another powerful influence for continuation of the traditional roles between students and teachers is the masculine bias at the heart of most academic fields, methodologies, and theories. This masculine bias is at the core of several factors that make it difficult for women students to participate fully in academic dialogue. Their whole experience in secondary and postsecondary education has succeeded in convincing them that their voices go unheard. Belenky, Clinchy, Goldberger, and Tarule (1986) state that colleges have been modeled after male institutions to give women an education that is "equivalent" to that of men and that little attention has been given to modes of learning, knowing, and valuing "that may be specific to, or at least common in, women" (p. 6). Furthermore, probably the "commonly accepted stereotype of women's thinking as emotional, intuitive, and personalized has contributed to the devaluation of women's minds and contributions, particularly in Western technologically oriented cultures, which value rationalism and objectivity" (p. 6). Belenky et al. charge that education, as traditionally defined and practiced, does "not adequately serve the needs of women." Research on sex differences reveals that girls and women have more difficulty than boys and men in "asserting their authority or considering themselves as authorities," in publicly expressing themselves so that others will listen, and in attaining respect of others for their minds and ideas. They simply feel that others do not listen and that they go unheard even when they believe they have important things to say. Any female nurse-faculty member in higher education who has participated in male-dominated committees has had this experience, regardless of today's consciousness regarding sexually based discrimination. This makes it more difficult to establish a class climate wherein participants have a dialogue together. Men in the class usually "catch on" and feel free to participate and more quickly immerse themselves in this kind of learning. All women understand a culturally communicated aspect of being female, that is, that women, like children, should be seen and not heard, and that there is something quite unfeminine about being viewed as intelligent. It is a difficult, but not impossible barrier to conversational education.

Another sex-related phenomenon is the female readiness to accept authority and the teacher's willingness to be that authority regardless of the teacher's gender. For women, authority may have a special meaning. Women, so often bereft of authority and shaped by a history of male-dominated majority culture, having now found a voice and having found some authority and a sense of worth and pride in what they know and can tell, are often very reluctant to give up that hard-won position. They like to be asked for information, and they enjoy giving help and answers and being viewed as intelligent, knowledgeable, and sharp. Being products of oppression and having survived the oppression to become *the authority,* there is often little if any notion about being oppressive themselves. They simply fail to see themselves in that role.

A Different Perception of Curriculum

At the heart of the paradigm shift from a behaviorist to a humanist-educative curriculum is a different perception of curriculum. Taba's pithy "essentially a plan for learning" (1962, p. 76) is a commonly accepted perception. In nursing there has been a custom of seeing curriculum as a series of objectives with the content outlines that are expected to achieve those objectives. Sometimes curriculum is "experiences" or even "learning activities." But for the model proposed in this book, curriculum consists of the transactions and interactions that occur between teachers and students and among students with the intent that learning occur. This definition, referred to many times in this book, places the emphasis not on plans, not on paper and pencil, not on goals and objectives, not on content outlines, not on programs of study or the attainment of behavioral changes, but on human interactions with learning intentionality. It rests upon the ability of teachers to set the climate for these interactions in ways that are educative. It follows that to be truly educative, the climate must be egalitarian, in that all are equal in worth, in rights to interact, and in rights to be treated as equals among equals. It also follows that to be educative in the truest sense, the climate must be fraternal/sororal so that all are brothers and sisters in the common search for skill, enlightenment, wisdom, truth, and expressive caring and compassion. For this to occur, the discussions must feature dialogue rather than polemics and must emphasize not so much winning as illuminating.

Different perceptions of curriculum lead to such different curricula that it is easily seen by contrasting the manifestations of these differences in teaching. Figure 4 illustrates this contrast. Once curriculum is viewed as interactions, then the way those interactions take place and

Figure 4
Comparison of Traditional and Educative-Caring Styles
According to Four Aspects: Manner, Climates, Characteristics of
Discussions, and Teaching Goals

TRADITIONAL	EDUCATIVE-CARING
MANNER	
AUTHORITARIAN MATERNAL/PATERNAL	EGALITARIAN SORORAL/FRATERNAL
CLIMATES	
OPPRESSIVE	LIBERATED
CHARACTERISTICS OF DISCUSSIONS	
POLEMICS WIN/LOSE	DIALOGUE ILLUMINATION
TEACHING GOALS	
BEHAVIORAL CHANGES MAINTENANCE LEARNING/ TRAINING	EDUCATION PARTICIPATORY-INNOVATIVE LEARNING

what they lead to become the essence of the curriculum. Traditional curriculum, in placing little emphasis on teacher–student and student–student interactions, is authoritarian with all the subsequently related factors. On the other hand, educative-caring curriculum is egalitarian with all the subsequent factors related to that characteristic.

Differing Teaching Goals

The goals of faculty development revolve around developing role changes that are liberating for faculty and students, that move the student into the mature areas on the maturity continuum, and that focus on educating for a profession.

Liberating students requires constant awareness about the ways teachers unintentionally oppress students and students participate in their own oppression. Few teachers deliberately oppress students. Oppression is a subtle, culturally accepted, and condoned way of conducting the educational enterprise. It is seen in the very arrangement of the classroom (see Chapter 6), wherein the teacher is expected to stand in front of the class, and students are arranged in rows facing front. Teachers are expected to give "permission" to speak and to place approval on the projects, papers, and other subjects that students wish to address. Negotiation and egalitarian operating procedures are not unknown in academia; they are just seldom used. The power that faculty have "over" students is strong medicine. The theme of power and oppression is discussed in Chapter 8. In that chapter, it is postulated that in such a shift, what must be held as first principle of change is that any and all changes in paradigm must in some way affect the liberation and empowerment of people—both students and teachers. Students and teachers are both empowered by the liberating force of Stenhouse's co-learnership (1975).

Oppression, which is the parent of powerlessness, can be escaped by what Freire calls the "critically transitive consciousness" (1976, p. 18). He speaks of the naive transitive consciousness as being characterized by oversimplification of problems, by nostalgia for the past, by underestimation of the common man (in this case of the usual student), by gregariousness or what might be called the herding instinct, by lack of interest in investigation, by fragile arguments, by emotionality, by magical explanations, and by polemics rather than by dialogue. This clearly characterizes students in immature modes of learning in oppressive teacher–student milieus.

On the other hand, Freire describes critically transitive consciousness as interpreting problems with depth, substituting causal principles for magical explanations, testing findings, being open to revision of ideas, avoiding preconceived notions when analyzing problems, accepting responsibility, rejecting passive positions, offering sound arguments, practicing dialogue rather than polemics, being receptive to new ideas for their worth (not for novelty), not rejecting the old just because it is old, and accepting what is valid in both the old and the new. He says that critically transitive consciousness is "characteristic of authentically democratic regimes and corresponds to highly permeable, interrogative, restless and dialogical forms of life—in contrast to silence and inaction, in contrast to the rigid, military authoritarian state" (Freire, 1976, pp. 18–19). It may be that critically transitive consciousness is only possible in liberated education. Clearly, the humanist-educative model, in order to be true to its philosophical roots, must have critically transitive consciousness as goal.

Where the behaviorist curriculum models have as teaching goals the accomplishment of specified behavioral objectives as *demonstrated by behavioral changes,* the educative-caring paradigm has as teaching goals such intangibles as creative and critical thinking, strategizing, methods of inquiry, learner maturity, and those things described in Chapter 4 under the learning types of syntactical, contextual, and inquiry. Where the former usually leads to learner immaturity and naive transitive consciousness, the latter leads to learner maturity and critically transitive consciousness.

New Teaching Approaches

The role change that occurs as a result of faculty development has reverberations not only in different perceptions of curriculum and different teaching goals but also as an inseparable aspect of those two changes, in the way the business of teaching is carried out. This change is so massive and so important that it is the basis for Chapters 5–7. The role change is one that shifts the whole approach in teaching from one of authority to one of co-learner, as mentioned above. Stenhouse (1975) suggests that teachers become expert co-learners and offers the following remarks about it:

> It follows that he [the teacher] must cast himself in the role of a learner. Pedagogically this may in fact be a preferable role to that of

the expert. It implies teaching by discovery or inquiry methods rather than by instruction.

The teacher is not free to cast himself in the role of the learner without regard to the learning of his students for which he must accept responsibility. What is required of him to make him a senior learner capable of offering something of worth to the junior learners with whom he works: Skills in finding things out, of course. But more than that: some hold on, and a continual refinement of, a philosophical understanding of the subject he is teaching and learning, of its deep structures and their rationale. (p. 91)

Stenhouse's proposal hits at the heart of teacher role changes with students. Its congruity with this model has much to do with the fact that teachers will then rely on the structures of knowledge, and the modalities of inquiry, of discourse, of finding things out, of seeking understanding, of, in fact, helping students to have a direct, not a mediated, relationship with the content. The only mediation is in suggesting methodologies, raising issues and questions, and teaching the critical examination of evidence, content, method, and results in ways consistent with nursing as a human science with a caring morality (see Fig. 5).

This means that in professional educational programs, there must be a changed relationship between teachers and students that gives rise to

Figure 5
Consequences of Faculty Development for Educative Teaching

HUMAN EXPERIENCE BASED
PHENOMENOLOGICAL TEACHING

COLLABORATION WITH   EXPERT AT DISCUSSIONS
CLINICAL SPECIALIST   AND DIALOGUE

NEW TEACHING APPROACHES

ALLIANCES WITH STUDENTS   EXPERT AT MODES OF
NOT CONTENT   INQUIRY *e.g.*, META STRATEGIST

CONTENT EXPERT *e.g.*
PHILOSOPHICAL UNDERSTANDING
OF SUBJECT AND DISCIPLINE
DEEP STRUCTURES

new teaching approaches wherein the teacher's role is one of meta-strategist. The meta-strategist is, of course, a strategist of strategies. As a meta-strategist, a teacher is seldom an information provider and often one who gives advice about strategies to find the answers. The teacher's strategies, then, are to help students find strategies that will find answers.

For example, two students have decided to study the nursing care of persons experiencing chronic debilitating pain. They come to the teacher asking for direction on how to go about it. The teacher does not say, "How do *you* think you ought to go about it?" That is most often of little help. The teacher might start raising some issues by asking such questions as: What have you done so far? How have you been thinking about approaching the study? What factors do you think would influence the nursing care in such patients? How will you ground your project in reality? What people are the most likely to be able to tell you something about the problems, needs, and care of people with this problem? What sources, in addition to people, do you think might shed some light on the subject? How can you be sure that your ideas are clinically sound? What will you do with the project when it is complete? Once the student's imagination is stirred, the teacher, as meta-strategist, might say, "One way to get started is to reflect and discuss these questions and devise at least three plans for approaching this study. You could then weigh the strengths and limitations of each plan. Next, attempt to combine the best elements from each into one plan. Then, before you start, it might be helpful to submit your plan and the criteria by which you think it could be evaluated to your classmates for criticism. After it has been criticized you may want to incorporate some of the class's suggestions in your plan."

What the teacher has done is help the students develop a strategy for developing a strategy for doing the plan. Built into the strategy is the safeguard of assembling other's ideas, of looking at several sources, of grounding the work in clinical reality, and of discussion and criticism. The teacher as meta-strategist does not leave the students to flounder but provides guidance about how they can go about working with the content. There is, of course, other work that would need doing. The class will want to explore what constitutes good criticism and possibly come to understand criteria. They may decide to work in small groups, so the whole class will not have to criticize each project. The point is that the teacher, as expert learner, guide, raiser of questions and issues, and meta-strategist, does not convey the content; the students find pathways to the content, and the teacher helps the students know how to find the pathways and what to do with the content.

A role change that enables teachers to see themselves in this different relationship with students requires that teaching approaches be phenomenological in nature. This, of course, means that the subject matter is based in students' lived realities. Earlier, this chapter addressed the necessity for curriculum to be clinically based. To be clinically based requires that teachers value the expert clinician, value collaboration with clinical staff, and work closely with them in the educational enterprise. Clinical grounding does not mean focusing exclusively on the here and now but in the students' lived realities. It is a phenomenological approach that includes the students' pain at the incompleteness, the imperfections, of the nursing care world. This pain and disappointment is part of the lived experience and enables teaching to move in the direction of future possibilities and historical roots. In the same vein, the phenomenological approach includes the students' joy in finding self as part of the transcendingly spiritual experience of helping, of being a positive force, of making an impact, of being a caring, humanizing force in a technologically impersonal world.

In a phenomenological approach to teaching, there is an indivisible unity of the person who is experiencing and the object or subject of that person's experience (Boyd, 1988). This unity must be explored and treated as whole and as experience rather than as intellectualization of experience. In educative-caring models of curriculum, teachers and other co-learners become part of the experience. In this way, co-learners vicariously gain the emotional and learning value of the actual experience.

In new models, clinical practice realities become the modality for study, and the approach is qualitative in methodology rather than quantitative. Phenomenology, hermeneutical analysis, poetics, and other qualitative methods discussed in Chapters 6–8 form the teaching–learning modalities. In these teaching modes, the stress is on humanness, on experience, and on an "intersubjective flow" (Watson, 1988, p. 63). Phenomenological methods stress living, and nursing is studying about living and its relationship to health. So, by definition, nurses must work with the experiences people have with health and health-related issues and problems.

One of the problems nurses face in a phenomenological educational approach is that the health care system is a world that has often surrendered its human-experience emphasis. For many, it has become a world not of people, of pain, of health and illness, and of experience but of technology. Phenomenological-caring approaches for teaching transmit to students a transforming-caring human science approach to nursing care. This conflict is at the very center of nursing's role in society. Reverby (1987, p. 1) calls it a "crucial dilemma in contemporary

American nursing;" it is the "order to care in a society that refuses to value caring." Indeed, nurses work in a society that values technology to the exclusion of humanity.

A teacher cannot teach phenomenologically without approaching subject matter in ways that focus on wholes, on patterns, on searching for truth—in other words, through the educative types of learning discussed in Chapter 4.

Therefore, if the role of the teacher is perceived differently, the role of the student must also be different, and out of these new relationships comes a new alliance between teachers and students. It must be an alliance that addresses content in both clinical and classroom settings and that uses learning methodologies that are qualitative rather than quantitative. These methodologies, phenomenology, hermeneutical analysis, poetics, and other qualitative methods based upon transformative education (all discussed in Chapter 8) form these teaching–learning modalities.

Tanner (1988) concludes her article, "The Curriculum Revolution: The Practice Mandate," by commenting:

> I do not think of developing more elegant and detailed formal models to be passed on to the next generation of nurses, for them to take and apply in their practice. Rather, I am struggling with ways in which the concerns of practice can truly be addressed by our educational activities, where classroom learning might be the application of practice rather than the other way around. (p. 214)

Benner (1984) states that expert clinical teachers can teach best through presenting paradigm cases. She states, "in order for students to learn from another person's paradigm case, they must actively rehearse or imagine the situation. Simulations can be even more effective because they require action and decisions from the learner" (p. 9).

What emerges in discussions of new teaching approaches is a concern for liberation, for active engagement of students, for collaboration with expert practitioners, for a commitment to reality and lived experiences, and for phenomenological teaching methods.

Deliberative Approaches to Practical Decision Making

Role changes not only involve how one relates to students and to one's teaching but how one relates to one's colleagues. Curriculum and teaching discussions are very often polemic in nature. Faculty bylaws often provide that parliamentary procedure is the accepted modality for business meetings. Parliamentary procedure is based on the premise that if one offers a statement, then the role of the "opposition" is to take exception, to object, or to disagree. And, in place of the statement or motion made, a counterproposal is offered. It is a procedure of polarity where all discussions immediately take the form of win/lose arguments. Long use of parliamentary procedure gives polarity to our faculty discussions, even in times when decisions are not at issue, and when ideas are being dissected ostensibly in a search for truth. One faculty member says, "I think students are not mature enough to handle the amount of freedom you are recommending." Another says, "Oh, I disagree, I think it is that very attitude that is patronizing and is used as an excuse to keep students powerless." The discussion immediately is shifted from a search for answers, from a clarification of the issues, and from an uncovering of meaning and intent to winning, to being right, to having the arguments lined up, to being aggressive in attack or refuting other's opinions. The only two postures available in polemics are attack or defense. Therefore, instead of listening with one's whole attention, one begins immediately to gather defenses and to prepare statements, arguments, disagreement, and opinion. If the goal of the discussion is to clarify problems, to find solutions, to question what the assumptions are that underlie certain positions, and to determine meanings, then polemics do not accomplish that.

Faculty development can focus on discussions that are highly charged and emotionally demanding with a coach to help people learn to say things that solicit alternative ways of perceiving a situation, that encourage examination of the issues under the issues, that examine incongruence in assumptions, that seek meanings, and that speak in terms of the inviting "I think" and "I feel" rather than the accusatory "you think" and "you feel." A discussion coach can encourage the development of ground rules for discussions that help faculties confront and solve the interpersonal problems that arise when faculties engage in curriculum work rather than avoid them or walk away from them unsolved or take them into halls and offices where they further the alienation and distrust rather than resolve it.

Faculty climate sometimes prohibits, by unspoken consent, curriculum discussions on specific topics from certain vantage points that differ from the accepted positions that faculty have agreed upon. Some ideas around this deserve mention. First, it is legitimate that faculty have vested interest agenda. To make it illegitimate is to force underground that which would be better openly discussed. If special interest agenda were made legitimate, faculty with these agenda could be encouraged to proselytize. This means that they could write their positions and support them with valid references. They would in turn read articles and position papers given to them and respond on the issues. This is a very active and rich way to pursue faculty development, and during the process enlightenment does occur especially if this is done in a manner that is a search for illumination and not a win/lose power war. How the game of persuasion is to be played is important because learning how to interact in ways that reveal assumptions and meanings helps faculties arrive at decisions that make for good curriculum; interacting in ways that exploit power bases and faculty personal loyalties masks the issues and meanings and often leads to poor curriculum planning.

Second, it is important to have no sacred cows. New faculty often feel that things are complete and that the older faculty that helped develop the curriculum are not open to any suggestion of changes. New faculty express this as "stepping on puppies" or "hurting the baby." They sense a defensiveness among the creators that does not allow further improvements or honest evaluation/criticism. All areas of the curriculum must be open for discussion, available for criticism, continually examined. It is territorially important for faculty to "meddle" with every aspect with which they are concerned. If this is not allowed, new faculty will never "own" the curriculum, and ownership is a significant aspect of membership in a group. People are, after all, in some respects like others of their fellow animals; one characteristic they have in common is territoriality. Dogs establish ownership by "peeing" on their territory. Making changes in the curricular materials is a teacher's way of "peeing" on it—establishing co-ownership of the curricular territory.

Practical Approaches.   Schwab (1978, pp. 287–383) proposes three forms of practical decision making. He distinguishes these from what he calls theoretical decision making. He believes the reliance on theory begs or ignores the real and practical problems of curriculum makers and that we must be diverted from theoretic pursuits into other modes of operation if we are to make progress.

To understand his position, we must explore his assumptions. Schwab believes that the theoretical deals with knowledge in general or universal statements that are warranted, confidence inspiring, and true. The theoretical statements hold good for long periods of time and apply to each member of a whole class of occurrences. In the theoretical, one expects a "truth" to hold constant from instance to instance and not be responsive to changing circumstances.

In contrast, the practical is "concrete and particular and treated as indefinitely susceptible to circumstance, and therefore highly liable to unexpected change" (p. 289). Practical curriculum problems deal with particular schools, particular courses, particular teachers, particular budgets, specific times of year, distinct types of students, and particular problems that "we wish were otherwise and we think they can be made to be otherwise" (p. 289).

Schwab believes that the theoretic and practical are radically different in method, in the origin of problems, in the subject matter (which is of a different character), and in the kind of outcomes.

Methods.   In methods, Schwab maintains that theoretic methods are those used directly in the pursuit of knowledge. They are characterized by one defining feature: control by a principle. The principle of theoretic inquiry determines the shape of the problem, the type and source of the data, how to interpret these data, and the possible conclusions. The investigator chooses the problem, how the problem will be formulated, and designs the experiment. But the direction in which the experiment is to go and what is to be done with the data are dictated by the guiding principle of the inquiry. The method of the theoretic is induction.

The practical method has no such guide or rule. Most of the time, we must clarify the problem and let it emerge as we examine the situation that seems to be awry and look, necessarily at random, for what is the matter. Problems may emerge with protracted examination. Then, as one searches for data, the search is slowly given direction by the gradual formation of the problem (there is interplay between the two). The method of the practical is deliberative.

Problems.   Theoretic problems are states of mind and arise from areas of subject matter regarding what we know and do not know about a given subject or discipline. Practical problems are states of affairs in relation to human beings, human lives, human living, and being. They arise from unfulfilled needs, unsatisfied desires, hurts, deprivations.

They are made up of conditions as noted above that we would like to be otherwise and believe can be made otherwise. Practical problems can be settled by changing either the state of affairs or the desires and needs. Solutions always involve change. These beliefs are human centered and phenomenological in nature and approach. They require a different relationship of faculty to their perceived problems and the way they work together to solve them. Parliamentary law and theoretical methods do not work for them.

Subject Matter. The subject matter of the theoretic is something assumed to be extensive, pervasive, perhaps even universal, and is investigated as if it were constant from instance to instance and not influenced by context and circumstance.

Practical subject matter is concrete and particular. It is treated as indefinite, influenced by context and circumstance, and bound by time and place.

Outcomes. Outcomes differ from the theoretical to the practical. The theoretical is knowledge, general or universal statements that are supposed to be true, trustworthy, and confidence-inspiring. They are held to be lasting, extensive, and applicable unequivocally to each member of a large class of occurrences or reoccurrences. The practical outcome is a decision, a selection, and a guide to possible action. Decisions are never lasting, trustworthy, extensive, nor do they apply unequivocally to all situations. They are not intended to be translated into general guiding principles for all time, placed in the minutes and used as touchstones for the rest of history. They are judged by their consequences as good or bad in afterthought. They have no great durability, no extensive application—and apply only to the case for which each was made. Wider applications proceed only from analogy and turn out to be good ones mainly by chance.

Quasi-Practical Approaches. Schwab's "quasi-practical is an extension of the practical methods and purposes to subject matters of increasing internal variety" (p. 291). The more internal variety, the more difficult it is to be effectively practical. For example, it is more difficult to be effectively practical in making wise choices for instruction of a heterogeneous group than a homogeneous group (one school or consortium or system).

In the quasi-practical, one may use the methods of the practical plus two special emphases:

1. Regarding the process of decision itself:
   a. It must identify the areas of variation.
   b. It must estimate the different directions and degrees of variation likely to occur among member groups.
   c. It must determine the ways in which different variations will affect the wisdom of its decisions.
   d. It must discern some of the ways in which its decisions ought to be modified or qualified in each specific application in order best to be applied to each varying context.
2. Regarding the formulation of decisions made:
   a. It must communicate the merely quasi-practical character of the decisions.
   b. It must point to some of the considerations that ought to be taken into account in translating these decisions into the practical.
   c. It must suggest some of the ways in which decisions can be modified in the light of item 2b.
   d. It must see to it that quasi-practical decisions are not mistaken for "directives" by those who make them or those who implement them.

One interesting note: Schwab believes that each group has its own set of practical problems (research is concerned with human talent, feasibility, utilization of space and equipment; recruitment of students has problems such as audiences to be reached and "messages" to be delivered). But it is part of our practical problem to discern the problem, and we do it well or badly to the extent that we keep our boundaries flexible and our terms fluid.

Another point Schwab makes is that when making decisions about specialty content, nonspecialists should be involved. Translated into nursing, content selection for such specialties as pediatrics, obstetrics, or psychiatric nursing cannot be left only to teachers of those specialties. The decisions about what subjects to include in the curriculum plans for these areas are affected by the kind of nursing required in a given setting or context and by how the material is presented. These matters affect the whole teaching program and cultural slant of the school.

Schwab places a special emphasis on the "cherishing of diversity" and the "honoring of delegated powers" (pp. 294–295). Seemingly unrelated faculty will be involved in discussions regarding decisions. Of these "unrelated faculty," Schwab says:

> He will be confronted by unfamiliar vocabularies. He will hear terms which he does not use brought to bear on "his" problems. Considerations which, in his framework, are alien and irrelevant will be raised and debated. His problem will be to listen, to master the new vocabularies, to appreciate the effect of new terms, and to begin to discern and honor the relevance of alien considerations to his problems and his interests. Eventually, his problem will be to discover that the diversity which poses these problems and obligations does, in fact, operate in his interest—since every additional factor taken into account in making a practical decision is one less factor which might otherwise frustrate the success of the ensuing action. (p. 295)

In such discussions, faculty who participate discover a world they know little of. For instance, each participant discovers the existence of numerous remote agencies and persons whose decisions affect his or her professional life. Each faculty member recognizes corporate deliberations as one of the few means by which the course of these remote agencies can be influenced. As a consequence of participation, of giving energy, time, and thought to deliberations, each faculty acquires an additional sense of proprietorship in one another's problems and in the group's decisions. As a result, there accrues a benefit that is in the best interest of the whole: the ultimate practical decision. That practical decision is then given to those delegated and empowered to carry it out. Subsequent to the reception of quasi-practical advice, the participants have a special moral obligation to honor the delegated powers.

Eclectic Approaches. The eclectic recognizes the usefulness of theory to curriculum decision, takes account of certain weaknesses of theory as ground for decision, and provides some degree of repair of these weaknesses. It has two major uses:

1. Theories are used as bodies of knowledge, thereby providing a kind of shorthand for some phases of deliberation and freeing the deliberator from obtaining firsthand information on the subject.
2. The terms and distinctions which a theory uses for theoretical purposes can be brought to bear practically.

Eclectic operations repair the weakness of theory in two ways:

1. They bring into clear view the particular truncation of subject characteristic of a given theory and bring to light the practicality of its view.
2. They permit the serial utilization or even the conjoint utilization of two or more theories on practical problems.

Schwab offers some basic precepts. He proposes that the practical arts begin with the requirement that existing institutions and existing practices be preserved and altered piecemeal, not dismantled and replaced. Changes must be so planned and so articulated with what remains unchanged that the functioning of the whole remains coherent and unimpaired. These necessities stem from the very nature of the practical—its concern with the maintenance and improvement of patterns of purposed action and especially its concern that the effects of the pattern through time shall retain coherence and relevance with one another.

Schwab's methodology for discourse or deliberation—as he calls it, practical decision making—offers real guidelines for those faculties whose goal is curriculum change. However, it provides little guidance for the emotional needs and overtones or for the power maneuvers that often characterize the politics of faculty meetings. Wheeler and Chinn, in their *Peace and Power: A Handbook of Feminist Process* (1989), hold more promise for that. In fact, feminist literature could be very helpful to faculties facing role changes in the interest of a paradigm shift in nursing curriculum. Wheeler and Chinn explore the idea of peace as intent and process. They have made an acronym of PEACE, which means *P*raxis, *E*mpowerment, *A*wareness, *C*onsensus, and *E*volvement. They offer feminist alternatives to the usual patriarchal meanings of power that would be helpful to faculty groups. The alternative power models include such ideas as the power of process, wholes, collectivity, unity, sharing, integration, nurturing, intuition, consciousness, diversity, and responsibility. The aspect of the book most useful here comes in some reality-based ideas about how to run meetings and accomplish group goals while meeting group needs in ways that are inclusive, confidence building, feminist, and healthful, while avoiding the usual politics of masculine business meetings. These methods address the sensitive political and emotional issues that all faculties struggle with in ways that develop and use each participant's skills, knowledge, ideals, and dreams. It also develops colleagueship, support systems, solidarity, and sorority/fraternity.

Valuing the Expert Clinician

Many things affect the devaluing of the potential contribution to education that can be made by clinicians who give daily direct care. Among them are three persuasive elements: the myth that education is the leader of innovation and expertise, the societal conditioning of women, and the tendency of the oppressed to squabble among themselves rather than coalesce in the endeavor to become free of the oppression.

Nurse educators have long suffered themselves to believe a myth of the larger society: that education is the forefront of new developments, that education creates new trends and society follows. In reality that seldom happens. Educational institutions do sponsor research, but that research most often occurs around societal needs and trends. Industry also sponsors research, and, because industry is reality, they often have need and innovation as the twin drivers. Education is more frequently reactive than proactive.

The schism that has separated nursing education from nursing service has led both camps into forgetting their common humanity, their common cause, their sorority and fraternity in service, and their membership in the society of caring.

The schism, along with its competitive, discounting stance, probably is part of the syndrome of oppression. Oppression commonly leads the oppressed to spend more time fighting among themselves than working together against the oppression. Nursing has reflected that as well as the common distrust and competitiveness with which society enculturates women. So with the syndrome of oppression, the distrust and competitive enculturation of women, and the mythology of educational leadership and responsibility in society, nurse educators have traditionally shied away from an intimate collaboration and peership with their colleagues in nursing service.

Benner, in both *From Novice to Expert* (1984) and along with Wrubel in *The Primacy of Caring* (1989), champions bringing expert clinical nurses into the mainstream of nursing education. She paints bright pictures of what expert practicing nurses carry embedded in their practice. Benner and Wrubel (1989) state:

We believe that we have much to learn from the best and worst of nursing practice. In the best practice, we discover selves of membership related to a common humanity and given over or defined by specific concrete concerns and human relationships. By being experts in caring, nurses must take over and transform the notions of expertise. Expert caring has nothing to do with possessing privileged information that increases one's control and domination of another. Rather, expert caring unleashes the possibilities inherent in the self and the situation. Expert caring liberates and facilitates in such a way that the one caring is enriched in the process. Instrumentalism, contract language, cost benefit analysis, social exchange, enlightened self-interest, and all the language of the autonomous self of possession misses the relationship of the person constituted by concerns and human relationships. (p. 398)

It is in nursing practice that we learn these things and from those who practice we can learn this and more. Nurses strive to be clinical experts and expert teachers, but those who labor daily in service agencies are far more familiar with and expert in care than most teachers can be. It is with these persons that we form new alliances for the benefit of nursing—new tripartite alliances, where teachers, clinicians, and students are co-learners together.

The tripartite alliance is more than a valuing that leads educators to include certain levels of service personnel to participate on committees. It leads them to full participation in the education of new nurses—a partnership with teachers and students to form the backbone of educative care. What one finds, once the barriers are down and the common denominator of caring is unearthed, is that the alliance is as eagerly sought by clinical experts as it is by students and educators.

The rational–technical models of care reflected in so much nursing literature and language—for instance, the language of nursing diagnosis and nursing process—comprise a language and practice of objectification, quantification, and decontextualization (Benner & Wrubel, 1989, pp. 398–399). And these models lead the managers and teachers of nursing care to seek ways to evaluate nursing care as a measurement of context-free performance. With a renewed valuing of and alliance with the clinical expert, nursing educators may be able to avoid passing on to future generations the rational-technical models and graduate, instead, those committed to caring practices, those committed to relationships comprised of caring communities of nurses with a sense of membership in, among, and with humankind.

The implications of this for curriculum is an intimate working relationship, especially in clinical settings, with clinical experts. Preceptorships, as designed and tested at Ohlone College under a grant from the Kellogg Foundation is one route (Limon, Spencer, & Waters, 1981). There are others. But without a role change and change in perception, a change in valuing, these new relationships—partnerships with service persons—cannot develop and influence curriculum.

THE GENERAL GOALS OR ENDS-IN-VIEW CLUSTER

According to Bevis (1989), the ends–means models of curriculum propose that all teaching centers around behavioral objectives and that these objectives are derived from the statement of philosophy and from conceptual frameworks. The conceptual frameworks originate from an analysis of the future and present health care problems and issues, problems and issues in society, and the needs of students. The objectives are behaviorally stated, and content flows from them. In this model, how to teach is much less important than what to teach. For what to teach is formulated as a *means* of helping students learn the specified behaviors (*ends*). This model requires that teachers have their basic commitment to what students are to learn, not how they learn it. Therefore, in most nursing schools it is the content of a course or a curriculum that absorbs faculty energy, and, according to behaviorist dogma, that content is best examined through an analysis of the behavioral objectives. The relationship of the teacher to the objectives then becomes an intimate one, in that failure of students to achieve those objectives becomes a failure in teaching.

How the purposes, goals, and objectives are perceived by the faculty, then, becomes a key influence cluster for faculty. If objectives are held dear, written in great detail and used as the driver of curriculum, then the teacher's role commitment remains in alliance with the content. And the role changes suggested earlier in this chapter cannot operate. The issue becomes one well expressed by Stenhouse (1975): "Can curriculum and pedagogy be organized satisfactorily by a logic other than that of the means–end model? Can the demands of a curriculum specification . . . be met without using the concepts of objectives?" (p. 84). In other words, are there other ways to derive content than by an analysis of objectives? This cluster of influence maintains that curriculum structure can be met by using general goals or ends-in-view accompanied by guides in the form of criteria for teacher–student interactions and criteria for selecting or developing learning experiences that are in keeping with educative-caring learning (see Fig. 6). Behavioral objectives are antithetical to liberating education and are an instrumentalist view of learning episodes. Peters (1966) holds that objectives are not necessary to content derivation and that content has its own intrinsic justification. He also holds that education involves taking part in worthwhile activities. These activities have their own inherent standards of excellence. Based on these ideas, he offers the suggestion that worthwhile activities can be appraised because of their intrinsic standards and because of what they lead to (p. 155). In the objectives model, the worth of an activity is not inherent but is in what it leads to (the objective). Peters goes on to say (p. 159) that skills do not have wide-ranging content. Skills are largely knowing *how* rather than knowing *that.* Knowing that is an understanding of things, is widely applicable, and influences the quality of living. Knowing how is a knack, a procedure that is mechanistic. Knowing that is education; knowing how is training. Instrumentalist learning activities are especially suited to knowing how.

Stenhouse (1975) argues that skills are "probably susceptible to treatment through the objectives model" (p. 85), but that the objectives model encounters real trouble when confronted with knowledge. He counsels that knowing how is procedural and prescriptive, whereas knowledge or knowing that is the focus of speculation, of understanding; it is not open to mastery. Stenhouse ties filtering knowledge through an analysis of objectives into oppression. He states:

> [This] gives the school an authority and power over its students by setting arbitrary limits to speculation and by defining arbitrary solutions to unresolved problems of knowledge. This translates the teacher from the role of the student of a complex field of

Figure 6
General Goals or Ends-in-View Cluster

GENERAL GOALS ENDS-IN-VIEW	
CRITERIA FOR TEACHER–STUDENT INTERACTIONS	CRITERIA FOR SELECTING/DEVISING LEARNING ACTIVITIES

knowledge to the role of the master of the school's agreed version of that field. (p. 86)

This point will be brought back into focus in subsequent chapters, and Stenhouse's position will be discussed further. The purpose for its occurrence here is that it highlights the problem in the general goals cluster. For curriculum models to change, the perception of the role of objectives in the curriculum must change; this influences the role of the teacher and the content and evaluation aspects of curriculum. If objectives as content-generators are used only for skill training (item, directive, and rationale learning), then how will the educative types of learning be derived and addressed?

The answer arises in an examination of Raths. Raths (1971) believes that "Activities may be justified for inclusion in the curriculum on grounds other than those based on the efficacy of the activity for specifically changing the behaviors of students" (p. 714). He proposes further that schools "should take as their major purpose one of involving students in activities which have no preset objectives, but which meet other specified criteria" (p. 714). In lieu of objectives, Raths suggests "criteria for worthwhile activities." He then provides some examples of these criteria. Peters (1959) suggests "principles of procedure," which, in effect, are similar to Raths' criteria for worthwhile activities.

Murray and Merrefield (1989) have generated criteria for selecting and devising learning experiences and for guiding teacher–student interactions (see Appendix I and Chapter 7). These criteria are in some respects goals: goals that teachers and students aspire to as ideal for guiding their learning both in content and in relationships. This makes possible a switch where criteria or principles of procedure are substituted for behavioral objectives as the drivers of education and content.

What then of objectives? In the educative-caring curriculum, general goals have a place, but objectives as behavioral specifics have no place except in relationship to skill training. It is possible to frame general goals or ends-in-view to point directions and to provide subjects or topics that become the rubric under which a wide range of content can fall. These, however, do not dictate specific content. What this does is to raise the level of ambiguity and uncertainty for teachers. For with general goals, ends-in-view, and criteria as guides for course work and curriculum development, the faculty is much less sure about what content goes where. As a result, what goes on between and among teachers

Figure 7
Content Cluster

PREREQUISITES	SOURCES OF CONTENT
CONTENT OF NURSING	
PROGRAM OF STUDIES	MISSION OF COLLEGE

and students grows less prescriptive in the interest in learning. Since it is less prescriptive, it is more liberating and more open to following where paradigm experiences lead.

Schwab (1978) argues for plurality in content, method, and inquiry. If nursing faculties are to relinquish behavioral objectives as guides to teaching and the selection of content and to adopt criteria and other sources, then there will have to be an increased tolerance of ambiguity. The certainty of prescriptive objectives gives way to the uncertainty of general goals and ends-in-view that leave teachers, in the final analysis, with only their expert knowledge, their experience in teaching, their commitment to liberating education, and their partnerships with fellow learners (students) as arbiters of what is worthwhile in the pedagogic enterprise.

CONTENT OF NURSING CLUSTER

The content cluster of influence has four aspects: the sources of content, the prerequisites, the resulting program of studies and the mission of the college or university. Figure 7 shows this cluster.

Prerequisites

One problem in finding widely applicable guidelines for deriving content exists as a result of the differences in the usual high school, public school, or gymnasium curriculum of a country and in the policies of a university or college regarding liberal arts courses prior to entering the major. In some countries, much more humanities or liberal arts are given in high school and in greater depth than in the United States.

And in some countries students are expected to choose a major and concentrate from the beginning of their college career on the courses specified as preparing them for that chosen field. This makes for career training and is unrelated to liberal arts education. In those countries, it is necessary to determine the amount of humanities and liberal arts acquired in secondary school and carefully select prerequisite requirements that enable the student to come to nursing with more than a biological and physical science background. The growing awareness of the role that philosophy, ethics, literature, art, music, and, of course, the social sciences play in nursing stimulates a reexamination of preprofessional curricula to ensure that the student comes to nursing major courses with this foundation.

Additionally, in places where medical influence is predominant in nursing curriculum structure, the prerequisites are laden with the biological sciences far beyond the normal needs of first-level professional nursing and are lacking in the psychosocial and humanities base of nursing practice. It has been traditional in collegiate nursing programs to concentrate on the sciences as prerequisites to the exclusion of all but a few of the humanities courses. Given that nursing is as much an interactive discipline as a scientific one, and given that it is developing as a human science rather than continuing in the traditional science posture it once pursued, the humanities should occupy as strong a place as the sciences. It is in humanities that one finds the vicarious paradigm experiences that teach us about beauty, suffering, violence, peace, and human connectedness.

The problem of attempting to prescribe a total package of prerequisites for students seems out of synchronization with the concept of student freedom of choice. Ideally, except for perhaps a few requirements, students might be trusted to work with advisers and to choose the prerequisites that will best help them attain a well-rounded education.

Mission of the College or University

Every educational program has a mission-and-goals statement that reflects the position of the parent institution that provides funds for conducting the program. Content responsiveness to the mission and goals of the parent institution is essential. This must be done so that the goals of the program reflect the values of the institution. In this way the faculty legitimizes the general direction supported by that agency. Some mission-and-goal statements are very general and sound much the same the world over. Some are highly unique to the particular school of nursing or university. Flagship universities usually have a mission that is more elitist than state colleges and universities. Some regional colleges or universities are designed to address the problems of upward mobility for minority or educationally disadvantaged groups, while others address the maldistribution of health providers. These missions influence content choices.

The Sources of Content

The sources of content, or how to derive content for the curriculum, is a problem in most curriculum models. Stenhouse (1975) simply suggests that one specify the content, "objects of study and some master concepts and . . . a specification of what the teacher is to do expressed in terms of principles of procedure" (p. 92). On reading his several books regarding the Humanities Curriculum Project and his works on curriculum, one can easily come to the conclusion that a master knowledge of the structure of the field of study being taught is one key ingredient of selecting content. Additionally, problems and issues within the society or within the field further define the content to be taught. Such vague and nonspecific advice regarding selecting content seems to beg the issue for a budding field of study such as nursing, because, as yet, no generally sanctioned structure for the nursing knowledge exists. It might be clearer to those involved in teaching mathematics, physics, or other subjects with a traditional structure for the content areas.

Content selection, however, is and will be for some time to come, an important issue in nursing at all levels. Indeed, most curriculum meetings, regardless of the level of education, are endlessly involved in content issues, ignoring what seems obviously the most important problems, socialization into nursing and the art and science of inquiry.

Baccalaureate and master's programs seem field-of-knowledge-oriented to the exclusion of other sources of content. The perception of the field and its structure differs vastly from country to country and, in most countries, from school to school. The variations in perceptions of the sources of content often exist because of traditional ties to other fields and because of differences in the usual high school or gymnasium curriculum. For instance, in countries where nursing is still more closely tied to the traditions of medicine, conditions may exist where medical curriculum and physicians' perceptions of nursing content may greatly influence curriculum structure. In some countries academic nursing schools are permitted by law only in universities where medical schools exist and are administratively placed under schools of medicine. In some of these settings physicians may control curriculum content and prerequisite courses.[1] The problem is not so much "power" as perception of nursing practice. In such settings, nursing content tends to be seen as deriving from medical content and appears as watered-down "doctoring" instead of nursing.

Generally speaking, nurses focus on the experiences that people have with health problems and issues while physicians deal with the etiology, pathology, diagnosis, and treatment of disease (see Fig. 8). These are two basically different areas of practice and lead to different sets of roles and functions. The two are complementary and not competitive. Some nurse time is spent dealing with etiology, pathology, diagnosis, and treatment of disease because these are some of the health problems and issues that people face. However, people face many health problems and issues that are not sickness, illness, or disease oriented. Even when the health problem is disease related, nursing problems may have little relationship to the diagnosis because nurses care for the *person* who is having an experience with a problem. It is the *experience* that becomes the issue with the nurse and client: the experience of not knowing what may happen, what the course of events may be and what life impact this may have, the shame or guilt that often accompanies some diagnoses, and such problems as despair, pain, fatigue, failure, hopelessness, helplessness, anxiety, and nausea. Experiences people have with health are the daily fare of nursing, the focus of caring, and form the bulk of the issues with which they deal.

Clarity regarding the differences in domain of practice of nurses and physicians is essential in all types of content derivation. Confusion about them is more striking where medical schools influence content selection. For instance, one usual way to select content is by using common medical diagnoses. This is inadequate because it is too easily skewed toward non-nursing problems. A multiple-source approach would provide a broader spectrum that is better balanced, more reflective of the culture of the people to be served, more reflective of the needs of the students, and more likely to lead to a program of study that is primarily nursing and not primarily medicine or some other kindred discipline.

"Content" is used here to mean the material used for teaching. It

---

[1] In countries in which this occurs, I have observed a very heavy emphasis upon such courses as histology and pathophysiology, sometimes requiring as many as 4–5 courses in each of these subjects.

Figure 8
Differences in Domains of Practice
Between Nursing and Medicine

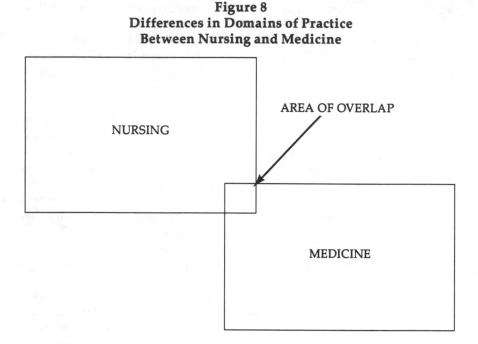

Nursing's Domain of Practice:
the experience people have around
health issues and problems

Medicine's Domain of Practice:
the etiology, pathology, diagnosis,
and treatment of disease

Differences are Complementary, not Competitive

---

includes both processes and ideas to be learned. The settings in which
"content" is taught spans all learning environments but depends greatly
on the clinical or practicum work of students.

The sources of content are the basis for its examination, for if these
can be identified, then content can be drawn from them (see Fig. 9).
The following basic sources of content for nursing might yield the kind
of curriculum needed to elevate nursing, increase its knowledge base,
liberate both teachers and students, and free the creative spirit of nursing as a human science.

Desired Qualities of the Graduates.   The American Association of
Colleges of Nursing's Project *Essentials of College and University Education for Professional Nursing* (1986) gave considerable thought to the

Figure 9
Sources of Content

PERCEPTIONS OF
NURSING PRACTICE

CULTURE OF   NEEDS OF
FIELD   SOCIETY

DESIRED QUALITIES   STRUCTURE OF THE
OF THE GRADUATES   KNOWLEDGE BASE

SOURCES OF CONTENT

NEEDS OF NURSING   HEALTH PROBLEMS

INTEREST/CHOICES   HISTORICALLY
OF STUDENTS   SIGNIFICANT ISSUES

FIELDS & DISCIPLINES CONTRIBUTING
TO NURSING

characteristics or qualities of graduates. These are not to be confused with measurable behaviors. They are qualities of the educated professional nurse, because (paradoxical as it may seem) true education makes behavioral outcomes unpredictable but at the same time makes the educative qualities or characteristics describable.

Some examples consistent with an educative-caring paradigm for curriculum are: reflection, creativity, criticism, use of knowledge regarding the structure of inquiry, analysis, uses of the structure of theory and theorizing, colleague interaction, judgment, deliberative thought procedures, logical progression, integration among ideas, consistency within a construct, congruence of examples with definitions and descriptions, use of cue clusters, ability to discern patterns, willingness to make intuitive leaps and take reasonable risks, use of research, and use of others' knowledge, experience, and expertise.

Structure of the Knowledge Base. Some examples of the structure of the knowledge base of a field as a source of content are the traditional ways of viewing and grouping content. Examples are the known cognitive and semantic maps; the conceptual constructs, concepts, propositions, theories, and values of nursing both in their present state and in their future possibilities; and the sanctioned ways of inquiry.

To seek to derive content from the structure of nursing assumes that the faculty each perceives the structure in the same way. It can easily lead to traditional (although not necessarily bad) medical model categories such as pediatric nursing, obstetric nursing, medical–surgical nursing, etc. Other sources of content could be from manifestations of disabilities, but this then stresses as Benner (1988) puts it, a "'pathological' or 'deficit' approach to human practices and concerns related to health, illness, disease and suffering and arrogantly recommends 'appropriate' responses in the process" (p. xiv).

Culture of the Field. The culture of the field and the relationship of this culture to the culture of the society in which it exists is another source of curriculum content. Nursing's rites of passage, cultural mores and folkways, and social norms for interaction and behavior are major content areas, as are the origins of these cultural modalities, their context, their desirability, the problems concerning them, and the societal conditions that support or inhibit them. The impact of feminism on nursing and the institutionalization of female values and norms in nursing are part of this content, as are the ways in which feminine practices work to enhance creative responses to society's attitudes toward women.

Needs of Society. Nursing is a social service and as such must continually tune into the problems, issues, trends, and needs of the society it serves. This includes the society of the community, the society of the nation, and the society of the world. Some countries, such as Sweden, are fairly culturally homogeneous; some, such as the United States and Israel, are very culturally diverse. The content selected must respond to the cultural needs of the people to be served by the program.

Since nursing is a humanitarian service profession, curriculum must include, as far as culturally normed values will permit, such universalities in content as caring. Compassionate service for the greater good of the people must override narrower, more confining political considerations when using societal needs as a content source. The difficulties in doing this are truly vast. Watson, in her book *Nursing: Human Science and Human Care* (1988), speaks of caring as the "moral ideal of nursing whereby the end is protection, enhancement, and preservation of human dignity" (p. 29). She says further that because this requires "a personal, social, moral and spiritual engagement . . . and a commitment to oneself and other humans, nursing offers the promise of human preservation in society" (p. 29). Watson represents a world view that is gaining in strength. Such a perception suggests transpolitical provision of care and services that has the force of moral commitment. Because of their unique role in society and their concern about the experiences people have with health, nurses transcend political ideologies but may be limited by those whose political ideologies transcend all else.

Needs of Nursing. Nursing's developmental level within a country and its need to grow and advance in order to fulfill better its societal roles are essential content areas. There are vast differences in the developmental level of nursing in various countries of the world. An essential aspect of the professional curriculum is an assessment of the content that will help graduates advance nursing in ways that are increasingly responsive to the caring needs of people.

Health Problems. One cannot plan curriculum out of context of the health problems that nurses will be called upon to face in the foreseeable future. Special emphasis must be given to content that will prepare graduates who are the highly educated, highly skilled scholar-clinicians capable of rising to the task of fulfilling the roles ascribed by the social mandate. Any movement for changes in nursing curriculum that fails to be attentive to these needs will render nursing impotent to deal with the needs of society and of the individuals that make up society. If this happens, nurses will be a footnote to history rather than among the main players. The curriculum must provide the graduate with the skills, tools, and creative thinking necessary to be autonomous, imaginative, inventive, flexible, caring, ethical professionals committed to the whole range of possibilities from national policy setting to patient care. From indicators currently available, the three major sources of health problems of the next 30 years are likely to be great increases in the eldest elderly, prolonged survival of more health-threatened people that will radically increase the numbers of the chronically ill, and large numbers of people with AIDS. These problems must be taken into account when deriving content for all of them are nursing care intensive.

Interest/Choices of Students. In a curriculum designed to liberate students and to be responsive to the uniqueness of individuals, the interest and choices of the student must play a part in content selection. Individuality of need, freedom of choice, and pursuit of private goals are educationally legitimate as a content source. Students are the soul of the curriculum; without the ability to pursue their private goals, the curriculum rapidly becomes mechanistic.

Some insights into the future must be formulated both by curriculum developers and by learners. Without a perspective into the future, the curriculum is instantly obsolete. Obsolescence built into the curriculum revives the old habit of the constantly revised curriculum. It keeps curriculum consultants busy and faculties despairing. The half-life of scientific information is about 2 1/2 years. One must plan so that obsolescence is held at bay. This is done in two ways: by planning for a future envisioned by faculty and students and by teaching the processes of nursing education as well as the content. The processes are the lasting aspects, the constants; the information is transient. Some information is obviously necessary but must be carefully chosen. Much of what was learned in nursing 30 years ago is now obsolete. Only the processes of education survive time's erosion.

Fields and Disciplines Contributing to Nursing.   Many other fields have influence on nursing content. According to Watson (1988), nursing must be understood in its "context and in its relationship to other subjects. Philosophy, the humanities, history, psychology, physiology, sociology, anthropology, and all the other social sciences affect—and are affected by—nursing" (p. 3). This puts nursing education in the position of having to rely heavily on helping students develop a semantic diagram or cognitive structure that makes the interconnectedness of all knowledge apparent. For nursing, more than the "pure sciences," exists in its real-life context, because nursing has a unique societal mission: caring for humans at their most vulnerable.

To do this and do it well, nursing education must help bring together, in its knowledge base and its practice, the best and most significant knowledge from the humanities and social sciences as well as from the pure sciences.

The historically significant issues and the events in nursing responsive to these issues form another source of content. Our past is an inescapable and valuable source of information regarding our traditional issues and what has been attempted regarding solutions and approaches to date. The important contributions of nurses and supporters of nurses provide more pegs for the cognitive structure developing in learners' minds and more models for the inspiration of their lives.

A PROGRAM OF STUDIES

Translating these sources of content into material which lends itself to being structured into courses and learning activities is simply a matter of finding some acceptable format that facilitates the conversion. Faculties can find their own method and begin to think of ways to facilitate content generation and ideas for learning activities that meet the criteria.

Regardless of the way this is done, the courses that are generated, or their descriptions and content, some general decision rules are helpful in the final selection of content. Below are some important considerations.

1. Content is the vehicle for developing the desired academic and personal qualities of students. Too rigid an outline of content can prevent the development of the desired qualities. Enough content flexibility must remain so that the learners, and for that matter the teacher, can follow the trail of developing inquiry, reflection, and interest. To rush off after a course outline and required content to be covered is one of the easiest ways to stymie educative learning.

2. The more "skill-oriented" the course content, the more content-laden (as opposed to process-laden) the course will be and the more item, directive, and rationale-learning-oriented the activities will be.

3. The use of behavioral objectives for course and activity development, while appropriate for item, directive, and rationale learning, is not helpful for syntactical, contextual, and inquiry learning.

4. Conversely, the more "educative" the course content, the less content laden the course will be and the more syntactical, contextual, and inquiry-oriented the activities must be.

5. Some content and qualities by their very nature build on other content. Some propositions, postulates, concepts, theories, and values may have a logical order, sequence, and hierarchy. This must be honored in designing the courses in a curriculum. However, the less course chaining and sequencing there is (such as required prerequisites), the more free and flexible the students' "selected" curriculum can be and, therefore, the more individualized the curriculum that each student can have. In advanced studies (doctoral and master's programs) there is less sequencing necessary and therefore more flexibility. However, in basic studies there is greater flexibility than usually recognized by content experts.

6. Some logic should be used in designing courses in the curriculum. This logic can be the structure of nursing and related fields, types of problems to be examined, natural groupings of program goals or

whatever conceptualization of natural or logical groupings of content and/or qualities of graduates appeal to the faculty's sense of order.

As Stenhouse (1975) points out, selecting content does not tell us "what students are to do with the content" (p. 90). Criteria for selecting and devising learning activities provide guidelines for this. Content as a list of topics to be covered can develop into a tyrant to which teachers and students alike become slaves. Lists of content can become detailed, long, and dull; it might be better to have some general categories and let teachers and students flesh them out as they explore the ramifications of real and simulated problems and issues of being in the world of nursing.

In conclusion, it seems apparent that the clusters each influence the other and act as a whole as faculty develop curriculum. There are no prescriptions, no formulas that are universally applicable. Faculties must work together in earnest dialogue, seeking not to win but to find a path that will enable students and faculty to have some freedom in developing their content as they go. For when all the rhetoric is summed up, curriculum remains, as defined earlier, as the interactions that occur between students and teachers and among students with the intent that learning takes place. These interactions take place around learning episodes, simulated nursing problems or issues, points of discontinuity, insights about self or the lived world, ideas, or curious events.

Teaching is the ability to capitalize on these things, to bring these things into focus; the ability to walk with students through nursing, knowing its power as a positive force for health and quality living; and the ability to help students learn how to use this power. This requires helping students shed naivete without losing the ideals and moral commitments that can keep them growing toward mature, skilled, scholarly, compassionate wisdom.

REFERENCES

American Association of Colleges of Nursing. (1986). *Essentials of college and university education for professional nursing, final report.* Washington, DC: American Association of Colleges of Nursing.

Belenky, M., Clinchy, B., Goldberger, N., & Tarule, J. (1986). *Women's ways of knowing: The development of self, voice, and mind.* New York: Basic Books.

Benner, P. (1984). *From novice to expert: Excellence and power in clinical nursing practice.* Menlo Park, CA: Addison-Wesley.

Benner, P., & Wrubel, J. (1989). *The primacy of caring, stress and coping in health and illness.* Menlo Park, CA: Addison-Wesley.

Bevis, E. (1989). *Curriculum building in nursing: A process* (3rd ed.). New York: National League for Nursing.

Bierce, A. (1958). *The devil's dictionary.* Mt. Vernon, NY: The Peter Pauper Press.

Boyd, C. O. (1988). Phenomenology: A foundation for nursing curriculum. In *Curriculum revolution: Mandate for change.* New York: National League for Nursing.

Freire, P. (1976). *Education: The practice of freedom.* London: Writers and Readers Publishing Cooperative.

Limon, S., Spencer, J., & Waters, V. (1981). A clinical preceptorship to prepare reality-based ADN graduates. *Nursing & Health Care, 2*(2), 267–269.

Murray, J., & Merrefield, S. (1989). Developing criteria for student–teacher interactions and learning experiences. In J. Murray, *Developing criteria to support new curriculum models for doctoral education in nursing.* Doctoral dissertation, University of Georgia.

Peters, R. S. (1959). *Authority, responsibility and education.* London: Allen and Unwin.

Peters, R. S. (1966). *Ethics and education.* London: Allen and Unwin.

Raths, J. D. (1971). Teaching without specific objectives. *Educational Leadership, 28,* 714–720.

Reverby, S. M. (1987). *Ordered to care, the dilemma of American nursing, 1850–1945.* New York: Cambridge University Press.

Schwab, J. J. (1978). *Science, curriculum, and liberal education, selected essays.* (Eds., I. Westbury & N. Wilkof). Chicago: The University of Chicago Press.

Stenhouse, L. (1975). *An introduction to curriculum research and development.* London: Heinemann Educational Books.

Taba, H. (1962). *Curriculum development: Theory and practice.* New York: Harcourt, Brace, Jovanovich.

Tanner, C. (1988). *Curriculum revolution: The practice mandate.* New York: National League for Nursing.

Tyler, R. (1949). *Basic principles of curriculum and instruction.* Chicago: University of Chicago Press.

Watson, J. (1985). *Nursing: The philosophy and science of caring.* Boulder, CO: The University of Colorado Press.

Watson, J. (1988). *Nursing: Human science and human care: A theory of nursing.* New York: National League for Nursing.

Wheeler, C. E., & Chinn, P. L. (in press). *Peace and power, a handbook of feminist process.* New York: National League for Nursing.

Zukav, G. (1980). *The dancing Wu-Li masters: An overview of the new physics.* New York: William Morrow and Co., Inc. (Bantam Books).

BIBLIOGRAPHY

Cohen, S. (1971). The forming of the common school. In G. F. Kneller (Ed.), *Foundations of education.* New York: John Wiley and Sons.

Committee on Curriculum of the National League of Nursing Education. (1937). *A curriculum guide for schools of nursing* (3rd ed.). New York: National League of Nursing Education.

National Council of State Boards of Nursing. (1988, July). Telephone conversation with staff regarding data for NCLEX.

6

Teaching and Learning: The Key to Education and Professionalism

Em Olivia Bevis

INTRODUCTION

There is a compelling splendor about both teaching and nursing that demands the highest forms of endeavor, for their ends are linked to the magnificent miracle of human thought and the quality of human life. They have a common core of caring about the human condition and an obligation to its improvement that confers a radiant beauty on the meanest of tasks in their service. They are a societal trust. And, for those who combine these two tasks into the teaching of nursing, there is a moral commitment to society's needs that requires industrious constancy in self-development efforts so that this trust will be steadfastly and excellently honored. It is to this trust that this chapter is addressed.

One of the key ingredients of the paradigm as described in Chapters 6 and 7 is the role of the teacher. This chapter concentrates on teaching learning as fulfulling the definition of curriculum, and expands on the position that it is the teacher's and students' transactions and interactions that constitute curriculum. To do that, this chapter will examine the social mandate for an emphasis upon education rather than training, explore what is meant by education and critical thinking, offer a criticism of the lecture-training model of teaching, present some ideas about the need for faculty development in changing perceptions regarding the teaching role, examine some of the issues involved in a paradigm shift, and propose caring as the moral imperative of nursing and nursing education.

A discussion of teaching and learning first requires a discussion of "teaching for what end in view?" If it were proposed that psychomotor skill is the primary purpose of baccalaureate nursing, the discussion of teaching and learning would take a tack quite different from the one taken by this book: that not being the case, the end-in-view is that graduates shall be educated as well as being skilled. Since I posit that only by being educated as scholar-clinicians can nurses be professionals who are responsive to the needs of society for compassionate, skilled nursing care, this chapter must explore those elements in curriculum that will lead inevitably in that direction.

THE SOCIAL MANDATE

Sakalys and Watson (1985) reviewed seven studies made in the 1980s. These were the Paideia Proposal (1982), Physicians for the 21st Century (1984), President Bok's Report to the Harvard Board of Overseers (1984), The National Institute of Education Report (1984), the National Endowment for Humanities Report (1984), the Institute of Medicine Report (1983), and the National Commission on Nursing Study (1981). They state that all seven reports make some similar recommendations. These are "a focus on process (vs. content) oriented educational aims, curricular reform, and a different quality of instruction" (p. 298). Among the recommendations culled from these reports are that additional emphasis should be placed on such items as:

1. Liberal arts.
2. Intellectual skills such as analytic, problem-solving, and critical thinking skills.
3. Attitudes and values.
4. Life-long learning.
5. Good teaching.
6. Active teaching modes.
7. Faculty development to promote learning of Socratic and other teaching strategies.

8. Increased faculty–student interactions as an aspect of teaching.
9. Revision of the reward structure to support good teaching (pp. 298–299).

These reports addressed both liberal arts and professional education. They all point to some kind of curriculum model that promotes education—critical thinking—creativity—engagement of learners' minds in issues and questions that will educate rather than or in addition to training. This seems to be a social mandate and as such requires an exploration of what this means to nursing in higher education.

EDUCATION: AN ELUSIVE CONCEPT

Education is an exclusive concept. A clear definition is impossible, for no clarity emerges from the literature. Therefore, rather than a definition there will be a discussion of characteristics and narrative depictions, which do not define education so much as describe it contextually. Such an approach can be justified. Smith (1987) says that lexical definitions are not precise enough to provide us with a sense of the whole, but that coordinated sets of sentences provide an implicated definition. He believes "this mode of defining brings our thinking closer to the observable and manipulatory level of experience than is possible by the classical form of definition where one abstract term is defined by reference to other abstract terms" (p. 14). So, by wandering about among those who discourse about education, we may grow closer to the idea of it and what it entails.

Despite much variety in perceptions regarding what education is, educators find common ground in the way they describe human beings who are educated and what they can do. And there is certainly a common perception that to be educated requires an immersion of the whole person in those things that mark the best and highest in human thought and endeavor: history, literature, poetry, art, architecture, music, philosophy, and politics. There further seems to be some agreement that these highest forms of human achievement must be dealt with in a context of real problems and issues that engage the educatee in ways that affect the modes of approaching not only the fields of study involved, but also normal life problems. There is also agreement that specialized education—narrowing down the fields of study or becoming expert—is done only after the liberal arts have given the mind the tools with which to learn, communicate, criticize, analyze, synthesize, create, and understand.

Norman Cousins (1985) says that one of the underlining features of being human is the "ability to create and exercise new options" (p. 2). He believes that the ultimate test of education is "whether it makes people comfortable in the presence of options; which is to say whether it enables them to pursue their possibilities with confidence." He thinks that education enables people not simply to survey experience but to preside over it. Some of his other characteristics of education are worth mentioning here:

1. The ability to deal with imponderables.
2. The capacity to innovate—to do something for the first time.
3. The ability to use words in order to move an idea from one point to another so that it can be understood.
4. The facility to think abstractly.
5. The skill to make correlations.
6. The imagination to anticipate the connections between causes and effects.
7. The ability to understand the function of qualifiers.
8. The wisdom to know that the most vital ingredient in decision making is sequential thought.
9. The confidence not to be intimidated by complexity.
10. The insight to identify compassionately with the mainstream of humanity.
11. The reverence to respect life.
12. The commitment to be concerned with the reality of human sensitivity and the need to refine it.

Whitehead (1929), in his classical essay on the "Aims of Education," describes education as the joy of discovery. What each person must discover is "that general ideas give an understanding of that stream of events which pours through his life, which is his life" (p. 2). By "understanding" he indicates that he means more than logical analysis, understanding in "the sense in which it is used in the French proverb, 'to understand all, is to forgive all'" (p. 2).

He speaks firmly for the usefulness of education and says, "Education is the acquisition of the *art of the utilization* of knowledge" (Whitehead,

1929, p. 4, emphasis mine). Among his other ideas about education, he speaks of what he calls the "most austere of all mental qualities." This he suggests is the sense of style, which he describes as "an aesthetic sense, based on admiration for the direct attainment of a foreseen end, simply and without waste" (pp. 12–13). Attainment and restraint mark style as does the love of a subject in itself and for itself. Style is clean and graceful and without waste. It is sheer elegance, economy. He calls it "the ultimate morality of mind" (p. 12). He believes that style is the fashioning of power and the restraining of power. In order to have style, one must be able to spot irrelevancies and not be distracted by them. He says "style" is always the exclusive privilege of the expert- specialist, a state that results from the cultured mind (p. 12). In other words, the cultured mind or educated mind must *precede* the expert-specialist. Whitehead's "style" seems very similar to Benner's (1984) description of the expert nurse except that Benner does not address the cultured mind or education.

Broudy (1972), in discussing esthetics education, speaks of the buff or connoisseur as the consequence of cultivation. His discussion throws light on education. He says that schooling should cultivate the student. Cultivation being intentional intervention, it leads one to be a specialist-expert, scholar, and connoisseur. He says it enables one to make fine distinctions and discriminations that result from analysis and lead to synthesis.

It is interesting to note that both the style of Whitehead and the connoisseur addressed by Broudy are results of specialist education that follows liberal arts education. The implications, for professional education such as nursing, are that the highest levels of expertise and the development of style with the ability to make fine distinctions, comparisons, and act with power and economy are consequences of specialist education based on a broad general education. This falls in line with the reports reviewed by Sakalys and Watson (1985) that recommend more emphasis on the liberal arts and may ultimately lead nursing in the United States to propose that true professional nursing can only come as a generic doctoral degree based on a liberal arts baccalaureate degree. The reasons for style being an outcome of specialist education based upon a liberal arts foundation may be found in the words of Greene (1986). In addressing informed awareness, she says that:

> recognition of the importance of interpretation and the many ways
> there are of constituting reality may lead individuals to recognize
> that their ordinary, conventional ways of seeing their own lived

worlds may exclude or obscure important dimensions of what is there to be known. (p. 496)

Education, then, provides the educated with more and different ways to view their world. This creates options. Furthermore, based on Merleau-Ponty's (1967) position that all humans are "condemned to meaning" (p. xix), Greene (1986) believes that educators must be concerned with empowering students to "make sense of, conceptualize, to develop perspectives upon, and perhaps to transform their actually lived worlds" (p. 496).

Transforming the lived world is the major theme of Botkin, Elmandjra, and Malitza (1979). They maintain that "innovative learning" (a term equivalent to educative learning used in this book) changes perception and its test is social response (pp. 20–21). They assert that grasping meaning is the pathway to understanding a problem and its significance and to envisioning solutions. They contend that meaning provides the criteria by which the individual makes sense of the overwhelming overload of information and by which they avoid the risk of alienation from society (pp. 21–22). They explain further that innovative learning cannot be a digestion of an input that results from an output or an additive process of connecting values to things. It must "enhance human capacity to act in new situations and to deal with unfamiliar events" (p. 23). They believe that innovative learning cannot be value free but must be "willing to question the most fundamental values, purposes and objectives of any system" (p. 14). This requires critical thought.

Speaking on the role of criticism and liberal education, Hanna Gray (1988), president of the University of Chicago, in her welcoming address to the class of 1991 supports the Botkin et al. (1979) position, although her words are quite different as she addresses liberal education. She claims, "The tradition of liberal learning and its methods, of liberal education and its ideals, has always been a tradition of criticism." She asserts:

> Liberal education will not make life easier but it will or should help to enrich and expand its possibilities. It will or should substitute independent thought, informed appreciation and critical judgement for dependent opinion, simplistic observation, and unthinking assertion. It will or should make intellectual integrity, respect for reasoned conclusions, and the willingness to make difficult decisions in the light of complex alternatives and relationships a goal and a responsibility that we refuse to evade.

This theme of responsibilities and the ability to deal with complex issues and creative alternatives is a major motif in Botkin et al. Although they address what they describe as maintenance and innovative learning (as two distinct types), and not education by name, in fact they are comparing training and education. Since they describe innovative learning by what it accomplishes, it is easy to conclude that their "innovative learning" is education. They describe it very simply as anticipation of problems and the ability to work with others in innovating workable, positive solutions (p. 12). They speak of "adaptation" as suggesting reaction—adjustment to external pressure. Anticipation, they posit, implies preparing for possible contingencies and considering long-range future alternatives. It is anticipatory learning and enables the use of forecasting techniques. It emphasizes the future tense (not excluding the past). It employs imagination but is based on fact. A second characteristic they attribute to innovative learning is participation and knowing how to participate responsibly and effectively. They describe this as more than decision sharing. It has the additional components of cooperation, dialogue, empathy, keeping communications open, constantly testing the operating rules and values, and rejecting those that no longer apply. They insist that these two elements, anticipation and participation, be tied together.

The literature on education is very extensive, and there has been no attempt to review it here, only to expose some thoughts about its general characteristics. There does seem to be agreement that education provides a critical thought process with all that it implies, including: a sensitivity and respect for life that denotes a compassionate identity with all humanity; an attainment of style with its power and restraint, that is, its elegance (for Benner's 1984 address of this in different words, see Chapter 9); an ability to anticipate and confront difficult and complex problems and participate with others in developing creative and flexible options; and the general moral obligation to act to improve global life. This implies mature wisdom, which includes such things as perspective, patience, historical views that help one see patterns and significance, and that last, tiny resident left in Pandora's box when all the ills of the world had escaped to plague us: hope.

Education as Emancipation

Education, to be any good at all to the educatee, must be emancipating. Emancipating or liberating education frees the intellect to range at will among the many ideas, problems, and issues that characterize life.

It enables one to perceive intellectually engaging phenomena and to master the skills necessary for investigating them. Additionally, emancipation means imbuing the spirit with:

- The clarity to see things seen every day but never really seen and to hear things heard every day but never really heard before.[1]
- The energy to pursue an idea wherever it leads.
- The vision to see beyond preconceptions and cultural conditioning and so enable departure from traditional bias.
- A love of reflection and contemplation.
- A trust of sensitivity and intuition.
- An enthusiasm for insights and meanings that requires detecting the assumptions that underlie assumptions.
- A fondness for strategizing.
- A commitment to search for that elusive thing called truth.
- A flexibility in generating and using options.
- And last, to infuse the whole with the moral ideal of compassion and caring.

CRITICAL THINKING

Stenhouse (1968) provides a transition from education to criticism. He believes that "the prime value in education is the development of individuality and creativity in relation to culture" (p. 58). He states further that "it is the central purpose of education to transmit culture through the symbols which make it accessible to criticism and creative thinking" (p. 58). All criticism is not critical thinking nor is all creative thinking critical. Criticism, in its true sense, is the purview of the expert and is linked to connoisseurship (see Chapter 9). In looking at thinking,

---

[1] This sentence was spoken to me in 1974 by a Cajun gentleman, Gordon Hebert, as the reason why he wanted to go home from the hospital once more before dying. He did go home so he could once again see and hear his beloved sights and sounds of the deep Cajun country of Louisiana with a sharpness, clarity, and appreciation he had never before experienced. He returned to the hospital as he said he would and died as he had lived: gracefully. Education can never achieve quite the vitality for living, seeing, and hearing with enhanced appreciation that dying can, but it can and does heighten the senses.

Meyer (1986), agreeing with Hunt (1982, p. 13A), posits that "we use our innate thinking abilities to categorize, generalize, and in other ways make sense of the world" (p. 11). This "making sense of the world" is a theme that runs throughout existential writing on thinking, critical thought, and education. Polanyi and Prosch (1975) propose that living things are "oriented toward meaning" and that man's "whole cultural framework, including his symbols, his language arts, his fine arts, his rites, his celebrations, and his religions, constitutes a vast complex of efforts—on the whole, successful—at achieving every kind of meaning" (pp. 178–179).

Botkin et al. (1979) assert that:

> The search for meaning—the desire to grasp a problem to under-stand its significance, and to envisage solutions—is central in the present world. One cannot make sense of the overwhelming over-load of information without the selective criteria provided by meaning. (p. 21)

They believe that learning is understanding and that "understanding is the context which bestows meaning" (p. 20).

Heidegger (1968, pp. 236–237) offers ideas that revolve around thinking as being a way of living—a search for truth. By "truth" he means revealing what is concealed (as opposed to truth as correctness or correspondence).

Undeniably, the search for truth, for revealing what is concealed, is characteristic of the educated person. It is more than a mere search, it is almost compulsion. The truly educated mind cannot inhabit the body of a couch potato. And that mind is active and critical about what it thinks—thus, the connection between education and critical thinking. The ability to think critically is an inevitable and important result of education.

Critical thinking, part of the null curriculum discussed in Chapter 4, is one of the stated goals of almost every academic program in nursing, particularly baccalaureate and higher degree programs. Its prominent place in goals and objectives would lead one to expect much more clarity regarding what it is and how it may be taught than is generally found among nurse educators. It is often equated with problem solving and is taught as such. Problem solving is not the same. Critical thinking, according to Meyer (1986), "is the ability to raise relevant questions and to critique solutions without necessarily posing alternatives" (p. 5). This definition differs quite drastically from problem solving wherein the point is instrumentality . . . to pose alternatives and make decisions among alternative choices.

Dewey (1933) defines critical thinking as "suspended judgment" and "healthy skepticism" (p. 74). He speaks at greater length on reflective thought and proposes it as promoting the use of criteria to examine beliefs. He suggests that a good belief is:

1. Clear and unambiguous (those who use it agree upon acceptable working interpretation).
2. Consistent with the facts.
3. Consistent with lived experiences.
4. Consistent with other beliefs that are well verified by experiences.
5. Utilitarian: It must be fruitful, lead to new suggestions, new hypotheses, more accurate observations, better discrimination between facts and propaganda, more reliable forecasts of probabilities for the future. It suggests other good beliefs.
6. Simple: It makes the fewest possible assumptions and is based upon the most obvious hypotheses.
7. Flexible: It admits to frequent change in the light of new thoughts, information, evidence, reflections.

Dewey's reflective thought differs from Meyer's critical thinking in that Dewey has a utilitarian component in number 5 of his list. However, a common thread in many writers on the theme of education is that education frees the human to look at new thoughts. It might be addressed as emancipation, liberation, flexibility, or creativity. However it is addressed, emancipation becomes a cornerstone of education.

Emancipation: A Consequence of Education

This, then, is emancipation, the gift of education: a release from the inhibitions of asking the unasked, an escape from the easy acceptance of the ready answer, a confronting of the social injustice of the oppressive classroom and a discontentment with passivity.

Without emancipation, education is an oppressive tool. It is an assembly-line industry producing nurse-workers who on the average follow the status quo. They may make waves, but they stay within the rules while living lives that are circumscribed by the inflexibility of large medical empire-bureaucracies and bear the inevitable stamp of banality and mediocrity.

This is how education has a claim on professional nursing education: One can attain a high degree of skill as a trained technician. And the greater the expertise in the skill, the more effective is the nurse. However, to attain the other characteristics listed above, one must become educated. In being educated one simply has more to give to life, to clients, and to the world. The problem arises in that the educated nurse is no longer content to be merely an institutional employee (Watson, 1988). The constraints of most health care institutions as they exist today have no place for the educated nurse. Unless educated professionals can transform hospitals into work places that support professional nursing care and that allow the emancipated mind to generate and use flexible alternatives, institutional employment for the educated professional nurse is not possible. There are powerful factors that mitigate against the possible transformation of mega-hospitals. It will take a critical mass of nurses educated at higher levels, working together and with other concerned professionals, to change that stable bureaucracy. Yet it is a challenge that must not be ignored. Nurses must not abandon the institution that gives care to those who are most vulnerable, most in need, and most critically ill. The critically ill and their families need the care and concern of the compassionate, scholar-clinician of the future.

FACULTY DEVELOPMENT

The mind is an awesomely powerful instrument. It can evoke memories that are as real and alive and full of feeling as the day of their occurrence. It can enact plans that are years in the making and complex in their execution. It can yearn, dream, imagine, envision, expunge, and intuit. It can follow a trail of clues so thin that there is hardly a smell of reality and leap through a chain of logic confounding in its convolutions. Its only limits are our inadequacy in its use, our unskilled handling of its superb potential, our waste of its vast abilities, our lack of vision of its limitless powers.

In classes, we teachers reduce it to its most elementary functions: absorption, memorization, and recitation. Those who challenge the mind never know where that challenge will lead, nor can they control its searching energy. It can give up today, only to reawaken unprompted tomorrow with answers for discarded questions. Faculty must develop strategies for releasing the power of the minds entrusted to them.

We thus return to faculty development—for the curriculum is, when examined for its essence, those transactions and interactions that take place between and among faculty and students with the intent that learning occurs. This learning must illuminate, must awaken, must liberate the human mind and harness its potential. Curriculum as interaction is a position that has been and will be repeated often in this book. And when viewed this way, the key element of the whole is not in the philosophy of the school, not in the curriculum plan or the program of studies, nor in the design of the buildings and grounds and the richness of the equipment, but in the quality of teaching, the imagination of the faculty for designing and selecting learning activities and in how faculty interact with students. Education requires teaching to be emancipating and liberating; to be active and thought provoking; to be reality grounded and deal with the sophisticated issues daily facing nurses; and to be imaginative, creative, and supportive of the imagination and creativity of others. And it must support learner-maturity, not dependence. Teachers of nursing therefore have a primary duty to develop the self. For teachers of baccalaureate and higher degree programs, the obligation is to be knowledgeable in content and to be expert learners so that they will elevate teaching to the degree that teachers are no longer lecturers who are merely knowledge and information brokers. Teacher development programs must help teachers learn to be liberating educators.

SOME OF THE ISSUES

Traditional Classroom Arrangements

The need to move from behaviorist-technical paradigms to educative-caring ones has been discussed extensively in the preceding chapters. However, it is not just behaviorism that has influenced the state of the art of curriculum, it is also traditional styles of teaching. Faculty in higher education are assumed to be able to "teach." Competence in the field, publications, research, and social acceptability are the requisites for employment as a teacher in higher education. No one investigates whether or not the person is a "good teacher." Therefore, most teachers in colleges have little or no training as educators. Teachers teach as they were taught. In elementary, secondary, and higher education, teaching mainly consists of the teacher as lecturer demonstrators and large group discussion leader. However, these discussions are, for the most part, forums where the teacher asks for information through some sort of question, and anyone who happens to know gives or guesses at the answer. Based upon the assumption that teachers are supposed to lecture to students, and sometimes to show them audiovisuals, the traditional classroom is arranged to support the teacher as lecturer. In a diagram, it looks like what is illustrated in Figure 1.

This traditional arrangement is based upon several assumptions:

1. The teacher needs to see all the students, the students do not need to see each other.
2. The teacher is the central and most important person, all the rest are of lesser importance.
3. The students need only interact with the teacher, whom they can see, not with each other, that is, their discussions will address the teacher.
4. The teacher is the authority (the classroom arrangement reflects this).
5. Listening is the main function of students; talking is the main function of teachers.

As one moves up the hierarchy in education to master's and doctoral education, there often exists the classroom seating arrangement for a "seminar" (see Fig. 2).

However, sometimes these are just that, a seating arrangement. Though there is often more discussion, there is seldom the enthusiastic, argumentative, brain-twisting, stimulating exchange necessary to engage the mind in an examination of information, principles, data, and assumptions that can arise from a skilled presentation of a problem or issue. Almost anyone looking at Figure 2 would envision the teacher sitting at one of the ends. The "end" of the table is the automatic

Figure 1
The Typical Classroom

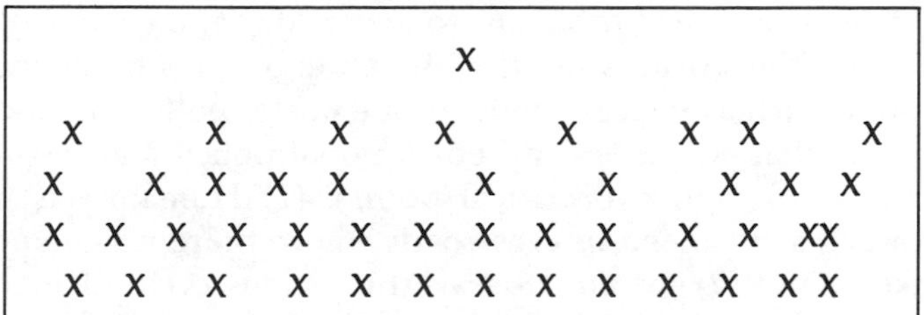

```
                         X

   X        X      X     X      X      X  X        X
   X      X  X  X  X          X      X      X  X  X
   X  X  X  X  X  X  X  X  X  X    X  X  XX
      X  X     X    X  X  X  X  X  X  X  X  X  X
```

Figure 2
The Seminar Classroom

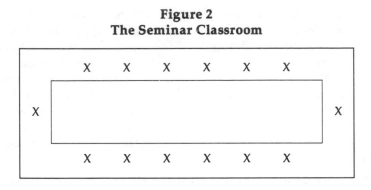

magnet to the teacher and presents a subconscious picture of authority placement. Such positioning gives a clear message about who is in charge, whose word is last, and when the discussion is over. These arrangements are politically inspired to maintain traditional power relationships.

Politics in the Classroom

In speaking of politics as an element of education, one must look first to Freire (1970, 1976), who writes primarily about liberating education being necessary in order to help people free themselves from oppressive governments. In reading his work, one becomes aware that classrooms and clinical areas are political microcosms, and what occurs in them is a reflection of the total society. The fact that the United States is a democracy often lulls us into thinking that all of our institutions are geared to democratic modalities and that our education results in liberated minds and creative persons. In his work, Freire proposes that teaching is often skill in persuasion, an insidious form of propaganda.

Botkin et al. (1979), in their report of international meetings over a 2-year period sponsored by The Club of Rome, support Freire's position. They suggest that education is a political tool that must be brought to bear on world problems to avert "doomsday" (p. 1). Their position is that the world is faced with "an enormous tangle of problems" in areas such as energy, population, waste, pollution, and food. They propose that educators and educational policy makers must be brought to understand two critical points: (1) Humanity is moving rapidly toward a "momentous crossroads where there will be no room for mistakes," and (2) we must break the vicious cycle of increasing complexity and lagging understanding while there is still time to avert catastrophe (p. 2). One solution they offer is education that supports integration rather than adaptation.

ADAPTATION VERSUS INTEGRATION AS A CONSEQUENCE OF SCHOOL POLITICAL CLIMATE

Botkin et al. (1979) believe that history shows that human learning (meaning societal learning as a whole) has been largely successful in adapting to its environment, for example, shaping its milieu in ways that ensured survival, well-being, improved the quality of life, and compensated for inhospitable climates or lack of resources. Of course, some cultures failed and largely disappeared. However, the authors express serious doubts about whether "conventional human learning processes are still adequate today" (pp. 9–10). Conventional human learning processes are referred to by them as "maintenance learning," which they describe as "the acquisition of fixed outlooks, methods, and rules for dealing with known and recurring situations" (p. 10). This type of learning requires an oppressive classroom climate and misuses of formal modes and procedural learning.

Gordon (1984), in her work on the use and misuse of formal models in nursing practice, discusses both the strength and weaknesses of such models. She lists 10 misuses of formal modes that are outcomes of her research on nursing practice (p. 242). One suspects that these misuses could be found in research of other practice fields, such as teaching, counseling, podiatry, physical therapy, etc. The 10 misuses uncovered by her research are the following: (1) "reification: equating the model with reality," (2) "an eclipse or devaluing of traits that cannot be formalized," (3) legislation of behavior so that it contradicts the goal of autonomy, (4) alienation and lack of challenge to the more experienced in favor of inexperience, (5) detailing so much that it overwhelms rather than helps, (6) oversimplification of complexity, (7) "demand for excessive conformity: using the same standard for all people may demand excessive conformity to a particular set of standards," (8) insensitivity to nuances in situations that will cause formal statements to be geared toward the typical rather than the particular, (9) confusion between following the rules and the need for judgment, and (10) mystification: speech becomes so slogan laden that it becomes trivial and narrow in meaning.

Gordon, in describing her research findings on the misuse of formal models, has clearly described what Botkin et al. (1979) seem to be saying when they characterize maintenance learning as "the acquisition of fixed outlooks, methods, and rules for dealing with known and recurring situations" (p. 10). They go further in their descriptions by saying that maintenance learning tends to disregard all values that are not in the status quo and to take for granted that those values in the status quo are the "best" ones. This book refers to Botkin's maintenance learning and Freire's adaptive learning as training. It is necessary to—but insufficient for professional nursing.

People who are trained and have maintenance learning are adaptive. The process of adaptation to change is one framework for viewing learning. However, according to Botkin et al. (1979), adaptive learning discounts human initiative. It implies a passive adjustment to external pressures. They state:

> Learning as adaptation implies that human beings can only react to follow new changes in a given environment, hurrying to catch up with uncontrollable mutations, having no power to forestall or even influence them. To be adaptable, i.e., to be able to change in response to changing circumstances, implies submitting to these circumstances and even succumbing to them. It is this reactive aspect intrinsic to adaptive learning that contrasts so markedly with anticipation. (p. 4)

Freire (1976, pp. 4–5) agrees. According to him, adaptation is adjustment to the existing context. The adaptive person is therefore passive in that the environment, culture, conditions, and contexts are accepted and adapted to. He suggests, on the other hand, that *integration* is the desired human goal. He defines integration as a distinctly human activity. It results, he says, from the ability to adapt to reality PLUS the "critical capacity to make choices and to transform that reality" (Freire, 1976, p. 4). In other words, adaptation is the ability to adjust to the existing context and integration is the ability to manipulate the environment/context/reality so that control is exerted over events and environment. The integrated person transforms his or her environment, culture, conditions, and context. The adaptive person is passive in that the conditions, environment, culture, and context are accepted. For instance, a dog in a cold, snowy environment finds a hollow log, digs a burrow, and perhaps grows a heavier coat—it is adapting to the environment. Humans, on the other hand, build a cabin and start a fire, thus transforming their immediate environment, controlling it and thereby making it more comfortable. These are the essential differences between adaptation and integration/innovation. As long as nursing uses behaviorist methods for education as well as for training, students are being supported in passivity, in adaptability, and not in being helped to develop creativity and integration.

The political implications for adaptation and integration/innovation in the classroom are also worth noting. The teacher as information giver, talker, lecturer, and authority person supports adaptability by the very nature of the limitation on the kinds of interactions that role imposes. Adaptation supports acceptance of authority, it supports not questioning commonly held beliefs, it supports low levels of initiative, it supports the adaptive-compliant position on the maturity continuum, and it compels teachers to be allied with the content rather than with the learner.

POWER

Power is always an issue in politics. When the teacher's role is information provider; arbiter of validity and truth; establisher of the rules and regulations of classrooms; and responsible for making the connections, analogies, explanations, assumptions, and implications around ideas and theories, then the teacher is the power. When the teacher is sole critic, evaluator, marker—the teacher is the power. When the teacher makes all the decisions, enforces the procedures and decides who shall speak, and when and what questions will be asked and answered—the teacher is the power.

Krishnamurti (1953) is suspicious of power as reflected in authority. He suggests that society teaches the obeying of authority by rewarding it and that the real problem with education is the educator. He also suggests the effects are crippling when students come under the influence of the authority of teachers who use their authority for "self-expansive fulfillment" (p. 36). In this light, he suggests that "both the educator and the child should be free from the fear of punishment and the hope of reward, and from every other form of compulsion" (p. 35); but, he suggests, compulsion will continue as long as authority is part of student–faculty relationships. He suggests that conventional education makes independent thinking extremely difficult and that it requires conformity, a conformity that leads to mediocrity (p. 9). Finally, he suggests that reward, punishment, compulsion, and conformity arise from the role of the teacher as authority figure and that only teaching based on mutual respect and affection can truly educate.

Freire (1976) has similar ideas, although they are cast in more revolutionary terms. He suggests that real teaching is the ability to dialogue with students in a mode of reciprocity. Actually, teaching requires more than Freire maintains. The real teacher has the ability to get students to have dialogue with each other in scholarly ways—to pose reality-based questions of such interest and import that the mind, the imagination, and the energy of students are engaged in active pursuit of possible answers and solutions, plans, and strategies. This should be the legacy of true democracy in the classroom. It is not that the teacher has no power—that would be artificial—but is that the power is restrained. The power is used to organize the class in such a way as to support educative learning. The power is that of expertise in content, in how to learn, in inquiry, and in scholarly pursuit. It is power that relies upon the consent of the learner and rests in mutual respect. It is dependent upon an alliance between the student and the teacher. The expert teacher has what Whitehead refers to as "style."

POLITICAL ALLIANCES

Political alliances are an important aspect of classroom politics. Alliances tell who is committed to helping whom do what. In classrooms they are not so much a written treaty as an understood one. In the traditional classroom, the teacher is allied with the content (see Fig. 3). The commitment is to the content; the teacher's responsibility is to see that the content is learned. It is in the interest of that commitment that the teacher chooses content that is perceived as important and makes sure the student "learns" the content. This content is usually provided passively through a required reading or through a lecture, and then the student is tested to see that the content is learned. It is this alliance that causes the teacher to feel responsible for students' learning and guilty for their failures. It is this commitment that makes the teacher want to ensure that all students have the same learning experience and to assume that if they do, then they have all learned the same thing. It is this alliance that makes the teacher fear to stray from the established field content as represented by the course outline. It is this alliance that makes passive learning attractive and active learning scary to teachers. Finally, it is this alliance that makes the teacher put so much content into a course that if the student breaks the point of the pencil with which he or she is taking notes, he or she is immediately a week behind.

Figure 3
The Teaching–Learning Process Alliance Diagram: Behaviorist

STUDENT—→   ←— TEACHER/CONTENT———→   LEARNING

If the alliance is changed and the teacher becomes allied with the student instead of the content (see Fig. 4), the whole political and educational climate changes.

In this alliance the teacher is still concerned with students' learning content—after all, processes of education (criticism, meaning seeking, pattern making, scholarly inquiry, etc.) are not taught in a vacuum but by using content. McPeck (1981) suggests that critical thinking varies from field to field because the essential ingredient of it is the epistemological knowledge of the field. One cannot think critically about nursing without a knowledge of the philosophy, theories, history, care models, and experiences of nursing.

The idea behind the shift in alliance is that the content is no longer sacrosanct. That being the case, the teacher is relieved of adherence to the lecture format and to long lists of "essential" content. That is not to say content is of *no* importance. Content is the vehicle for providing an education—it is what is acted upon by the actors, that is, teachers and students in alliance. Content is the raw material. What is made of the content depends upon what one does with it. Content changes as the social, physical, biological sciences, and nursing change. It changes when societal needs change, when faculty come and go, when the calendar is altered, and when the field of study grows. Furthermore, while the half-life of scientific information is $2^{1}/_{2}$ years, the educative processes are timeless; they mature and develop and people grow in their ability to use them. In essence these educative processes serve the person for a lifetime. Therefore, the responsibility the teacher has for helping students to learn scholarship, critical thinking, and the arts of the mind are exceedingly

Figure 4
The Teaching–Learning Process Alliance Diagram:
Educative–Caring

STUDENT–TEACHER————→   CONTENT————→   LEARNING

great. If the content (information, directions, rules, and rationale) is in error or does not apply in a given situation, it is the nurse who can think critically, who knows the right questions to raise and how to find the clues, cues, information, ideas, and models to help determine the accuracy and appropriateness of the content, and who will be the safe, effective, caring, expert nurse all teachers long to graduate.

Content is not diminished in importance; it simply takes a different role and position. It is to be looked at from every angle, questions about it are posed, assumptions are examined, and thinking becomes the road to learning—not memorizing—information. Teachers and students, students and students, interact, and the curriculum comes to life.

So, in the new alliance, the teacher sees questions as the key to learning, the key to motivation, the key to reflection, the key to critical thinking—in short, the key to education.

FACULTY DEVELOPMENT FOR NEW ROLES

The first paragraph of this chapter proposed that society's need for quality nursing care requires "industrious constancy in self-development efforts." This industrious constancy must address itself not only to the specialty content that is so often the subject of workshops, but also equally to education. Teachers are not born—the strategies teachers use are most often those they were themselves subjected to. There is a whole movement in nursing education *away from education* as a choice of functional specialty. Nursing, once again, wishes to follow in the footsteps of other academic fields that assume that if you know your specialty area, you can teach it. The assumption is fallacious and the position discounts one of the most important functions of any academic field—that of educating others in the field's content, culture, inquiry, modes, and practice. This discount of the study of education also assumes that the way we were taught is the way everyone should be taught and that teaching comes naturally. To follow this pathway away from nursing education as an option in graduate progress will do far more damage to nursing than any other of the false trails nursing has ever embarked upon.

Teaching and Instructing

There is a difference between teaching (as used in this book) and instructing. Technically, teaching is the generic term. It includes instructing. However, the distinction in what instructing is and all that teaching includes is an important distinction here. A teacher (as contrasted to an instructor) is what has been described earlier: a person who structures for learning; a meta strategist; one who helps learners explore the scholarly modalities of a field of study; who poses questions and provides the climate that supports the student's struggle to find answers or possibilities; and who provides guides, criteria, standards, and information when needed.

Instruction is quite different. By its very meaning, it has information as its primary content and acquiring information as its learning intent. Information is part of the essential material of thought—it is part of content. But content is more inclusive than information. Content must encompass the methodologies of scholarship. There are some things that cannot be told and must be experientially learned. "Telling" novice learners that they should look for assumptions is like telling city dwellers they should not starve in the woods. Just as a woodsperson must work with a city dweller on how to obtain food in the wild, teachers must work *with* students to help them see beyond statements to assumptions and to peek underneath the surface to see the assumptions behind the assumptions.

Roles of Teachers

Since educative learning for professional nursing practice demands more than the prescribed training of behavioral-objectives-structured curricula, a faculty member must change his or her role from the one who gives information, prescribes the lecture content, "regulates the outer phenomenon," and controls the educational setting (instructing) to the one who is an expert in learning and content, helping novice learners find their way into the "deeper structures" (Stenhouse, 1975, p. 91) of the field of study in order to see the patterns, meanings, assumptions and implications of the content (teaching).

The message is clear: We must dispense with the idea of teacher as information-giver either in the classroom or in the practicum. We must restructure teacher perceptions of their roles (see Table 1). The teacher's main purpose, beyond the minimal activity of ensuring safety, is to provide the climate, the structure, and the dialogue that promote praxis. The teacher's role is to design ways to engage the student in the mental processes of analysis of cues until patterns are seen that provide paradigms for practice. Furthermore, the teacher's role is to raise questions that require reading, observation, analysis, and reflection upon

Table 1
The Teacher's Roles

Purposes: To Ensure Safety and to Provide the Climate, the Structure, and the Dialogue that Promote Praxis

Roles

1. Become a co-learner/expert learner
2. Design ways to engage the student in analyzing cues until patterns are seen that provide paradigms for practice
3. Raise questions that require reading, observation, and reflection upon patient care
4. Initiate the learner into the culture of the area or field (mores, folkways, customs, ethics, and politics)
5. Help find inquiry modes appropriate to the field
6. Act as meta strategist
7. Nurture the learner
8. Nurture the ethical ideal
9. Nurture the caring role
10. Nurture the creative drive
11. Nurture curiosity and the search for satisfying ideas
12. Nurture assertiveness
13. Support the spirit of inquiry
14. Nurture the desire to seek dialogue about care
15. Interact with students as persons of worth, dignity, intelligence, and high scholarly standards

patient care. The teacher's role is to nurture the learner: to nurture the ethical ideal, to nurture the caring role, to nurture the creative drive, to nurture curiosity and the search for satisfying ideas, to nurture assertiveness and the spirit of inquiry together with the desire to seek dialogue about care, and to be available for that dialogue. The teacher's role is to interact with students as persons of worth, dignity, intelligence, and high scholarly standards.

Nursing education graduate programs in teaching do not usually support these roles. If faculty have any courses in nursing education at all, they are usually within the Tyler legacy. What they know is training, not education. Curriculum development in the traditional sense just rearranges things and, if one is lucky, improves the flow of content. It does nothing at all for teaching, and it is teaching that makes the curriculum.

In the classroom and in practicums, teachers must begin to see themselves as what Stenhouse (1980) calls expert learners. As expert learners their primary role revolves around helping students, as novice learners, learn how to learn—how to be scholars—how to think critically—how to gain insights and find meanings—how to see patterns—and how to capitalize on their paradigm experiences. Teachers must see their role as structuring learning activities that will help achieve these ends. This role is one of meta strategist—developing strategies to help others develop strategies for caring expertise and scholarship.

In essence the teacher's main problem is not what to lecture on, or how to organize that lecture. The teacher's main problems are two: what learning activities to select or design that will promote the type of learning desired and what kinds of teacher–student transactions will best promote educative learning.

Solving these two problems must become the central issues in any professional curriculum development paradigm. To do that, teaching roles must alter.

As with any educational problem, giving teachers *information* about the needed changes is insufficient. Faculty development must occupy a dominant place in faculty life and must itself be in a mode of active learning. Hospitals and health care agencies have long been required by accreditation standards to have full- or part-time staff development persons. Staff development is an accepted position within the organization, and budgets are established to support the developmental programs. Faculty development must occupy the same accepted position in academic nursing, and full- or part-time faculty must be employed to conduct such programs. In curriculum development for an educative paradigm, experts must work with faculty to help them develop the strategies of teaching through small group learning that focus on educative dialogue about the essential aspects of nursing. Only when that has occurred is the faculty ready to open the curriculum to the possibilities that are available. In fact, once faculty have switched roles, curriculum development follows naturally.

TEACHING'S MORAL IMPERATIVE

Classroom Culture

Stenhouse (1968), in discussing his theories of curriculum as they are manifested in the classroom (pp. 70–89), relates a successful teaching episode and then remarks, "The key problem seems to be: what kind of culture should we try to generate in the classroom? This is the problem of the design of a curriculum and its interpretation to the pupils" (p. 88). He presents a view of curriculum as culture rather than as knowledge. Of this he says, "it [curriculum] must function as a basis for communication and thinking in the class as a group" (p. 88). He then offers the idea that critical standards and a sense of quality are absolutely necessary for such a curriculum and concludes, "A good curriculum is one which makes worth-while standards possible" (p. 89). One can assume standards of scholarship, of consistency, and of relevancy and validity. One can assume that the standards of teaching reflected in the criteria generated by the research of Murray and Merrefield (1989) can be applied and used to direct curriculum. I wish to go beyond that and look at the culture of the curriculum as the moral responsibility of faculty.

Classroom Culture as Faculty Attitude

The culture of the classroom begins with the culture of the faculty and the general expectations of the faculty for the curriculum. The curriculum plans reflect this culture. Plans that are merely courses, descriptions, sequence, and outlines communicate a coldness that becomes the climate of the school. Culture is reflected in the faculty's attitude toward each other, toward new members, toward students, and toward their occupation. This culture manifests itself in standards of conduct for the faculty. What standards do faculty accept and expect from each other? Is it colleagueship that is sharing, concerned, and caring, or colleagueship that is protective, jealous, tense, and isolating? Are dual standards of conduct tolerated? Is there one standard for interacting with students and another for faculty? Some teachers are very nice to colleagues or superiors but unfair and gamey with students or conversely charming, witty, wise, and caring with students and competitive and destructive with colleagues. *These faculty climates—cultural norms—create the school climate and filter into the teacher–student interactions and thus become curriculum.* Stenhouse (1967, p. 68) goes so far as to say they are curriculum. Therefore, choosing a culture and creating it becomes of primary importance in the faculty developmental program. Often this takes the form of permission giving, practice, and group approval for the normal warmth, concern, caring, and moral rectitude that characterize most nursing teachers. A climate of validation of self-worth; of wholeness; of perfect person; of good intent; of respect for the needs, integrity, life choices, and styles; and personal and professional values is created in agreement and effort together. It is created with shared responsibility for the climate and acknowledgment of everyone's participation in setting and maintaining that climate. Climate is much too important to allow it to be part of the hidden curriculum. These verbal and nonverbal messages and the condoned intrafaculty and faculty–student interactions must be raised into awareness and become part of the legitimate curriculum.

Women's Ways of Knowing as Legitimate Basis for Shaping Classroom Culture

Women make up a disproportionately large percentage of nursing class enrollments. Women still comprise between 97 and 98 percent of nurses, and that majority is usually reflected in classrooms. Beyond the perspective of the large plurality of nurses being women, women numerically dominate the field of teaching in elementary and secondary schools. Feistritzer (1983) claims that 83 percent of elementary teachers, 49 percent of secondary teachers, and 68 percent of all teachers are women. Since the 19th century, teaching in the United States has been considered women's work (Feiman-Nemser & Floden, 1986, p. 518). Only in higher education do men outnumber women. There, the traditional masculine ways of being and thinking traditionally dominate. Historically, until quite recently, higher education was exclusively male. It is, however, not numbers that make either nursing or teaching feminine fields. It is the nature of the field itself—the fact that women numerically dominate is probably a complex social phenomenon.

The feminine status of nursing and teaching require some comment upon the way women think as an aid to those who are their co-learners and expert guides in the educative process and who set the climate for the classroom.

The classroom climate for both teaching and nursing must reflect the feminine nature of the fields and the students. Belenky, Clinchy, Goldberger, and Tarule (1986) have described their research regarding women's ways of knowing. Their study grouped women's perspectives on knowing into five epistemological categories. Some understanding of these categories may give the teacher insights into the different perspectives women have for viewing reality and drawing conclusions about what they learn. They paint a picture of struggle for women acquiring power over their own minds and "making it" in educational institutions that traditionally value only masculine ways of knowing. They say, "In spite of the increase in the number of women students in higher education and professional schools, faculties, usually predominantly male, argue against a special focus on women students and resist open debate on whether women's educational needs are different from men's" (p. 5). Major researchers in the field (Gilligan, 1979, 1982; Keller, 1978, 1985) argue convincingly that there is a masculine bias reflected in most academic disciplines. This includes their methodologies and theories. Academic disciplines, even today, after more than 20 years of feminist research and literature, give little attention to women's modes of learning, knowing, and valuing (Belenky et al., 1986, p. 6). Feminine literature on knowing becomes an important issue because, regardless of age, gender, or progress on the educational ladder, students, by the nature of their role are in the process of defining or redefining themselves and their view of the world. They reflect on the context and conditions that influence their self-perception, understanding, and definition. Only in so far as this process is successful will students come to define themselves as "professionals" and to develop the self-confidence, direction, structure, and maturity to be the "new nurses" that are required by society. Although some may reason that most self-definition work is completed by the individual prior to higher education, that is not the case.

A side issue that helps underline the process of continuing self-definition is to note the work done on the influence of formal higher education on moral reasoning. Felton and Parsons (1984), in a study on female senior baccalaureate nursing majors and graduate students who had completed 18 semester hours in six schools in the Southeastern states, found that education had a significant impact on overall ethical/moral reasoning levels. Among other substantiating data, it was found that graduate students' D mean score was significantly higher than that of undergraduate students. This supported previous research findings reported by Rest (1979) that education is a significant variable in the development of ethical/moral reasoning. Additionally, participants' socioeconomic level and years of work experience were not significantly related to ethical and moral reasoning (D scores). Furthermore, findings support that stabilization of ethical/moral development occurs at the point at which one leaves formal education and that the educational experience may counteract socioeconomic level and work-experience-influenced moral and ethical reasoning. Ethical and moral reasoning is at the central core of defining the world, viewing the self, and establishing the self as a scholar. If ethical and moral reasoning are school-related, I think it fair to say that students are in the process of defining and redefining their world and themselves by virtue of the fact that they are students.

Since, as discussed earlier, women constitute a majority of nursing majors, since these students are in the process of growing in their view of the world and in developing their ethical and moral reasoning, and since they are changing their ways of knowing, it becomes necessary to comprehend something regarding the ways women know. Belenky et al. (1986) contribute important perceptions in a teacher's search for understanding women's knowing and through rich descriptions give the reader the feel of how the women came to those places in their lives. For real information, a description of the categories (as listed below) is insufficient. The descriptive material within the study about participants, often in their own words, enriches insights and shows the way to understanding. Belenky et al. list the following categories:

Silence is a position in which women experience themselves as mindless and voiceless and subject to the whims of external authority. They are among the most oppressed and the most socially, educationally, and economically deprived of women.

Received knowledge is a perspective from which women conceive of themselves as capable of receiving, even reproducing, knowledge from the all-knowing external authorities but not capable of creating knowledge on their own.

Subjective knowledge presents a perspective from which truth and knowledge are conceived of as personal, private, and subjectively known or intuited; truth resides within the person and is more powerful than the answers the outside world offers. The authors offer the idea that subjective knowledge is an important growth step for women. It is an adaptive move that leads to strength, optimism, and self-valuing on one hand and to stubborn rejection of other forms of knowing that can isolate them and make them impatient and dismissive of other persons' ideas.

Procedural knowledge is described by the authors as "the voice of reason." It bears examining in some detail here because it is, in the world of academia, very important. No paradigm for curriculum development, no insights about learning can ignore or discount it. Procedural knowledge is basic to strategizing, to inquiry, to standard approaches to content, to understanding and knowing. Additionally, it is having a thorough knowledge of standard procedures that allows one to create unique combinations and even new ways to inquire into the nature of things. It is in this category that women are invested in learning and applying objective procedures for obtaining and communicating knowledge. It tends to be a masculine modality. Women in this category "think before they speak; and, because their ideas must measure up to certain objective standards, they speak in measured tones" (Belenky et al., 1986, p. 94).

Procedural knowledge is about "knowing how" and according to the authors, borders on the term coined by feminist theologian Mary Daly (1973), *methodolatry*. Methodolatry is methodology taken to the point of tyranny. And when that happens, according to Daly (p. 11), it hinders new discoveries because it prevents one from raising questions that do not fit into preestablished "boxes and forms." She suggests that basing decisions upon form or methodology implicitly dictates content because a particular methodology in the research supports or "outlaws" questions that cannot be answered in that fashion. (Obviously, good researchers attempt to find a form or method to fit the questions, not the reverse.) One point worth underlining regarding this category is that procedural knowledge is very attractive because the knowledge yielded by procedures provides a person more control and makes the world, though more complex than the previous ways of knowing, more orderly, and more manageable. The problem comes, not in the kind of knowledge that procedural knowledge is in itself, but in its "dogmatization" in education. It is an invaluable part of knowing, but it is only one way and one part and becomes a liability only when it becomes "methodolatry."

Constructed knowledge is a position in which women view all knowledge as contextual, experience themselves as creators of knowledge, and value both subjective and objective strategies for knowing. It is in this position that women integrate all of the ways of knowing. Compared to other positions, there is a capacity at the position of constructed knowledge to attend to another person and to feel related to that person in spite of what may be enormous differences. Theirs is a capacity for "attentive love" and an empathic potential that is maternal in constructivist women. Theirs is the ability to be sensitive to the inner life of others, to imagine that life is part of women's constructivist knowing. Constructivist knowing brings it all together—received, subjective, and procedural—and brings it to bear on all problems. This must be the goal of all education for women—but for nurses and teachers, because of their unique position in society, it is essential.

Longing after Good

If women are to develop constructed knowing, the classroom climate and politics must support it and provide a legitimacy for the "attentive love" and empathy Belenky et al. construe as part of the essential feminine knowing. Most authors refer to this as caring. Watson (1988, p. 34) maintains that persons are caring when they somehow respond to a person as a unique individual, perceive the other's feelings, and set apart one person from another and from the ordinary. Murray and Bevis (1977) assert that caring "impels one to create an environment for loved ones that enables them to fulfill themselves" (pp. 127–128). This becomes then the moral imperative of nursing education: to create the climate, give the permission, model the affirmations, establish the role models, and build into both the learning activities and the teacher–student interactions the fabric of feminine knowing and feminine ethics that is caring. Without it education becomes rhetoric—and the educated are moral paupers.

Noddings, in her book, *Caring, a Feminine Approach to Ethics and Moral Education* (1984), states, "human caring and the memory of caring and being cared for . . . form the foundation of ethical response." She suggests that the masculine view of ethics and moral reasoning that has dominated the literature has failed to listen to the feminine voice. By this she means that it emphasizes a mathematical appearance and is hierarchal. She acknowledges that philosophers have recognized the difference between "pure" or logical reasoning and "practical" or moral reasoning, but she maintains that both concentrate on the establishment of "logical principles and their exceptions and uses such language as justification, fairness, justice." The feminine (as distinguished from "women," i.e., not necessarily the private ground of women but representative of feminine approaches to the world) approach begins with the "moral attitude or longing for goodness and not with moral reasoning" (p. 2). It is not that women cannot use logic or that they discard it, only that their approach is different. She illustrates this point with the story of Abraham offering Isaac as a sacrifice at God's command (p. 43). She points out that Kierkegaard interprets Abraham's action as supra-ethical and that that immoral act was justified by being derived from duty to God. She says that for the mother, the relation to one's "children is not governed first by the ethical but by natural caring." In other words, a woman would not have been so obedient to God's command but would have responded to her natural ethic of caring for her child. Noddings goes on to say, "We love not because we are required to love but because our natural relatedness gives natural birth to love. It is this love, this natural caring, that makes the ethical possible" (p. 43). Her point is that caring—loving—is fundamental to the ethical ideal and that ideal sustains us as caring persons toward the good that is longed for.

Based on this she suggests, "Our efforts must, then, be directed to the maintenance of conditions that will permit caring to flourish." This makes us dependent upon the ethical ideal, and one outcome of that is to emphasize moral education. She states unequivocally, *"The primary aim of all education must be nurturance of the ethical ideal"* (p. 6).

Noddings (1984), in carrying this point forward, uses such terms as receptivity, relatedness, responsiveness, and subjectivity. She suggests that this does not mean that logic or empiricism be discarded but only that there is an alternative to the usually offered objective logicism, which is that one begins with a moral attitude of longing for goodness and not with moral reasoning.

Some of Noddings' terminology is central to any attempt to increase our awareness of some of the ways we need to recast education—in an ethic appropriate to nursing. Noddings speaks of *receptivity* as an attempt to grasp or to receive a reality rather than to impose it. Her term *relatedness* is much as it sounds—to have a caring relationship or to view organisms in relation, striving to maintain the relation as a caring one or to transform it from noncaring to caring. It embodies the idea of reciprocity—that there is an exchange of positive energy and a commitment to good for and by each other. *Responsiveness* is a natural consequence of receptivity and relatedness, and her term *subjectivity* means a willingness to risk and use one's feeling abilities as well as one's cognitive abilities. Receptivity, relatedness, responsiveness, and subjectivity are all involved in *confirmation*—of the better self, the higher ideal, the best possibility.

Van Manen, in his article, "Edifying Theory: Serving the Good" (1982), speaks of "truth in the Greek sense" and says it "refers us to the disclosure of the essential nature, the essence of the good of things" (p. 44). He also explores the etymology of "theoretical" and says it derives from the same root as theatre. It is a place for "beholding and presenting." He says, "The theoretical as theatre is a place where in the midst of everyday life we find the possibility of contemplating, beholding, and presenting the good; and the possibility of thus having a transforming experience—in the edifying sense of 'inspiring,' 'making pure,' 'enlightening,' and 'uplifting spiritually.'" He agrees with Noddings in saying that "some theorists have been eager to show rigor by adopting a mathematical logos and such control-oriented techniques. But mathematical logic belongs to the being of things, not to the being of beings" (p. 46). He proposes that theorists need to rid themselves of the ideal that theoretically prepared rationality or ethic furnishes the means, standards, and criteria for "a more rational practice." He also maintains that norms, values, and principles that have not been embodied in our spiritual or individual life histories will fall short of our ways of being with students. Such rationality, void of the spiritual (not religious), is incapable of "minding the good" (p. 46).

TEACHING NURSING AS A MORAL ACTIVITY

Teachers of nursing have more cause than most to nurture the ethical ideal in students. Nursing is a deeply moral activity. Nurses perform the most difficult drudgery that human misery generates and some of the most sublime activities that one person ever has the opportunity to do for another. Nursing is intensely intimate and touches people at the times in their lives when they are most vulnerable; when they are threatened, in pain, afraid, hopeless, and often isolated from friends, family, and familiar environments and routines. If we are to entrust society to their hands, teachers must do all that is possible to engender the moral ideal of caring so that that caring will compel nurses to act in ways that are positive for these vulnerable individuals and families that are their trust. Nursing teachers must keep that primary aim of education, the nurturance of the ethical ideal, first in their minds, first in their plans, and first in their interactions and transactions with students.

I do not want to enter the argument of Meno and Socrates (Plato, 1952) regarding whether or not virtue can be taught. If it can be—and it probably can—it can only be taught in a climate that lives the ideal of caring so that it pervades all interactions: learning activities, teacher–teacher, teacher–student, student–student, and nurse–patient.

Noddings (1984) asserts, "When the attitude of the one-caring bespeaks caring, the cared-for one glows, grows stronger, and feels not so much that he has been given something as that something has been added to him" (p. 20). This is affirmation at its most beneficial.

If one accepts the proposition that caring is the moral ideal of nursing (Watson, 1988), then teaching caring becomes the moral imperative of nursing educators. It motivates nursing educators' curriculum planning, triggers the drive for self improvement and faculty development, and governs teacher–student interactions and the climate of schools and classrooms. Caring is as essential to educative teaching as water is to human life.

Therefore, it becomes the moral responsibility of nursing educators to study theories of caring, read the literature on caring, and practice caring, making it as natural to their lives as breathing.

With this imperative in the forefront of the mind, it is legitimate to move on to some of the other ideas that may support educative learning. For without caring, these other theoretical constructs become mechanistic techniques for classroom and student manipulation.

If we are to rewrite the script for nursing education and cast it in humanitarian caring, ethical, and professionally educative terms, we must uphold the legitimacy of caring as a philosophy and ethic of nursing.

Teachers of nurses have a special responsibility as do nurses who practice in settings where students learn. These nurses can be instrumental in being the students' mirror, revealing to the students things about themselves that will nurture the ethical ideal or destroy it. The ethics of nursing practice, education, and research first flows from Noddings' "moral longing." "Longing for good" will support educators in knowing how to do good. Educators must part with their anthropological and sociological colleagues who claim that morality is based on common human character traits and needs, and, therefore, an objective morality is possible. We nurses must be expert ethicists, because nurses in practice encounter more complex ethical and moral issues in a month than most other people do in a lifetime. We can agree with anthropologists that morality is perhaps grounded in some common human needs, feelings, and thoughts, but to conclude, therefore, that objectivity is possible is a non sequitur.

Nurses deal with people who are subjects, not objects, and a subjective ethic provides the flexibility and allows the feelings and sensitivities that cannot be found in the rule-driven rigidity of objective ethics. Noddings (1984) translates this into some ideas about moral education. She states that the teacher has two major tasks in moral education. These are to expand the student's world by presenting an effective and accurate selection of that world and to work cooperatively with the student's struggle toward competence in that world—and in doing this the teacher's highest priority is to nurture the student's ethical ideal. It is easy to recognize the merit in what she says; it is not so easy to find ways of accomplishing those high goals. Our usual ways have fallen short, *for no code of ethics, no list of injunctions, no fear of punishment or hope of reward, and no rules or logical decision tree will effect these tasks of moral education. Only a mentor/preceptor/teacher modeling a humanistically caring ethic and having dialogue with students that underscores constructed knowing and encourages them to be personally related to the ethical issues involved can facilitate and enhance students in their moral development for life and for nursing.*

Teachers must make deliberate attempts, through learning activities and teacher–student interactions, to move the student into ways of knowing that are most useful to students and helpful in furthering their ability to respond caringly and effectively to client needs.

REFERENCES

Adler, M. J. (1982). *The Paideia proposal: An educational manifesto.* New York: Macmillan.

Belenky, M., Clinchy, B., Goldberger, N., & Tarule, J. (1986). *Women's ways of knowing, the development of self, voice, and mind.* New York: Basic Books.

Benner, P. (1984). *From novice to expert: Excellence and power in clinical nursing practice.* Menlo Park, CA: Addison-Wesley.

Botkin, J., Elmandjra, M., & Malitza, M. (1979). *No limits to learning: Bridging the human gap.* New York: Pergamon Press.

Bok, D. (1984, May/June). Needed: A new way to train doctors (The President's Report to the Harvard Board of Overseers for 1982–83). *Harvard Magazine,* 32–71.

Broudy, H. S. (1972). *Enlightened cherishing, an essay on aesthetic education.* The 1972 Kappa Delta Pi Lecture. Chicago: University of Illinois Press.

Cousins, N. (1985). The options of learning. *Creative Living, 14*(4), 2–4.

Daly, M. (1976). *Beyond God the father.* Boston: Beacon Press.

Dewey, J. (1933). *How we think* (rev. ed.). Boston: D. C. Heath.

Feiman-Nemser, S., & Floden, R. (1986). In M. Wittrock (Ed.), *Handbook of research on teaching* (3rd ed.), pp. 505–526. New York: Macmillan.

Feistritzer, C. (1983). *The American teacher.* Washington, DC: Feistritzer Publications.

Felton, G. M., & Parsons, M. A. (1984). *The effect of education on the ability to resolve ethical/moral dilemmas.* Unpublished manuscript.

Freire, P. (1970). *Pedagogy of the oppressed.* New York: Herder and Herder.

Freire, P. (1976). *Education: The practice of freedom.* London: Writers and Readers Publishing Cooperative.

Gilligan, C. (1979). Women's place in man's life cycle. *Harvard Educational Review, 47,* 481–517.

Gilligan, C. (1982). *In a different voice: Psychological theory and women's development.* Cambridge, MA: Harvard University Press.

Gordon, D. R. (1984). Research application: Identifying the use and misuse of formal models in nursing practice. In P. Benner, *From novice to expert:*

Excellence and power in clinical nursing practice. Menlo Park, CA: Addison-Wesley.

Gray, H. (1988). The aims of education. *The University of Chicago Magazine, 80*(2), 2–8.

Greene, M. (1986). Philosophy and teaching. In M. Wittrock, *Handbook of research on teaching* (3rd ed.). New York: Macmillan.

Heidegger, M. (1968). In J. G. Gray (Trans.), *What is called thinking.* New York: Harper and Row. (Original work published 1954).

Hunt, M. (1982, May 12). Do you know how you think? *Minneapolis Star and Tribune,* p. 13a.

Institute of Medicine, Division of Health Care Services. (1983). *Nursing and nursing education: Public policies and private actions.* Washington, DC: National Academy Press.

Keller, E. F. (1978). Gender and science. *Psychoanalysis and Contemporary Thought, 1,* 409–433.

Keller, E. F. (1985). *Reflections on gender and science.* New Haven, CT: Yale University Press.

Krishnamurti, J. (1953). *Education and the significance of life.* San Francisco: Harper and Row.

McPeck, J. (1981). *Critical thinking and education.* New York: St. Martin's Press.

Merleau-Ponty, M. (1967). In C. Smith (Trans.), *Phenomenology of perception.* New York: Humanities Press.

Meyer, C. (1986). *Teaching students to think critically.* San Francisco: Jossey-Bass.

Murray, J., & Bevis, E. (1977). Caring: Process and practice. In E. Bevis (1982, 1989), *Curriculum building in nursing: A process.* New York: National League for Nursing.

Murray, J., & Merrefield, S. (1989). Criteria for teacher–student interactions and learning experiences. In J. Murray, *Developing criteria to support new curriculum models for doctoral education in nursing.* Doctoral dissertation, University of Georgia.

National Commission on Nursing. (1981). *Initial report and preliminary recommendations.* Chicago, IL: The Hospital Research and Educational Trust.

Noddings, N. (1984). *Caring: A feminine approach to ethics and moral education.* Berkeley, CA: University of California Press.

Panel on the General Professional Education of the Physician and College Preparation. (1984). *Physicians for the twenty-first century.* Washington, DC: Association of American Medical Colleges.

Plato. (1952). In R. M. Hutchins (Ed.), *Great books of the western world.* Chicago: Encylopaedia Britannica.

Polanyi, M., & Prosch, H. (1975). *Meaning*. Chicago: The University of Chicago Press.

Rest, J. (1979). *Manual for the defining issues test: An objective test of moral judgment* (rev. ed.). Minneapolis: University of Minnesota.

Sakalys, J., & Watson, J. (1985, September–October). New directions in higher education: A review of trends. *Journal of Professional Nursing*, 293–299.

Smith, B. O. (1987). Definitions of teaching. In M. J. Dunkin (Ed.), *The international encyclopedia of teaching and teacher education*. New York: Pergamon Press.

Stenhouse, L. (1968). *Culture and education*. New York: Weybright and Talley.

Stenhouse, L. (1975). *An Introduction to curriculum research and development*. London: Heinemann Educational Books.

Stenhouse, L. (Ed.). (1980). *Curriculum research and development in action*. London: Heinemann Educational Books.

Study Group on the Conditions of Excellence in American Higher Education. (1984). Involvement in learning: Realizing the potential of American higher education. U.S. Department of Education. *The Chronicle of Higher Education, XXIX*(9), 35–49.

van Manen, M. (1982). Edifying theory: Serving the good. *Theory Into Practice, XXI*(1), 44–49.

Whitehead, A. N. (1929). *The aims of education and other essays*. New York: The Free Press.

Watson, J. (1985, 1988). *Nursing: Human science and human care, a theory of nursing*. New York: National League for Nursing.

Watson, J., & Bevis, E. (1988). Nursing education: Coming of age for a new age. In N. Chaska (Ed.), *The nursing profession: Turning points*. New York: McGraw-Hill, in press.

BIBLIOGRAPHY

Bennett, W. J. (1984). To reclaim a legacy: Text of report on humanities in higher education. *The Chronicle of Higher Education, XXIX*(14), 32–71.

Dunkin, M. J. (Ed.). (1987). *The international encyclopedia of teaching and teacher education*. New York: Pergamon Press.

Gagne, R. (1970). *The conditions of learning* (2nd ed.). New York: Holt, Rinehart and Winston.

Piaget, J. (1976). *Psychology of intelligence*. Totowa, NJ: Littlefield Adams. (Originally published 1947).

Stenhouse, L. (1983). *Authority, education and emancipation.* London: Heinemann Educational Books.

Tyler, R. (1949). *Basic principles of curriculum and instruction.* Chicago: University of Chicago Press.

7

Making the Connection: Teacher–Student Interactions and Learning Experiences

Joyce P. Murray

Through dialogue, the teacher-of-the-students and the students-of-the-teacher cease to exist and a new term emerges: teacher-student with students-teachers.

Freire, 1971

INTRODUCTION

The key thesis of this book—that curriculum is the transactions and interactions that occur between student and teacher and among students with the intent that learning takes place—by its very nature places emphasis upon two things: (1) the nature of the interactions that occur between teachers and students and among students and (2) the type of learning experiences that comprise the curriculum. This central concern creates the differences between the products of curriculum development in behaviorist curriculum models and this humanistic-educative one. While among the products of curriculum development, the behaviorist paradigms have a philosophy, conceptual framework, and behavioral

objectives, this one concentrates on the nature of teacher–student interactions and the devising and selection of learning experiences.

This chapter concentrates on teacher–student interactions and
learning experiences and ways they may be translated into curriculum.
Methods of generating criteria to devise, select, and critique teacher–
student interactions and learning experiences are explored. In order to
be able to interact in different ways and to structure learning differently, faculty development becomes key to the success of this paradigm.
This change may be anxiety producing and unsettling for faculty, and,
therefore, the change may be subject to sabotage. This chapter will also
explore ways in which curriculum development may be sabotaged.

TEACHER–STUDENT INTERACTIONS AND
LEARNING EXPERIENCES AS CURRICULUM

Curriculum in the educative-humanistic paradigm is defined as the transactions and interactions that occur between student and teacher and
among students with the intent that learning take place. This definition
provides us with information concerning the elements that must be examined to create a curriculum. Intentionality is a key component. It means
that something is purposefully designed to accomplish a goal or an end. In
this definition, it means that teacher–student interactions and learning
experiences are purposefully designed so that students may learn; however, intentionality is different from preselected behaviors. The goals or
ends-in-view may be as specific as students learning to think deductively
based on pattern recognition or as vague as creating a climate in which
students learn how to interact with teachers as colleagues.

Consideration of the intent to learn leads one to devise, build, or
select learning activities that are likely to provide the student with successful learning experiences. Selecting teacher–student interactions
that are educative, caring, and egalitarian increases the chances of accomplishing learning of educational and nursing value and worth. In this
regard, devising, building, or selecting learning activities and teacher–
student interactions are the most essential components of this paradigm.

PHILOSOPHICAL BELIEFS AND
DEFINITIONS OF TEACHING

Teaching is an idea or concept that has been broadly defined and takes
many forms. Literally thousands of articles have been written covering

such areas as the capacities, thoughts, and actions of students and teachers, the activities of teaching, the milieu in which teaching occurs, and content, including the purpose for which it is taught (Shulman, 1986). An examination of related research and writings offer support for the idea that teacher–student interactions comprise the heart of education and learning. Through this examination, patterns emerge, ideas are offered related to specific types of interactions and the types of learning they support, and connections between philosophical beliefs and types of interactions are made. The literature may be thought of as a stimulus for thinking about the types of teacher–student interactions that make up a curriculum. Philosophical beliefs, definitions of teaching, the intent for learning, and content are all variables influencing teacher–student interactions.

Defining teaching requires one to think about the intentions in which teaching begins, the values that are espoused, and the ends that are to be accomplished (Greene, 1986). The philosophical basis of one's beliefs will impact how one thinks about what is being done in the act of teaching. Philosophical discussions with respect to differences between teaching, learning, indoctrination, training, and education can be found throughout the educational literature. Most contemporary philosophers view teaching as intentional activities or complexes of activities aimed at moving others to take cognitive and perhaps imaginative or creative action on their own initiatives (Greene, 1986).

A philosophy of teaching will assist teachers to reflect upon their definition of teaching, their values, and the ends desired. Greene (1986) stated:

> to examine philosophy with respect to teaching is to be concerned with clarifying the language used in describing or explaining the practice of teaching, to penetrate the arguments used in justifying what is done, and to make visible what is presumed in the formulation of purposes and aims. (p. 479)

Wissot (1979) suggested that teaching is an art form based on the natural compulsion in teaching to control the qualitative features in the classroom. He stated that the driving force of art is particularization, and the aim is to make statements about the specific subjective response to the physical world.

Gage (1984) offers a description of teaching. He describes it as an instrumental or practical art, rather than a fine art. Being an instrumental art means that teaching departs from recipes, formulas, and algorithms. It requires improvisation, spontaneity, the handling of a vast array of considerations of form, style, rhythm, and appropriateness in very complex ways.

Klein (1969) does not question that there is such a thing as teaching. He considered searching for a real definition as a trap because no one definition will suffice. He enumerated the propositions upon which he believed teaching is based. These were: (a) teaching is a goal-oriented activity; (b) teaching is only one of several activities with a goal of learning; (c) teaching is a pattern of action that must be repeatable, public, and intelligible; (d) teaching involves interaction between human beings as persons, as free and rational agents. He perceived the last two presuppositions as the most important in differentiating teaching from other activities, such as indoctrination and conditioning. Klein's propositions offer support for the idea that teaching is goal oriented with an intent that learning take place, involves interactions between human beings, and is different from indoctrination, conditioning, and probably training. The idea that it must be repeatable could be stifling or constrictive if teaching is an art. Interactions with students may have the same intent; however, with each student it will be varied and unique based on the context, content, and the individuals involved.

TEACHER–STUDENT INTERACTIONS

The idea that teacher–student interactions are critical to the success of teaching and education can be found throughout the literature. Many research studies have included teacher–student interactions as components of the effects of teaching. These studies offer clues and ideas about the types of teacher–student interactions that are effective in facilitating students' learning. They provide rich sources for faculty as they begin identifying teacher–student interactions that are likely to accomplish the type of learning desired or intended. Several research studies have been selected for review to demonstrate their usefulness in identification of possible teacher–student interactions and related learning that seems to occur.

For example, Gaff and Wilson (1971), in a study commissioned by the Project to Improve College Teaching, conducted a research-based analysis of college environments from the perspective of college faculty. The effects of college policies and practices concerning teachers and teaching, the characteristics of students and faculty–student relationships, and the characteristics of faculty colleagues and colleague relationships were examined. Although one must consider the tenor of the times in the late 1960s and early 1970s, the findings related to faculty–student interactions support the importance of these interactions to students' education. Faculty perceived that students had little meaningful interaction with their teachers, that lack of continuing contact between students and faculty contributed to students' unrest and was detrimental to students' learning and to faculty's satisfaction with teaching, and that the amount of contact with students reflected faculty's educational philosophies. Two groups of faculty emerged from this study. There was a high-contact group and a low-contact group. The high-contact group believed that students learn best if teachers take a personal interest in them, that emotional and personal development is as important as intellectual, and that college education ought to affect students' values as well as develop their minds. The low-contact group was less interested in affecting the student in noncognitive areas. As faculty begin exploring possible types of teacher–student interactions, differences in values and beliefs will emerge and will need to be considered. Within their own situation, faculty may find similar groups of high- and low-contact preferences.

As stated earlier, identification and selection of criteria will need to reflect the makeup of the faculty, and differences will need to be legitimized and valued. Faculty strengths in terms of content and types of interactions become key issues in faculty assignments.

In another study within the same period of time, Chickering (1969) generated hypotheses about the effects of teacher–student relationships. He described seven major vectors of student development and six major aspects of the college environment that operate and influence these vectors. College students develop competence, learn to manage emotions, develop autonomy, establish identity, engage in freeing interpersonal relationships, and develop purpose and integrity. One of the aspects of the college that influence this development is faculty and administration. Chickering found support for his hypothesis that when student–faculty interaction is frequent, friendly, and when it occurs in diverse situations calling for varied roles, then development of intellectual competence, sense of competence, autonomy, and purpose are fostered. All of these characteristics are desired in nursing students at all levels of education and provide the intent or desired learning goals for these teacher–student interactions.

Few studies on teacher–student interactions have been conducted in nursing; however, two studies focused on student–instructor relationships and interaction techniques of faculty in clinical areas (Griffith & Bakanauskas, 1983; Wang & Blumberg, 1983). Griffith and Bakanauskas

(1983) compared the student–instructor relationship to the therapeutic relationship of nurse-client indicating that students could benefit from a relationship that provides open, honest communication
based on trust and support, and that they could more readily learn the
therapeutic approach essential to nursing. Professional socialization,
self-actualization, self-fulfillment, and self-concept are affected by interpersonal relationships, interactions with others, and the ability of the
nursing instructor to meet the students' learning needs. Caring attitudes, demonstrated by an admired, respected instructor who acknowledges students' strengths and weaknesses, are significant to students'
lives and their learning. Caring is as central to the teacher–student
relationship as it is to nursing. Noddings (1984) described teachers as
having a very special and more specialized caring relation. Caring must
be enacted for it to be experienced and learned.

Wang and Blumberg (1983) studied the interaction techniques that
nursing faculty are using in clinical and field settings. Observations in
the clinical area were made throughout the clinical day. Data were then
grouped into high- and low-level interactional techniques. Low-level
interactions and questions included asking leading/direct questions,
summarizing statements, and verbal exchange of a factual or procedural nature. High-level interactions and questions demanded analysis,
synthesis, evaluation, and included comparing and contrasting. Findings indicated that low-level interactions predominated at the sopho-
more, junior, and senior years. The authors thought it possible to infer
that faculty might lack the skills in the use of higher-level interactions
and this might indicate a need to improve clinical teaching interaction
skills. Not only does this study identify desired teacher–student interactions, it also recognizes the value and need for faculty development as
one of the methods for improving or changing teacher–student interactions to increase student learning. Several questions arise from this
study: (1) How will teacher–student interactions vary according to the
level of the student? (2) What teacher–student interactions are most
appropriate for the behavioristic paradigm as opposed to the humanistic? (3) What teacher–student interactions are needed in clinical to promote learning of the technical and mental skills desired?

Although not a research study, the writings of Noddings on moral
education and caring offer valuable clues and suggestions on how teachers and students interact. Noddings (1984) described the relationship
between the teacher and student in moral education. In this relationship,
the teacher seeks the involvement of the student. For example, when questioning a student and a student responds, the teacher receives not just the

"response" but also the student. The student's answer matters whether it is right or wrong. Students are not discounted because of giving a wrong answer. The teacher uses the student's response to probe gently for clarification, interpretation, and contribution. The teacher recognizes that students learn what is most meaningful and what pleases them. Although students may be forced to respond in certain ways, they eventually will find their own way and apply effectively that which has meaning for their own lives. Noddings (1984) suggested that students reward teachers with their efforts, comments, and cooperation. She supports the practice that the relationship between student and teacher is mutually beneficial and that the teacher cannot nurture the student intellectually without regard for moral education.

Inherent within the idea that curriculum is the interactions that take place between teacher and students with the intent that learning take place is the underlying message that teaching interactions are designed by faculty members. Faculty own and develop the curriculum, and, therefore, desired types of interactions must be devised, selected, and critiqued by faculty. These interactions become the curriculum; therefore, they are broad and take on many forms. Interactions may be nonverbal, written, or oral. The development of these interactions will reflect the faculty's definition of teaching, will reflect their philosophical beliefs about teaching, and will be related to their purposes and aims desired for the education of the students.

Criteria that may be used to devise, critique, and select teacher–student interactions become a useful tool for faculty in structuring the curriculum. These criteria can become guidelines for faculty development and evaluation, curriculum critiques, and for increasing awareness of the connection between the interactions and the goals or ends-in-view. An example of types of teacher–student interactions can be found in Appendix I (Murray & Merrefield, 1989). Methods to assist faculty to develop such a list of criteria will be explored later in this chapter.

DEFINITIONS OF LEARNING AND EDUCATION

In this section, definitions of learning and descriptions of education and the role they play in determining the type of learning experiences teachers choose for their students are examined. The goals of these chosen learning experiences will reflect the teacher's definitions and beliefs about learning and education.

Learning activities in the Tyler behaviorist models spell out exactly what is to be accomplished in the behavioral objectives. For true education, this is too confining and narrow. It limits what is valued and what is to be learned. In the humanist models when curriculum is described as the interactions between and among teacher and students, it is significant that the intended learning is not specified. This is not to say there isn't a learning agenda; however, it is a minimalist agenda. Learning that takes place is valued and has meaning for the individual. It is positive learning and, therefore, has positive social and personal value.

In the 1930s, Dewey (1938) defined education as "the reconstruction and reorganization of experience which adds its meaning and which increases ability to direct the course of subsequent experiences. The increment of meaning corresponds to the increased perception of the connections and continuities of the activities in which we are engaged. . . . An educational activity makes one aware of some of the connections which had been imperceptible" (pp. 89–90). Dewey supported the position that learning is an active process and that a person learns by being able to relate the learning to some personal experience.

Krishnamurti (1953) described what education is not: "It is not merely a matter of training the mind. Training makes for efficiency, but does not bring about completeness. A mind that has merely been trained is the continuation of the past, and such a mind can never discover the new" (p. 13). He continued by saying that education is not merely acquiring knowledge, gathering, and correlating facts, but it is seeing the significance of life as a whole, discovering lasting values, understanding ourselves, and creating human beings who are integrated and therefore intelligent.

In support of parallel lines of thought, Burton (1962) offers a more concrete explanation of learning by stating, "learning is far more than the mastery of the so-called fundamentals" (p. 26). To be successful in teaching and learning, a teacher must utilize principles of learning as a basis of teaching. Burton believes that some of the factors that lead to successful learning are: (1) utilizing principles of learning as a basis of teaching, (2) having insight into the way knowledge originates, (3) understanding how individuals learn, (4) obtaining knowledge into the nature of the types of individual and society that are desired as a result of learning and educational growth, (5) understanding the relation between personality and organized society, and (6) having available methods to determine whether desirable learning has taken place. He reports his definition of learning as: "Learning is a change in the individual, due to interaction of that individual and his environment, which fills a need and makes him more capable of dealing adequately with his environment" (p. 26).

It is appropriate to acknowledge that the literature is full of definitions of learning arising from the two major families of contemporary learning theories. The behaviorists' definition of learning will include changes in behavior as a measure of learning while the gestalt field psychologists will define learning in terms of reorganization of the learner's perceptual or psychological world (Bigge, 1976). An educator's acceptance and beliefs about learning will be reflected in choices of learning theories used to support teaching activities and development of learning experiences. Inherent within the definitions of learning reviewed are clues about types of experiences or activities that lead to successful learning.

Review of recent literature elicited a frequently used phrase closely related to learning. This phrase is *ways of knowing*. If an individual learns, how do they learn or know? Eisner (1985), editor of *Learning and Teaching the Ways of Knowing*, presented writings of well-known figures in the field of curriculum and education centered on modes of knowing and the implications for educational practice. Eisner contributed an article on the esthetic modes of knowing describing how esthetics serve as a source of experience and understanding. He explored the ideas of form, coherence, knowledge of, knowledge through, and stimulation as they relate to the fields of fine arts, literature, and scientific inquiry. He asked and addressed the question of what needs to be taught in each of the areas students study to help them understand the role that esthetics play in a particular field. Related to learning experiences and curriculum, Eisner (1985) stated, "the curriculum is a mind-altering device, and when content and tasks are selected, one has defined the kind of mental skills that will be cultivated" (p. 34). Questions that must be raised related to Eisner's writings are: (1) What are the types of mental skills that will be needed by nurses now and in the future? (2) What content is essential and what learning activities will lead to the development of these mental skills? (3) What role do esthetics play in nursing practice, education, and research?

As mentioned in Chapter 5, a 5-year phenomenological study conducted by Belenky, Clinchy, Goldberger, and Tarule (1986) offered a model of "ways of knowing" utilized by women. This study has important implications for nursing, which is approximately a 97 percent female profession. An intensive interview/case study approach was used to explore with women their experiences and problems as learners and knowers, as well as to review their past histories for changing concepts of the self and relationships with others. One hundred thirty-five women with varied demographic characteristics were interviewed. Ninety of the women were enrolled in one of six academic institutions, and 45 women were from "invisible colleges," which were family agencies that deal with clients seeking information about or assistance with parenting. The mixture of the group allowed for exploration of learning and knowing in formal education settings as well as settings organized and staffed by women that focused on the traditional maternal role. The first phase of analysis was centered on the section of the interview designed to elicit information on the woman's assumptions about the nature of truth, knowledge, and authority. Blind coding and contextual analysis were techniques used to analyze the data. The data analysis resulted in the grouping of women's perspectives on knowing into five major epistemological categories. These categories were the following:

1. Silence, a position in which women experience themselves as mindless and voiceless and subject to the whims of external authority.
2. Received knowledge, a perspective from which women conceive of themselves as capable of receiving, even reproducing, knowledge from the all-knowing external authorities but not capable of creating knowledge on their own.
3. Subjective knowledge, a perspective from which truth and knowledge are conceived as personal, private, and subjectively known or intuited.
4. Procedural knowledge, a position in which women are invested in learning and applying objective procedures for obtaining and communicating knowledge.
5. Constructed knowledge, a position in which women view all knowledge as contextual, experience themselves as creator of knowledge, and value both subjective and objective strategies for knowing (Belenky et al., 1986, p. 15).

The implications of this research project according to the researchers are pointed at women's development as the aim of education. Educators can assist women in developing their own authentic voices. This can be accomplished by focusing on "connected teaching." Learning experiences that emphasize connectedness over separation, understanding over assessment, collaboration over debate, that allow time for knowledge to emerge from firsthand experiences, and encourage students to evolve their own patterns of work based on the presented problems are needed for this "connected teaching" to occur. How might faculty develop learning activities that will hopefully lead to the types of experiences needed by nursing students to move through the different ways of knowing and to provide the connectedness needed for women's (nurses) development? Noddings described connected teaching as caring. Within this caring relationship, the teacher attempts to look at the material from the student's perspective and is totally and nonselectively present to each student. The relation between student and teacher is not necessarily a lasting, time-consuming personal one, but, however brief it may be, it is a total encounter (Noddings, 1984).

In another approach to "ways of knowing," Carper (1978) wrote about fundamental patterns of knowing in nursing. These fundamental patterns were identified from an analysis of the conceptual and syntactical structure of nursing knowledge, and are distinguished according to logical type of meaning. They were designated as (a) empirics, the science of nursing; (b) esthetics, the art of nursing; (c) the component of a personal knowledge in nursing; and (d) ethics, the component of moral knowledge in nursing (Carper, 1978). Approaching learning experiences from this framework broadens perspectives with which one can consider the phenomena of health and illness. Incorporation of these patterns into designed learning activities will provide the student the opportunity to struggle and think about nursing from these perspectives.

As indicated in this discussion, definitions of learning, education, and descriptions of "ways of knowing" hold many implications for the construction of learning experiences for students. Consideration of implications, found in the literature, directs the teacher in terms of setting goals and aims and the development of desired learning experiences in the student's educational process. Implications, such as developing learning experiences that focus on connectedness over separation; collaboration over debate; that provide for an interaction with the environment; that define and include practice of the types of scholarly skills desired, are examples that serve as a basis for criteria development.

GOALS OF LEARNING EXPERIENCES

Meaningful learning experiences shape a student's learning and education. Structuring learning experiences are at the heart of teaching and creating an educational process for the student. Learning experiences are the second major component of curriculum in this paradigm and, therefore, are keys to its success. The intent of the curriculum is that learning take place. The writings on learning experiences offer goals, and the possibility of developing criteria that might be used to guide designing, selecting, and critiquing of learning experiences. Examples of writings that reveal these possibilities are presented.

Burton (1962), whose definition of learning was offered earlier, posed the idea that learning has two basic overall characteristics. These were integration and the effect of the learner's perceptions. The integrating aspect of learning requires learning experiences that were (a) unified around one central purpose, (b) continuous and simultaneous, and (c) interactive with the environment. Learning is also affected by how the learner perceives the goals, other persons, self, and the situation.

Other ideas for criteria can be found in the works of Chickering. Chickering (1969) generated two hypotheses related to types of learning experiences found in curriculum, teaching, and evaluation. Hypothesis A stated:

> When few electives are offered, when books and print are the sole objects of study, when teaching is by lecture, when evaluation is frequent and competitive, ability to memorize is fostered. Sense of competence, freeing of interpersonal relationships, and development of autonomy, and identity, and purpose are not. (Chickering, 1969, p. 148)

Conversely, hypothesis B stated:

> When choice and flexibility are offered, when direct experiences are called for, when teaching is by discussion, and when evaluation involves frequent communication concerning the substance of behavior and performance, the ability to analyze and synthesize is fostered, as are sense of competence, freeing of interpersonal relationships, and development of autonomy, identity, and purpose. (Chickering, 1969, p. 148)

What Chickering did not say here is that writing is another way to develop the ability to analyze, synthesize, and communicate. Chickering provided data to support his belief that curriculum, teaching, and evaluation are linked together and that the approach to each has implications for the development of the student in the areas of intellectual competence, cognitive behaviors, sense of competence, development of emotional and instrumental independence, identity, interpersonal relationships, and clarifying purposes. This research is supportive of developing learning activities that provide for choice, flexibility, and evaluation that includes frequent communication. These types of learning activities foster the mental skills of analysis and synthesis and lead to growth in the student that reflects competency, healthy interpersonal relationships, and development of autonomy, identity, and purpose.

In support of the learning activities criteria position, Raths (1971) put forth three major arguments that exist in education today. He challenged the basic assumption that the primary purpose of schooling is to change the behavior of students in specific predetermined ways. He also asserted that activities may be justified for inclusion in the curriculum on the basis other than that of efficacy for changing behavior. He further stated that schools should take as their major purpose one of involving students in activities which have no preset objectives but meet other specified criteria. Raths advanced a list of 12 criteria for identifying activities that seem to have inherent worth. A similar task must be undertaken by faculty choosing to use the paradigm being developed throughout this book.

In a similar stance, Peters (1973) discussed the aims of education from his point of view. He believed the many disputes about the aims of education are disputes about principles of procedure, rather than about "aims" in the sense of objectives, to be arrived at by taking appropriate means. The crucial question to be asked related to aims is "what procedures are to be adopted in order to implement them?" (p. 129). In other words, what types of learning activities are needed to implement the goals or ends-in-view identified by faculty? What needs to occur to accomplish the intent of the learning desired?

Another goal or aim of education with suggested activities can be found in the writings of MacDonald (1974), who proposed that centering is the aim of education and called for the completion of the person or the creation of meaning that utilizes all the potential given to each person. He believed that activities that develop the aim of centering must be sought. For example, what kind of activities provide for the opening up of perceptual experiences, for facilitating the development of patterned meaning structures, or for organizing knowledge to enlarge human potential through meaning?

A major contribution to the literature on learning from an international perspective was published in 1979. This publication mentioned frequently in other chapters was the report of a learning project sponsored by the Club of Rome and was written by authors from socialist and Third World countries, as well as countries in the West. The purpose of this project was to focus primarily on the human element in relation to such global problems as energy, communications, cultural identity, and the arms race. The human being was perceived as the key to the world's future. The world must come to understand two critical points: (a) Humanity is rapidly moving toward a crossroads where there will be no room for mistakes, and (b) the vicious cycle of increasing complexity and lagging understanding must be broken while it is still possible to exert influence and some control over our destiny and future. The human gap, which is the distance between growing complexity and our capacity to cope with it, and the potential for learning to help bridge the gap was examined in this report. Botkin, Elmandjra, and Malitza (1979) defined learning as:

> . . . an approach to knowledge and to life that emphasizes human initiative. It encompasses the acquisition and practice of new methodologies, new skills, new attitudes, and new values to live in a changing world. Learning is the process of preparing to deal with new situations. It may occur consciously or often unconsciously, usually from experiencing real-life situations, although simulated or imagined situations can also induce learning. (p. 8)

Every individual in the world, whether in an educational setting or not, is learning; however, probably no one is learning at the level, intensity, and speed needed to cope with the complexities faced in modern life. The authors describe two types of learning, one that is presently occurring in society and one that society must pursue for long-term survival (Botkin et al., 1979).

Maintenance learning is traditionally found in societies today and is described as "the acquisition of fixed outlooks, methods, and rules for dealing with known and recurring situations" (Botkin et al., p. 10). Problem solving is geared toward given problems, and it is this type of learning that maintains an existing system or established way of life.

Innovative learning has two primary features—anticipation and participation. It is this type of learning that will prepare individuals to act together in situations. Anticipatory learning prepares individuals to use techniques such as forecasting, simulations, scenarios, and models. It encourages consideration of trends, planning, and evaluating for future consequences, examining possible side effects of present decisions, and recognizing the far-reaching side effects of these decisions. Participation is more than the formal sharing of decisions. It is characterized by an attitude of cooperation, dialogue, and empathy. It means keeping communication open, constantly testing the operating rules and values, while retaining relevant ones and rejecting those that are obsolete. The types of learning activities that allow students to become involved in participative learning are critical to nursing. Nursing currently operates in a troubled, fast-changing health care system. Technological advances are rapid and challenge learned rules and values. Nursing faculty must assume the responsibility of creating learning activities that provide direction for students in developing critical thinking skills, in making judgments about relevant rules and values, and in maintaining personal and professional integrity while rejecting obsolete, outdated rules, values, and beliefs.

Support for different approaches to learning are even occurring in the field of instructional development. Low (1980) describes this shift that seems to be happening. This shift is from the behaviorist approach to that of cognitive learning theory. If teachers adopt the assumptions represented in information processing and schemata representation approaches to learning, how would testing, objectives, instructional strategies, instructional taxonomies, and analysis be affected? He describes information processing as a model of knowledge acquisition and the use of schemata to organize knowledge. If cognitive learning theories are utilized, alternative learning experiences and instructional strategies will be needed.

The idea of organizing knowledge is one to be considered when creating learning activities. Weinstein (1989) supports this idea when he states,

> the difference between an expert and a novice is not just the amount of knowledge they possess but also, and perhaps even more important, the way that knowledge is organized. It is the difference between storing one thousand folders by throwing them in the middle of the room versus storing them by some meaningful organization in filing cabinets. (p. 8)

Assisting the student to organize information around personal or meaningful experiences, to lead the student from the familiar to the unfamiliar, and to aid the student to develop the ability to conceptualize are organizing techniques to be built into learning activities.

Benner's (1984) study is having tremendous influence on nursing education and practice. The study was aimed at discovering knowledge embedded in actual nursing clinical practice, at understanding the differences in clinical performances, and at situational appraisal of beginning and expert nurses. Benner (1984) stated that "such knowledge has gone uncharted and unstudied and that what is needed is systematic observations of what nurse clinicians learn from their clinical practice" (p. 1). To obtain this data, paired interviews were conducted with beginning nurses and nurses recognized for their expertise. The pairs were interviewed separately about patient situations they had shared and that had significance for them. The aim was to determine if there were distinguishable differences in the novice's and expert's description of the same clinical incident. Additionally, 51 experienced nurse clinicians, 11 new nurse graduates, and 5 senior nursing students were interviewed and observed to further delineate and describe characteristics of nurse performance at different stages of skill acquisition. Utilizing the Dreyfus model of skill acquisition and the analysis of interviews and observations, it was possible to describe the performance characteristics at each level of development, and to identify, in general terms, the teaching–learning needs at each level. These five levels are novice, advanced beginner, competent, proficient, and expert. Several implications for types of learning experiences and education of professional nurses arise out of this study. These implications are:

1. A situation-based interpretive approach to nursing care is more effective than the linear nursing process model currently being utilized. This linear process model can actually obscure knowledge embedded in clinical nursing practice.

2. Strategies that include content, context, and function are necessary to incorporate the relational aspects of nursing.

3. The accomplishments and characteristics of expert nurse performance can be observed and described in narrative, interpretive form.

4. Exemplar cases of nursing practice offer the advantages of identifying nursing competencies that include actual performance demands, resources, constraints, and provide a rich description of nursing practice.

5. Educational nursing programs must provide the background knowledge necessary for advanced skill acquisition. Descriptions of actual nursing practice can provide a basis for realistic curriculum planning.

6. Understanding the process of acquiring advanced knowledge and skills will teach students and graduates how to go about becoming expert practitioners.

These are only a few of the educational implications that can be derived from this research project. Embedded in this research are valuable ideas that can contribute to the development, selection, and critique of learning experiences.

Writings in current educational literature also seem to reflect the concern around changes that are needed in education and learning. Weimer (1988), editor of *The Teaching Professor,* spoke of the idea that there is almost a constant tension between the way things are in education and the way some educators believe they should be. She interviewed Christopher Knapper, coauthor of *Lifelong Learning and Higher Education,* who proposed a change of what might actually come to be in the future. In the interview, Knapper stated that teaching approaches used today are not particularly effective in fostering autonomy, creativity, integration, and other skills perceived as so important. Didactic teaching is not very effective in producing autonomy and creative problem solving. He proposed that the strong orientation to content prevents the teacher from focusing on the development of high-level cognitive skills, such as writing, speaking, conceptual thinking, problem solving, and decision making. He advised teachers to clearly think about the knowledge and skills desired in students that will serve them well the rest of their lives, examine what can be done to best achieve this learning, and consider ways to enable students to become responsible for their own learning. He believed that the individual teacher will be the one to effect the changes that need to be made—not the institution. Knapper's writings are supportive of the idea of the teacher becoming allied with the student rather than the content. It is the knowledge and skills desired in the student that need more consideration when developing learning activities. The content becomes the vehicle around which scholarly skills are developed.

As illustrated, the literature offers many ideas and clues about criteria for learning experience for this new paradigm; however, this is only one source from which faculty can begin identifying possible criteria. A sample list of criteria can be found in Appendix 1 (Murray & Merrefield, 1989) that is based in the literature, personal teaching experiences, and dialogue with colleagues. The next section of this chapter discusses in more detail generation of criteria for teacher–student interactions and learning experiences.

GENERATION OF CRITERIA TO DEVISE, SELECT, AND CRITIQUE TEACHER–STUDENT INTERACTIONS AND LEARNING EXPERIENCES

The generation of criteria for teacher–student interactions and learning experiences requires a search for sources of information about these interactions and experiences and consideration of several major models and ideas of the humanistic-educative paradigm. The movement of the student along the learner maturity continuum, the types of learning desired, the acquiring of a different perception of curriculum, the alliance of the teacher with the student as opposed to the content, and the importance of faculty development and role change will be considered as the criteria for teacher–student interactions and learning experiences are developed. Acceptance of the definition of curriculum for this paradigm compels faculty to develop criteria that reflect their beliefs and values about the most effective ways to move the student along the learner maturity continuum, to accomplish the types of learning required, to indicate an alliance with students as opposed to content, and to reflect their changes in their perceptions of faculty roles. Exploration of

Figure 1
Sources of Information on Teacher–Student Interactions and Learning Criteria

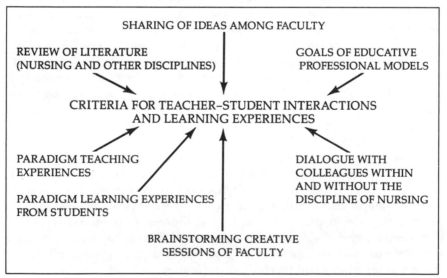

sources of information about teacher–student interactions and learning experiences (see Fig. 1), the dynamic process of developing criteria, the selection of and methods of critiquing criteria will be discussed in this section.

SOURCES OF INFORMATION

As with the development of any idea, a starting point is frequently the current and classical literature. Much has been written about teacher–student relationships and about learning experiences and activities. Some of the literature reviewed earlier in this chapter are examples of the types of information found in the literature. The literature reviewed included research studies with findings that are valuable and helpful in developing criteria. The descriptions of the types of teacher–student interactions and learning experiences found in the literature can become the basis around which faculty begin the development of their criteria. The review of the literature might result in a beginning list of criteria that could be rated according to faculty's perceptions about its value and usefulness.

To continue the development of this list, faculty might be asked to describe paradigm teaching experiences. (Paradigm teaching experiences are those that stand out in our minds, those when we know we have connected with students and that the learning was meaningful for both student and faculty.) Faculty could tease out the types of teacher–student interactions and the qualities of the structured learning experiences that were present. The descriptions of these paradigm teaching experiences are rich sources of information for identifying types of teacher–student interactions and learning experiences in which faculty have been successful and therefore illuminate faculty strengths. Teacher–student interactions and learning experiences identified can be added to the list that faculty have begun to compile.

Students also can provide valuable information about the types of teacher–student interactions and learning experiences they have found contribute to their learning. Students may not have experienced educative-professional curriculums and their knowledge may be limited; however, their paradigm experiences would be an important source of information.

Frequently in nursing, we isolate ourselves and have limited contact with colleagues in other disciplines. Review of the literature in education reveals that similar ideas of change are affecting education, teaching, and learning in other disciplines. Arranging opportunities to dialogue with colleagues in other disciplines can lead to the sharing and creating of ideas about effective teacher–student interactions and learning experiences. In addition to working with faculty outside of the discipline, nursing faculty can keep a running file of those teacher–student interactions and learning experiences that seem to work. This file can be shared to check out and modify as it is used. It is also helpful to keep an open mind and remember that teacher–student interactions and learning are not limited to any specialty area such as psychiatric or medical–surgical nursing.

As discussed in another section of this book, when teacher–student interactions and learning experiences are being considered, it is essential to review the goals of the humanistic-educative models. If students are to be scholarly clinicians with the ability to think critically, derive meanings, examine the whole, search for patterns, be responsible for own learning, etc., then teacher–student interactions and learning experiences that contribute to this happening are essential.

Review of these many sources for information provide faculty with a growing list of possible teacher–student interactions and qualities for learning experiences. As the list grows, it can be examined for repetition and commonalities that may also result in a set of categories including all or most of the items identified. As with the Murray and Merrefield lists of criteria, four major categories emerged for both teacher–student interactions and learning experiences. The four broad categories for teacher–student interactions were the following: (a) creativity; (b) style of presence; (c) reciprocal interactions; and (d) teacher–student interactions that support contextual, syntactical, and inquiry learning. For learning experiences, the categories were the following: (a) introduction, (b) working phase, (c) culmination, and (d) resolution. This is provided only as an example of how faculty might categorize and conceptualize their teacher–student interactions and qualities of learning experiences as their lists begin to come alive.

CRITERIA DEVELOPMENT AS A DYNAMIC PROCESS

There exists a danger as faculty develop these lists of criteria for teacher–student interactions and learning experiences. As with the multitude of behavioral objectives currently in nursing curriculum, there is the danger of committing ideas to paper and seldom referring to them until evaluation time. These lists of criteria need to be living and dynamic. As faculty try out new ones or find that some do not work, the list is modified and kept up to date. The list is not filed and therefore not used as faculty implement a new way of approaching curriculum. It becomes an essential tool for faculty in the process of implementation and faculty development.

The issue of faculty development has been addressed in many places in this book. It is the key to success in the paradigm. Perceptions of the role of the teacher and role change can be addressed as the generation of criteria for teacher–student interactions and learning experiences occur. As criteria are identified and developed, faculty will recognize their areas of strengths and weaknesses in terms of interacting and developing learning experiences with goals from the new paradigm. Questions of how to assist faculty to develop the role of teacher as expert learner with responsibilities will arise.

Creating ways in which the lists are reviewed, updated, and critiqued become important. Activities such as keeping files of those teacher–student interactions and learning experiences that work, utilizing the teacher–student interactions in role-playing situations with each other, discussion and debate around the criteria, periodic review of the literature, and setting up research projects around criteria for validation are only a few suggestions that would assist faculty in maintaining involvement with the criteria. Faculty workshops centered on the use of the criteria would keep faculty involved and assist with the role change and faculty development needed to successfully implement the paradigm. The list of criteria is viewed as a temporary working list that is changing and is up for review. The process of working and developing criteria can provide faculty with the opportunities to interact with each other, to recognize the strengths of their colleagues, to encourage dealing with the issues at hand, and to begin to legitimize differences that exist among faculty groups.

FACTORS TO CONSIDER WHEN SELECTING CRITERIA

The major goal or overriding factor to consider when selecting criteria for teacher–student interactions and learning experiences is the goal or intent of the learning to take place. These interactions and experiences make the connection to the goal or intent of learning. Examination of the criteria in this light increases the chances of success in learning for the student. Questioning the possibilities and relationships between the intent of the learning and teacher–student interactions and learning experiences becomes a critical factor to consider in the selection process. How might certain teacher–student interactions lead to growth in selected scholarly skills and growth in the student? What will the learning experience require that leads the student in the direction of the intended learning?

The learner maturity scale has been addressed earlier and is a factor to consider when selecting criteria for teacher–student interactions and learning experiences. Interacting with the student in ways that reinforce the student's positions of charming, anticipatory-compliant, and resonating would stymie the student's movement to the mature positions of reciprocating and generating. What specific types of interactions are needed to interact with students who assume these positions on the scale? What are the types of teacher–student interactions and learning experiences that will facilitate the student's movement along the continuum and lead the student in the direction of the intended learning? Which criteria would allow the teacher to structure the course with the types of teacher–student interactions and learning experiences that require students to be at the reciprocating and generating position from the very beginning of the course? Do the criteria address the ideas of reciprocal relationships, mutual respect, the role of the teacher as expert learner with responsibility, dialogue and debate among teachers and students, and the types of scholarly skills required in educative learning episodes? Answers to questions such as these can become guidelines as faculty make choices and selections among criteria related to the learner maturity scale.

The learning model plays a role in the selection of teacher–student interactions and learning experiences. Although active learning is possible with all types of learning, each type will influence the choice of teacher–student interactions and the structure of the learning experiences. If the intent of the learning is focused on item, directive, or rationale learning, approaches that foster memorization, use of rules, and providing reasons or the whys of practice are selected. Teacher–student interactions and learning experiences will provide more structure for the student on exactly what is to be learned and practiced. Most of the learning will be behaviorally based and measurable. However, when syntactical, contextual, and inquiry learning are desired, teacher–student interactions and learning experiences direct the student to develop meanings and insights, to look at wholes, to examine practice and theory as they influence each other, to participate and become enculturated in the caring profession of nursing, and to use a variety of inquiry skills to investigate, theorize, predict, etc. Teacher–student interactions and the selection of learning experiences of students become quite different when the intent of learning is focused on these three types of learning. Criteria are developed from which teachers are able to choose in order to accomplish the intent of the learning.

As discussed earlier in the book, there is a synergism among the models in the paradigm. This synergism results in the development of criteria to build, select, and critique the teacher–student interactions and learning experiences that will make up the curriculum.

CRITIQUE OF CRITERIA FOR TEACHER–STUDENT INTERACTIONS AND LEARNING EXPERIENCES

The critique of the criteria for teacher–student interactions and learning experiences is an important task for faculty. In a large sense, it is a critique of the curriculum. Methods for critique have been discussed in other parts of the book. This section will provide several ideas or ways in which faculty might begin thinking about the process of critique.

The ability to critique is a tool used by scholars to improve understanding, provide feedback and information about what exists, and to lead to desired improvements. A critique of criteria can be related to ideas such as the effectiveness or the effects desired in students, an incorporation of the major models or ideas in the paradigm, and consideration of other ideas such as caring, feasibility, efficiency, etc.

One method for critiquing the effectiveness of the criteria is to create a safe caring environment in which faculty might practice in simulated situations and be critiqued by colleagues. This allows the opportunity to get feedback and support from colleagues while obtaining information on the effects of the teacher–student interaction and the structure of the learning activity. Similar to this, interactions can be videotaped in role play or actual situations and then critiqued.

As faculty begin to critique their lists, there may emerge an imprimatur for the graduate of the program. The desired hallmarks of graduates may be debated and discussed among faculty. Another approach is to choose a graduate that is an exemplar or choose several graduates and develop a composite that is realistic. This composite will contain elements of idealism that will assist in transforming nursing. Such an approach will move nursing toward idealism while being reality-focused. This may clarify for faculty the ultimate goals desired in the curriculum and may lead to a critique of teacher–student interaction and learning experience criteria in relationship to these goals. The evaluation and effectiveness of the curriculum will be directly related to the success of selected teacher–student interactions and learning experiences.

WAYS TO SABOTAGE THE IMPLEMENTATION OF
THE NEW PARADIGM

Periods of change and transition are often characterized by endings, periods of confusion, and new beginnings (Bridges, 1980). When faculty decide to use a new paradigm for nursing education, it may mean an end to the old ways of doing things, being not quite sure of what to do differently, and finally realizing there are new beginnings or different ways to accomplish the task of preparing nurses for tomorrow's world of nursing.

Letting go has never been an easy task for nursing. Examination of nursing curriculums today show evidence of this. Content that students are never likely to encounter remain in the curriculum. Letting go of sacred content and becoming aligned with the student is necessary for the success of any educative paradigm. A willingness to do this by learning to recognize and value the components of the model is essential.

As stated earlier, the behaviorist models are useful to nursing for selected types of learning; however, to educate the kind of nurse needed and desired for the future, nurse educators will need to let go of the rituals of their teaching and develop different ways of interacting and structuring learning. Without a willingness and a decision to commit to such change, the possibility of sabotage is present. It is hoped that an exploration of how sabotage might occur will raise faculty's awareness to the level that will lead to an active response to prevent its happening.

The decision to move forward with the implementation of the new paradigm is considered a faculty prerogative. Faculty own the curriculum and therefore reserve the right to make this choice. If faculty become divided on the issue and are not committed, it creates a situation in which sabotage is inherent. Faculty generally have responses and ways of interacting with each other when differences arise. If faculty are able to work through such situations and come to a decision, then a commitment to change can occur. A divisiveness within the faculty may lead to time and energy being spent on attempting to gain resolution and as a mechanism for preventing change.

Faculty–faculty interactions become important as criteria for teacher–student interactions are being developed. Poor communications, noncaring behaviors, and unwillingness to talk or dialogue about the issues sap the energy of faculty and lead to poor morale. If faculty interactions with each other are poor and unhealthy, students will lack the healthy role modeling that is such a powerful learning tool. Power plays and political maneuvers may be used to convince other faculty to one side or the other. Unresolved issues of the past may rise up and become entangled in the present situation of curriculum change. Being unclear and unwilling to talk straight and honest leave faculty with their wheels spinning and not making progress in any direction.

Faculty may, usually out of awareness, bring students into gamey situations to elicit support for their issues. For example, asking students to talk about and judge new teaching approaches being tried out by other faculty and then asking faculty to defend what they are doing, sets up unpleasant situations for all involved. This may be carried further when faculty play the game of blemish and find fault with any of the new approaches. Paying lip service to offer support of the change and then becoming passive-aggressive creates ill feelings among faculty and leads to mistrust. This mistrust affects all aspects of the program, especially major curriculum change.

I once heard a comment that if nursing faculty can survive major curriculum changes intact and friendly, it is a strong faculty. All of this is not to be pessimistic about the process but to increase faculty awareness of issues involved in a paradigm shift and to encourage the active development of ways to support and care about each other during the process. Accepting endings and change and working through the periods of confusion lead to exciting new beginnings.

THE SIGNIFICANCE OF TEACHER–STUDENT INTERACTIONS AND LEARNING EXPERIENCES

The quality of faculty interactions with students and the goal of learning experiences selected or devised for students make or break the curriculum in this educative-caring paradigm. The strongest and weakest parts are the teachers. This is true in any paradigm, but if there is such a thing as something being more true, then it is more true for this paradigm. Without the rule-driven focus or list of behavioral objectives, a major portion of curriculum is left in the hands of teachers.

REFERENCES

Belenky, M., Clinchy, B., Goldberger, N., & Tarule, J. (1986). *Women's ways of knowing, the development of self, voice, and mind.* New York: Basic Books.

Benner, P. (1984). *From novice to expert: Excellence and power in clinical nursing practice.* Menlo Park, CA: Addison-Wesley.

Bigge, M. L. (1976). *Learning theories for teachers* (3rd ed.). New York, NY: Harper & Row.

Botkin, J. W., Elmandjra, M., & Malitza, M. (1979). *No limits to learning.* Elmsford, NY: Pergamon Press.

Bridges, W. (1980). *Transitions: Making sense of life's changes.* Reading, MA: Addison-Wesley.

Burton, W. H. (1962). *The guidance of learning activities.* New York: Appleton-Century-Crofts.

Carper, B. A. (1978). Fundamental patterns of knowing in nursing. *Advances in Nursing Science, 1* (1), 13–23.

Chickering, A. W. (1969). *Education and identity.* San Francisco: Jossey-Bass.

Dewey, J. (1938). *Democracy and education.* New York: Macmillan.

Eisner, E. W. (1985). *The educational imagination* (2nd ed.). New York: Macmillan.

Freire, P. (1971). *Pedagogy of the oppressed.* New York: W.W. Norton, p. 67.

Gaff, J. G., & Wilson, R. C. (1971). The teaching environment. *American Association of University Professors Bulletin, 57,* 475–493.

Gage, N. L. (1984). What do we know about teaching effectiveness? *Phi Delta Kappa, 66,* 87–93.

Greene, M. (1986). Philosophy and teaching. In M. C. Wittrock, *Handbook of research on teaching* (pp. 479–499). New York: Macmillan.

Griffith, J. W., & Bakanauskas, A. J. (1983). Student–instructor relationships in nursing education. *Journal of Nursing Education, 22,* 104–107.

Klein, J. T. (1969). Presuppositions of teaching. *Educational Theory, 19* (3), 299–307.

Krishnamurti, J. (1953). *Education and the significance of life.* San Francisco: Harper & Row.

Low, W. C. (1980). Changes in instructional development: The aftermath of an information processing takeover in psychology. *Journal of Instructional Development, 4,* 10–18.

MacDonald, J. B. (1974). A transcendental developmental ideology of education. In W. Pinar (Ed.), *Heightened consciousness, cultural revolution, and curriculum theory* (pp. 85–116). Berkeley, CA: McCutchan

Murray, J., & Merrefield, S. (1989). Criteria for teacher–student interactions and learning experiences. In J. Murray, *Developing criteria to support new curriculum models for doctoral education in nursing.* Doctoral Dissertation, University of Georgia.

Noddings, N. (1984). *Caring: A feminine approach to ethics and moral education.* Berkeley, CA: University of California Press.

Peters, R. (1973). Must an educator have an aim? In R. Peters, *Authority, responsibility, and education* (pp. 83–85). London: George Allen and Unwin Ltd.

Raths, J. D. (1971). Teaching without specific objectives. *Educational Leadership, 28,* 714–720.

Shulman, L. S. (1986). Paradigms and research programs in the study of teaching: A contemporary perspective. In M. C. Wittrock (Ed.), *Handbook of research on teaching* (pp. 3–36). New York: Macmillan.

Wang, A. M., & Blumberg, P. (1983). A study on interaction techniques of nursing faculty in the clinical area. *Journal of Nursing Education, 22,* 144–151.

Weimer, M. G. (1988). What should future teaching be like? *The Teaching Professor, 2* (2), 1–2.

Weinstein, C. E. (1989). How are you storing files? *The Teaching Professor, 3* (4), 6.

Wissot, J. (1979). Teaching as an art form. *Educational Forum,* March, 265–278.

8

Teaching and Learning: A Practical Commentary

Em Olivia Bevis

Teaching is knowledge beyond the given. It is allegorical knowing, knowing of the possibility of a situation, of the potentiality of a child, of the manner in which this potentiality may be actualized, the ways in which its *logos* may be brought to our presence. . . . Teaching, then, like art, is making the way open for the Being of beings to unconceal itself as truth—which, after all, is what teaching is all about. When authentic, teaching is a mode of being through which unconcealedness—that is, truth—takes place.

Ignacio L. Goetz, Heidegger and the Art of Teaching

INTRODUCTION

Teaching as "unconcealment" of truth is no easy task. Telling what one thinks is "truth" is much easier than opening a way or seeing the possibilities of a situation. The difficulties for teachers lie in visualizing the potential of a situation and exploiting that potential until excitement and imagination converge into knowledge. Excitement and imagination are necessary ingredients to education and permeate

217

both teaching and learning. Whitehead (1969) comments about this as one of the justifications for a university:

> The justification for a university is that it preserves the connection between knowledge and the zest of life, by uniting the young and the old in the imaginative consideration of learning. The university imparts information, but it imparts it imaginatively. At least, this is the function which it should perform for society. A university which fails in this respect has no reason for existence. This atmosphere of excitement, arising from imaginative consideration, transforms knowledge. A fact is no longer a bare fact: it is invested with all its possibilities. It is no longer a burden on the memory: it is energizing as the poet of our dreams, and as the architect of our purposes. (p. 93)

Imagination is not to be divorced from the facts: It is a way of illuminating the facts and investing them with meaning. It works by eliciting the general principles that apply to the facts, as they exist, and then by an intellectual vision of a new world that goes beyond or departs from the facts, and it preserves the zest of life by the suggestion of satisfying purposes.

The purpose of this chapter is to illuminate teaching—to provide some ideas about active learning and how to teach so that students are engaged in the self-discipline of learning. This is not a recipe chapter. Recipes never work, because teaching is as individualistic as art and as disciplined as science. What this chapter provides is some guidelines, some ideas that the teacher can use to help structure classes and clinical experiences in ways that support active, educative learning; that marry excitement, imagination, love of learning, intuition, and freedom; and that unconceal truth.

TEACHING AS ART AND SCIENCE

Imagination, as implied by Whitehead, is as much a requisite of good teaching as it is of good art—perhaps because teaching is an art form. It is not that teaching nursing lacks science; it is a human science and as such is imbued with art. Goetz (1983) says that, like art, teaching deals with world, truth, beauty, and being. He also says that calling teaching an art is a metaphor for what is essentially indescribable. Teaching as art is worth investigating briefly, because teaching perceived as a traditional science rests upon assumptions that reduce its capacity to

Table 1
Comparison of the Characteristics of Art and Science

Mission	
Science: The Explanation and Regulation of Outer Phenomena	Art: To Remain Faithful to Personal Emotional Experience Through Aesthetic Form

Characteristics	
Logical-objective	Emotional-subjective
Observable-concrete	Intuitive
Outer-physical	Inner-spirit-geist
Regular-laws-empirical	Phenomenological
Generalizable	Specific-unique
Discovered	Revealed
Cause-effect	Coexisting-mutually interactive
Predictable	Unpredictable-context-situation-guided

transform the quality of human life. And both nursing and teaching have life quality as a primary responsibility.

The theoretical basis of the position that art and science have different roles has its origins in the nature of art and science (see Table 1). Science's mission, according to Wissot (1979), is the explanation and regulation of outer phenomena. To be accepted as truth, something must be empirically validated. It has characteristics of being logical, objective, concrete, outer-physical-oriented, regular, and governed by reliable laws. It is predictable, it has cause and effect relationships, and it concerns facts that can be discovered and from which generalizations can be made. On the other hand, Wissot describes art's mission as to remain faithful to the personal, emotional experience through aesthetic form. Art has the characteristics of being emotional, subjective, intuitive, inner-spirit-geist-oriented, phenomenological, and specific-unique. Its truths are revealed and coexist with mutually interactive factors that are ambiguous. Art is unpredictable and context-situation-guided.

TEACHING AS A HUMAN SCIENCE

The question arises: If teaching is an art, and if its characteristics are emotional, subjective, intuitive, phenomenological, specific-unique, revealed, unpredictable, and context-situation-guided, can discipline then be imposed upon it? The answer is "yes," an unequivocable "yes." How then? The answer lies in the metaphor—as art is a metaphor for teaching, as Goetz reminds us—for describing the indescribable. But the indescribable must be described, and art seems to be the metaphor and poetry the language. This may tempt one to romanticize teaching for there is such a temptation. This is possibly because, as Denton (1974) says, "Perhaps the language of teaching is similar to the language of love in that it is about an experience so holistic, so immediate, and so close to us that we can't say what it is" (p. 93). It is indescribable. However, the question need not be addressed as asked, for teaching is not all art; it is also science. Art is necessary but not sufficient, just as science is necessary but not sufficient. Neither can they be combined unchanged. Thus, teaching, like nursing, is a human science . . . both art and science . . . but different from either, a combination of art and science so mixed as to be alive with possibilities for working with persons and greater than the addition of the two elements.

A human science is a science of, for, and about humans. It is a science with a humanistic base that is rooted in art, compels logic and reason, exacts discipline, respects intuition, necessitates critical thinking, requires creativity, demands a world view of person as irreducible whole, and has caring as its ethical imperative. The term *human science* was coined by Giorgi (1970) in an attempt to differentiate those types of psychology that were traditionally scientific, such as behaviorism and psychoanalytic, from those that study the person as a whole. Although Giorgi was not the first to favor the concept, he was probably the first so to name it. Actually, for modern times, Jan Smuts (1926), the South African statesman and botanist, brought the term *holism* into popular usage to signify the indivisible unity of living things and ideas. Alfred North Whitehead, in his book entitled *Process and Reality* (1969), laid the philosophical basis for a world of wholes, working in creative synthesis to bring forth unique new wholes. Giorgi's creation of the term *human science* was a natural step in evolving terminology for human service fields. The term was created to apply to those fields that (1) are practice oriented, (2) deal primarily with the life experiences of persons, and (3) see their domain of responsibility as the whole person. In the past few years, nurses have come to use the term to describe their domain of study. This is due primarily to the work of Watson (1988). Many educators write of teaching as if it were a human science but neither the term nor the idea has yet achieved popular usage. On the other hand, since the early part of this century, educational writers have spoken about the "whole" child. The "whole" child movement is precursor to the idea of teaching as a human science. Wholeness is not the only "truth" at stake in a shift of terminology. Watson (1988) maintains that a human science accepts the position that there are multiple realities, that the parts are interrelated in such a way as to make separation not only difficult but dangerous—study of them as separates provides an erroneous picture.

Behaviorism, empiricism, and other "scientific" positions see reality as being single and having parts that one can separate out and manipulate in context-free ways. However, human science sees reality as context dependent. Furthermore, traditional science sees objectivity as desirable, necessary, and attainable. In science, that which is studied—even persons—are seen as objects. Human science sees objectivity as impossible and the inquirer is related to the studied persons through the process of inquiry, which in turn influences the inquiry. When persons are studied they are subjects, not objects; the relationship is subject-subject, not subject-object. A human science relies heavily on meaning, understanding, intuition, creativity, and human values as pervasive. Traditional sciences struggle to be value free.

Once one gains this insight, it is possible to understand the strain possessing modern education. Most of its research remains in the traditional scientific paradigm, while most of its practitioners operate in the human science paradigm. This creates a dissonance between its theory and its practice, between its science and its art, that can only be resolved by working with both the research and practice of teaching as a human science.

SOME THEORETICAL MODELS FOR GUIDING TEACHING

The Passive-to-Active Continuum

Teachers create the climate of the course—its contextual reality. It is they who determine whether the learner will be active or passive, whether their realities will be context free or context based, and whether they will view wholes or parts. It is in active learning that students find their own truth, find "unconcealment." The strategies the teacher uses to effect learning determine the degree and extent of learner involvement in the learning enterprise. This involvement can be plotted on a continuum from passive to active (see Fig. 1).

Passive learning is acquiring facts, ideas, and information through

Figure 1
The Passive-to-Active Continuum

Passive   Active

\ —————————————————————————————————— /

inactive means. It involves reading, listening, and watching. Passive learning is a spectator sport and involves few higher cognitive operations. This does not mean that important things cannot be learned passively. Observation, reading, and listening can impart information and can *lead to* reflection, analysis, synthesis, insights, and meanings. Analysis, synthesis, insights, and meanings, however, are *active* cognitive processes that can be triggered by passive learning. The usual products of passive learning have to do with recall and not with patterns, significance, and meaning. The higher cognitive processes are most profitably triggered by active involvement in the learning process: by being engaged in examining an issue, solving a problem, or determining a strategy. Listening seldom results in engagement. Most often in passive learning, ideas, facts, information, and data are dripped into the psychomotor system through a funnel and go through a neuropathway to a pencil and onto paper. At some later time (preferably before a test), it is siphoned back up from the paper through the eyes into the head, where it is placed in short-term memory until after the test.

In active learning, information is needed, dissected, analyzed, rearranged, examined for underlying assumptions, used to project implications, compared with other known data, turned inside out and upside down, and used or discarded for that issue or problem . . . but in the process, it becomes part of the system of knowledge that is owned by the student. A very effective form of active learning involves dialogue with others: argument, debate, challenge, and taking a position and defending it with peers. These scholarly forms of interactions force a close and disciplined examination of facts, data, ideas and their relevance, validity, and accuracy for given problems.

Learning has degrees between passive and active; all teaching strategies can be placed somewhere along that continuum. Lecture and reading are very passive. Computer-assisted instruction is somewhere further along the continuum on the passive side, while interactive computer-assisted instruction is more active. Small group problem solving using a relevant and real problem is at the far right on the active continuum.

The secret is how "hooked" the students are—how engaged their minds and imaginations. No one strategy works all the time for every student. Therefore, the skilled teacher, the real artist, has many tools and many strategies and tactics with which to work, varying the methods depending upon the students, the subject matter, the timing, the environment, the equipment, and the group's needs. In general, the postulate is: the more active the student, the greater the engagement; the greater the engagement, the more learning takes place.

The Three Aspects of a Learning Episode

Goetz (1983) says, "Teaching is a praxis, not a theory. Whoever wants to know what teaching is must look not at the theories and definitions, but at the actual teaching" (p. 7). Praxis, however, requires the examination of the interaction of practice and theory and how each influences and shapes the other. It is ineffectual to look at actual teaching without also looking at learning and the effect of theory on teaching and learning, and vice versa. It is possible for learning to take place without teaching, just as it is possible for lecturing to take place without learning. But it is probably not possible for educative teaching to take place without learning. The reason for this is in the nature of educative teaching.

Teachers who educate do so by devising learning episodes. A learning episode is a natural grouping of events in which students engage in the process of acquiring insights, seeing patterns, finding meanings and significance, seeking balance and wholeness, and making judgments or developing skills (see Chapter 4). Each educative learning episode has three aspects (McDonald, 1966). As seen in Figure 2, these aspects are called information, operation, and validation. Until all three aspects have occurred, the learning episode is not complete. If all three aspects have occurred, something will be learned, although it may not be what the teacher thinks will be learned. There are, of course, some exceptions. If the student has already milked the ideas around which the learning episode is structured, and the interactions are banal, there may be no learning. However, on the whole, given a reality-grounded problem devised to hook the interest of the learners and plans that include all three aspects of a learning episode, learning will occur during the activity as well as being rounded out when the learning episode is complete.

The three aspects of a learning episode—information, operation, and validation—need not occur in any given order. Nor must the aspects

Figure 2
The Three Aspects of a Learning Episode

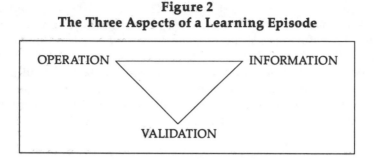

occur in any given time period. Retroactive integration allows the human mind to gain insights and make connections over very wide time ranges. For practice fields, such as nursing and teaching, however, all three must occur or the episode is not complete.

Operation. Operation is an *active learning* part of a learning episode. It is the opportunity to engage the mind in ways that motivate and spark interest. The operational phase is an issue, a problem, a puzzle, or a conundrum. The teacher's ability to invoke reality *imaginatively*, to simulate a problem, and to raise real and relevant questions and issues around the educative types of learning (contextual, syntactical, or inquiry) is the key ingredient of this aspect of a learning episode. This is called the "hook" and can make the difference between joyful, enthusiastic learning and "ho humming" through class (see Appendix II for examples).

The operational aspect is usually done in simulation, as reality is too risky or too expensive. Reality, by its very nature of being real— involving real people dealing with real issues and problems—is validational. Operational aspects are safe, so that students can deal with them without shame, fear of failure, fear of damaging patients or students, or waste of equipment.

The operational aspect is most effective when students are given some structure in the amount of time to spend, the types of questions to be answered, and the kinds of issues to raise and are left to struggle with it in very small groups of three to five persons without unrequested teacher consultation. Devising the "hooks"—structuring the operational aspect of a learning episode—requires educated imagination.

Information. The informational aspect is usually *passive*. The student is acquiring data that relate to the issues and problems that either were raised in the operational phase or will be raised, depending upon the sequence of events. If no informational aspect occurs, the students flounder in nescience; and if this lack of information flows over into the discussions and dialogues that frequently characterize the operational aspect, the students pool their ignorance rather than their knowledge. Information, facts, findings, documentation, and data are the elements that make learning take on new meanings, provide for analysis and synthesis, and shed new light and provide for new dimensions. In active learning, information is not given without the students' needing and wanting it. Active learning requires that the students be engaged with an issue or with problems that require them to need information in order to solve the problem (see Fig. 4); the learning map provided later in this chapter shows this. Students who are required to acquire information without a need and who must take on faith that this information is important are reduced to memorization and recall, rather than moved to finding meaning and insights.

Information is most often acquired in several ways. In group discussions among prepared students, information is a shared commodity. When it is needed, someone comes up with it. Sometimes the teacher, circulating in a room in which small group discussions are occurring, is stopped by one or more groups and is asked to be a consultant and thereby provides guidance and information. (This represents the reciprocal position on the learner maturity continuum.) Sometimes the students read, watch a movie, listen to a tape, watch an audio-film strip presentation, or watch instructional television. Sometimes they utilize a computer-assisted instructional program, and most often they listen to a lecture. Sometimes the information is culled from an operational activity. For instance, students may be asked to watch a television clip regarding an interaction and to list principles of communication that were used or violated in the clip. In this way they compile a list of principles from what common sense tells them about good communications. For example, a teacher can give an injection to a lemon, and students can list the techniques they think were violations of safety (deliberately included), using only what they know of sterile technique as guides. In ways like these, students can generate the informational sequence. However, the most common way is to read, watch, or listen. In fact, there are some things one can only learn in these ways.

Validation.   Validation is the *testing* aspect. The test need not be formal, graded, or evaluated. Validation is, at least for the student, a form of reality. Validation occurs when they see what they can do. Any practice done in reality is validating for the student. Written tests are simulated realities—no one dies or is hurt, no supplies are wasted, and no emergencies occur in such simulated validations. The only irretrievable errors are those generated by policies that prevent the student from trying again and again. It is inevitable that the time comes in courses in which tests are used and when students may not try again. However, for the student, tests—regardless of how they come—are part of the validation sequence because they are reality itself or because they are grade-laden. The operational sequence need not always be the "hook." Interest is often first sparked clinically, and reality brings things into focus for students so significantly that teachers can use reality as the key to the course content. However, once the situation is encountered clinically, the safety of classrooms or clinical conferences for operational work helps students to be able to confront problems and issues in a protected context.

The most useful validations are clinical. A second very useful one is that in which students must write a paper or take a position and defend it. Simulation can help a student become competent—therein lies the use of an operational phase—but confidence only comes with reality validation.

It must be noted that validation is part of the *learning* episode. It is not considered only a test and to have no learning consequences. Learning is an inevitable aspect of validation.

The Use of the Three Aspects of Learning Episodes in Planning Curriculum

In most curricula there are three kinds of courses: those that are in classrooms—misnamed "theory"—which are usually lectures; those in the clinical area in which students "practice"; and those in laboratories that are usually for nursing "arts" or "fundamentals" skills that are usually demonstration-return demonstration (sometimes using media).

What happens in these curricula is that in most instances, students only experience two of the three aspects of a learning episode. They get the informational aspect in a lecture and the validational aspect in clinical practice. Students are expected to translate information into the ability to give nursing care without ever having the opportunity to try it out in ways that are safe practice runs, that help them own the ideas or make them real. Having no operational phase robs the student of the danger-free interaction of simulated trials in which ideas, models, principles, data, and information can be squeezed for their relevance to reality-oriented problems. Students are cheated of the insights, meanings, and other educative learning that operational phases provide in a safe manner. Educative curricula organize their courses in such a way as to allow the students to acquire information—almost always a passive activity—through assignments of reading, television, slide-tapes, and some (minimal) lectures and to use the time in class for valuable student–student and teacher–student interactions structured around realitylike simulated problems and issues. This maximizes learning.

Factors Influencing Complexity

Complexity is a factor in all teaching. How to strike a given level of complexity for learning episodes is a difficult problem. To say that the curriculum is planned from "simple" to "complex" provides little help to teachers attempting to determine what is simple and what is complex. Every course contains a gradation of learning episodes. The course begins with the more simple and moves to the more complex. Every new subject must be introduced at a level that students can understand and yet does not insult their intelligence or bore them. It must challenge without being too difficult. Clinical experiences present the same problems as classrooms that use active learning as the mode. But clinical experiences furnish a reality and enable students to develop confidence in a way that simulation cannot. On the other hand, reality can be extremely threatening to students in a context in which simulation is safe for learning. Lectures, although much easier to gauge, also must be planned and delivered with the level of the student in mind and geared to the appropriate level of complexity. Although there are no formulas that work for this problem, Bevis (1989) offers some help by providing a list of five factors that influence complexity and can be used to make adjustments in teaching (see Table 2). At the suggestion of students, one more has been added.

These six factors come into play each time a student and teacher interact. Most of the time, expert teachers consider these factors unconsciously or intuitively. By monitoring students' interactions, their questions, their expressions, and their postures, teachers perceive the

Table 2
Six Factors that Influence
Complexity

The number of variables
The amount of structure
The degree of familiarity
The students' characteristics
The degree of intensity
The level of theory

operating level of the students and make adjustments in their teaching. Raising this process into awareness and giving it structure helps the learning episode to be more realistically commensurate with the students' level.

The factors cannot be reduced to formula. When one factor alters, the others must alter. For instance, if the students in the clinical area or in a problem-solving discussion are dealing with many variables at one time, the teacher may wish to give them more structure, for example, in the form of some direction about how to arrange priorities. If the level of theory is very high or the ideas abstract, the teacher may wish to give more time to decrease the intensity. In fact, each factor can be placed on its own continuum and manipulated by the teacher to affect complexity (see Fig. 3).

The Number of Variables.   The number of variables with which the student must deal at one time can be controlled only in some instances. If the problem is simulated, the teacher can increase or decrease variables and thereby make the situation more complex. In the clinical area teachers control the variables by setting limits on what the student will be responsible for on specific days. However, sometimes clinical situations that appear simple can get complex rapidly because the variables multiply. Large numbers of tests can be ordered for a patient, medications can change, conditions can alter rapidly, visitors can get upset, fire can break out . . . the possibilities are endless.

Figure 3
The Six Complexity Factors Continua

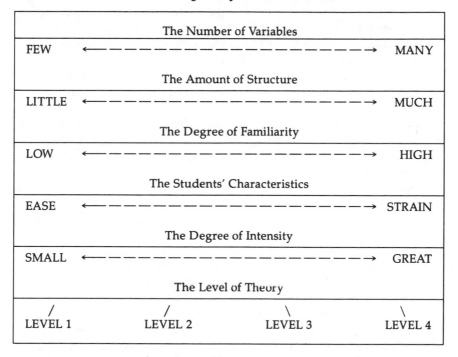

The Number of Variables		
FEW ←— — — — — — — — — — — — — —→ MANY		
The Amount of Structure		
LITTLE ←— — — — — — — — — — — — —→ MUCH		
The Degree of Familiarity		
LOW ←— — — — — — — — — — — — — —→ HIGH		
The Students' Characteristics		
EASE ←— — — — — — — — — — — — —→ STRAIN		
The Degree of Intensity		
SMALL ←— — — — — — — — — — — — —→ GREAT		
The Level of Theory		
/ / \ \		
LEVEL 1 LEVEL 2 LEVEL 3 LEVEL 4		

The Amount of Structure.   The amount of structure depends upon the setting, the teacher's directions, the course materials, and the availability of materials. Structure exists in some instances simply because there are walls that limit intrusion from extraneous sources. That is why community health visits in the home can be complex. Structure is inherent in having policy and procedure manuals that provide guidelines and directions. Structure is most often provided by the teacher by giving explicit directions. A learning episode is simple for students when the teacher says, "Write a four-page paper on one possible postpartal complication and cite at least two research studies on the subject. Use APA style. Follow the attached outline." A learning activity is much more complex when the teacher says, "Submit a scholarly project regarding perinatal care."

The Degree of Familiarity. Things seem simple when familiar. Elderly people who can move around their cluttered rooms in the dark tend to trip and fall in uncluttered rooms in unfamiliar environments. Paragraphs in legal instruments that seem clear to a lawyer may be difficult for lay persons to understand. Regardless of how complicated a pattern, a maze, a plan, or a mechanism is, it seems simple to the initiated—the expert. Unfamiliar things seem complex by way of their strangeness; once the strangeness is overcome, they seem much more simple.

Teachers have little control over initial familiarity or strangeness of situations, equipment, or settings in structuring learning episodes. But they can allow the time or provide experiences that will quickly familiarize students with things alien. Teachers can also use familiar things as similes when making explanations. This is why fundamentals courses usually begin with bedmaking and bathing patients. Most students have made beds, slept in beds, and have bathed themselves.

The Student's Characteristics. Culture, previous life experiences, developmental level, maturity level, poise, self-confidence, cognitive style, and other characteristics such as one's usual way of approaching problems all influence the ease or strain with which a student approaches learning situations. If a student tends to approach problems with confusion, low self-confidence, or fear, other factors need to be manipulated initially so that the student will have an opportunity to get beyond the initial response. Some situations have different meanings for students. Differing culturalities change meanings and can either make something more simple or more complex depending upon the impact of the meanings on the student. A student may have great difficulty coping with aging, and aging clients might then be more complex for that student than would children or young adults.

The Degree of Intensity. Intensity is a powerful influence on complexity. If the speed of a student's work affects a person's life, as in cardiac resuscitation, recognition of arrhythmias, or other emergency measures, then the very fact of the significance of the consequences acts as a complicating factor. If what the student does affects the job of another person—as in assisting someone else change a dressing, sew a wound, or implant chest tubes—it affects the complexity. The unskilled person is conscious of the other person's waiting, and that creates pressure for a competence that is not possessed. This contributes to the perception of complexity: The more intense a situation, the more anxious the student will be and the less likely to learn quickly. In these situations, adding structure in the form of coaching or decreasing the variables enables some control of complexity.

The Level of Theory.   The influence of the level of theory on complexity is directly related to the level of the student. Using Dickoff, James, and Wiedenbach's (1968) classical article on the levels of theory, one can easily see how theory level influences complexity. Dickoff and his colleagues propose four levels of theory: factor isolating, factor relating, situation relating, and situation producing; each succeeding level is more complex than the previous one.

Level 1 (factor-isolating theories) consists of naming, labeling, and simple classifications or categorizations. Being the lowest level, it is equivalent to item learning in the learning typology (see Chapter 4).

Level 2 (factor-relating theories) consists of descriptions or depictions that show how one named thing relates to another named thing. These are simple relationships of individual factors or items. Anatomy, in its simplest form, is factor relating.

Level 3 (situation relating) is much more complex. It is predictive theory. It is concerned with causal relationships or correlations. It is involved in anticipating the consequences—in knowing what will influence a situation.

Level 4 (situation producing) are theories that are related to creating the circumstances and conditions that will produce the situation desired. This requires the imaginative use of knowledge of all the other levels of theories. It is the ordering of events in the right sequence, and the arrangements of logistics, time, persons, and equipment.

These levels, already arranged on a complexity continuum, influence the complexity of a learning episode through governing the order and sequence of concepts taught so that no level is omitted. In any new practice-oriented field, teachers begin with factor-isolating theories and move to situation-producing theories.

A Map for Planning Learning Episodes

Learning theories vary tremendously, and each "camp" of theorist lays claims to being incompatible with all others. Those of us who are teachers, that is, practitioners of learning theory, know that all theories work under certain circumstances, with certain students, and with particular content. In the absence of a unifying theory about learning, it may be helpful to have a practical map that helps the teacher thread a way through teaching in ways that are reliable for helping students think creatively and critically, that is, educative learning. If in building or choosing learning activities, one were to approach the problem in logical ways, following such a map, then the teacher could recognize where the student is in the process and raise questions appropriate to the student's progress on the map. The dangers to avoid in such a map are in using it rigidly or in letting it become a formula. It must be used only as a general guide to provide clues about where the student is and where one might want to guide the student next. By no means must teachers approach using the map as if it were a sequential process. The human mind, like human experience, does not lend itself to consistently ordered sequences of thinking, for it flexibly bounces around from category to category on the map as logic, inspiration, insights, and questions take it. One of the assumptions of this curriculum development paradigm is that learning occurs more readily if students have a problem to pit their minds against, and so that belief is reflected in the map. Each teacher, whether or not it is in awareness, uses a learning map that is based in beliefs about how learning takes place.

Learning maps aid teachers gain a view of the process of how educative learning occurs so that teaching strategies and learning activities can be selected or constructed in ways that increase the potential for learning. It is important to keep in mind that a learning activity is not a learning experience. A learning activity is something the teacher plans for students to participate in. The experience the learner has is individual and may not necessarily coincide with what the teacher planned or hoped the experience would be. Learning is tied to the experience, so learning activities are constructed with the *intent* of influencing the student's *experience*. Maps help in this enterprise. A learning map assumes an underlying theory and every theory can be translated into a map. For instance, Gagne (1970) gives eight "conditions of learning," each being prerequisite to the next and, therefore, forming a sequential map for constructing learning activities. The stimulus-response-associationist map is also well known. It is laced with such words as "stimulus," "response," and "reinforcer." The Hull-Dollard map (Dollard & Miller, 1960) is less well known but perhaps more closely approaches what is intuitively used in nursing, especially for skill teaching.

There is no one theory of learning that guides the educative-learning types (see Chapter 4) addressed by this map, but one could be derived from the map if it were necessary or important. Probably any number of theories could be inserted at appropriate points on the map. However, the map is devised as a practical tool only—not as a means for generating theory. It should be used as a guide if it is helpful; any parts of it can be used or omitted as desired without destroying the usefulness of the rest.

Following is a suggested "map" for educative learning. Note that it is not as sequential as it appears. The fact that it is in "map" form makes it seem that it "should" be followed in serial order. In reality one may start with one problem, and, in the light of information, reflection, meanings, ideas, etc., the perception of the problem changes. When that happens, one has to recover some ground. One moves back and forth between cues and information, criteria for criticism, search for meaning, synthesis, and trials. To be actually sequential would be entirely artificial and improbable.

Whether or not a teacher uses a map, teachers struggle with the questions of how to help students learn, especially types four, five, and six of learning, and how to help the student become that "expert learner" espoused by Stenhouse (1975). Regardless of the content—nursing, history, music, or philosophy—the approaches of the scholar to the content have great similarities. The nature of the trials and the nature of the simulations alter because nursing is a practice field, but the basic elements of approach to content are similar.

Teachers must devise ways to raise questions and issues with students and to establish realistic nursing problems to be approached so that these elements of scholarship can be learned. To do this, teachers need a clearer idea of the ways open to them to facilitate syntactical, contextual, and inquiry learning. Some clues can be found in examining learning modalities and heuristics of scholarship.

MODES AND HEURISTICS

The educated person routinely uses common modes and heuristics of scholarship to approach problems and issues. Without them they muddle about. Nursing's traditional model, called "nursing process," is insufficient as the usual heuristic for educating professional nurses. Problem

Figure 4
Learning Map for Educative Learning

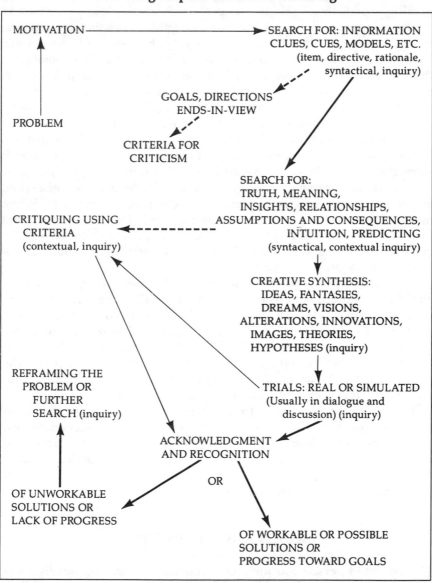

solving, in most nursing curricula, is approached not as inquiry but as if it were item and directive learning. Modes and heuristics are neither taught nor mentioned. For instance, teachers expect students to be able to "analyze" and tell them to do so without ever having taught them what it is and how to do it. Analysis is a process and has an accepted approach. The old analogy about swimming holds here. There is no need in telling the man overboard to swim if he does not know how.

The following list of scholarly modes is by no means exhaustive; it does provide a partial list of the scholarly modalities that are marks of the educated nurse. Using such a list, teachers can assume the role of expert learner and guide the student beyond looking for the "rationale" behind an approach to nursing care. Looking at "rationale" is necessary and is part of type three (rationale) learning and characteristic of high levels of training. The "beyond" is educative learning for professional nursing.

The focus of the teacher's role is that of an *expert learner* who, as such, teaches the student to be a more expert learner. It is the modes and heuristics, well and appropriately used, that characterize an expert learner.

Scholarly Modalities

It is not enough to have categorized nursing into types and separated them into training and professional categories. Nor is it sufficient to have a "map" for devising learning activities. Indeed, one must have clarity regarding the scholarly modalities that enable educative learning. These modes enable the learner to cope with syntax and inquiry (types 5 and 6), and they enable all the other types to make sense to the learner. If teachers recognize the value of these modes, they can raise issues and questions that provide the subject matter for teacher–student interactions that require the student to use the modes and the heuristics in the learning process.

Examples of Scholarly Modes

- Analysis.
- Critiquing.
- Recognizing insights.
- Identifying and evaluating assumptions.
- Inquiring into the nature of things.

- Projecting, futuring, anticipating, predicting, or hypothesizing.
- Searching for structural or organizational motifs (patterns) or building them.
- Engaging in praxis.[1]
- Evaluating: assessing merit using criteria and expert judgment.
- Viewing wholes, not just parts in relation to each other.
- Acknowledging paradigm experiences and cases in ways that enable them to be useful in practice and theorizing.
- Finding meanings in ideas and experiences.

Expert learners use these modes both in training and in education. However, it hardly bears remarking that all learners have insights, find meanings, anticipate, project, structure, and so on. It is the frequency, the habitual approach, the valuing of these modes, and the expertise of their use that mark educative learning. Furthermore, it is the types of conclusions, ideas, and insights that are derived from these modes and the quality of abstractions that can be elicited from them by the student that distinguishes the educated mind.

Educational Heuristics

In order to facilitate students in learning these scholarly modes, the teacher must help students develop learning tools (heuristics) so that the ways of approaching modes, ideas, content, and practice can be learned. For instance, if a teacher is attempting to help a student find meanings in ideas and experiences, the teacher might ask the student to write a paper using an experience that the student identifies as a paradigm experience and ask that propositions, postulates, or hypotheses be derived from the experience and that the significance and meanings, both personal and professional, be presented. Since the purpose of the paper is not to evaluate the student's ability, but through writing to help the student learn to think through the significance and meaning, one would engage in criticism but not in evaluation for grading. Dialogue and debate among students and/or between students and faculty would be another mode of arriving at the same search for meaning.

---

[1] Praxis can be defined several ways. One way to think of it is enabling theory and practice each to inform and shape the other. Another is Goulet's definition (1976, p. vii): "the precise symbiosis between reflective action and critical theorizing."

The following is a nonexhaustive list of educational heuristics frequently used by expert learners.

Examples of Educational Heuristics

- Reflection.
- Incubation (letting an idea or thought lie fallow until it emerges of its own volition more fully developed than when it initially came into awareness. This may take minutes, hours, days, or years).
- Discussion, dialogue, and debate.
- Fantasizing, imaging, imagining, and envisioning.
- Intuiting, hunching.
- Trials (simulated, imagined, or real).
- Tracing logical pathways.
- Writing in which one uses scholarly modes such as formulating propositions, postulates, and hypotheses and supporting or defending them; or in which one traces logical pathways,[2] explores insights, or describes interaction conclusion.
- Reading analytically.

Teachers engaging in educative teaching are sometimes unsure about how to teach something the teacher does so expertly that it is natural. It helps to call the heuristics by name. For example, a teacher might use the fantasy heuristic by prompting a student with "fantasize what it would be like . . . if . . ." Students soon begin to coach each other in the same manner.

It helps to have a preconceived idea about the structure of some of the modes, so that teaching them can be a simple matter of helping

---

[2] Writing is an essential educational tool. To write is to make commentary on oneself, on lived as well as imagined life; to battle with cause, effect, and correlation; to defend, determine, make assessments, and find meanings. And in the end, it is to attempt to balance merit, compassion, justice, and need. To write is also both to mask and reveal ourselves in layers of meanings that are often unanticipated, building on steps of assumptions and illusions, sometimes unidentified, often unilluminated. This is what enables writing to be a great tool for unraveling mystery and seeking feeling tones that hide in logic's shadow. Writing stretches the inner resources as does nothing else. It is too often used as an evaluative tool and too seldom as a learning one.

students walk through the process and use it until they own it for themselves. When that happens, students will begin to modify the modality in ways that make it more useful to their own uniqueness. The following are a few examples of processes required for two of the modalities, analysis and criticism.

Examples of Aspects of Two Intellectual Modalities

Analysis

- Identifying elements or factors.
- Sorting these into conceptual categories that are consistent, hierarchically congruent, and more mutually exclusive than inclusive.
- Devising an organizational structure for the categories and elements that relates the elements in logical ways; surfaces structural patterns among the elements; provides a framework for insights and understanding of the elements; enables criticism of the elements, the categories, and the structure; and connects to other structural groupings, data sets, or conceptual constructs.

Critiquing

In criticism, all elements listed here may not be appropriate to everything subjected to criticism. One would need to choose the appropriate elements. For clarity, three sets of elements of criticism are listed as examples.

General:

- Internal consistency.
- Congruency of definition (inherent or explicit) with examples used.
- Logical development.
- Conclusions are consistent with and supported by the data.
- Assumptions are valid (do not violate known or suspected world).
- Legal.
- Ethical.

When one is examining data (fourth item above), the following elements are considered:

- Relevant to issue or problem.
- Valid.
- Competence of methods for gathering data.
- Necessary to support conclusions.
- Sufficient.

When one is examining solutions, teachers guide learners in critiquing whether or not the solutions are:

- Feasible (can be done).
- Efficient in time, effort, energy, material.
- Efficacious (effective in solving the problem).
- Safe for the nurse, the client, the agency, and others.
- Culturally acceptable, ethical, and moral.
- Legal.
- Caring, humane, and compassionate.

Reaching clarity on such things as criticism and analysis and what they entail helps the teacher formulate questions that are useful to raise in discussions with students when examining rational, syntactical, contextual, and inquiry issues. It is the skill the teacher has in establishing an intellectual climate of mutual searching after knowledge, understanding, and expertise that enables a truly scholarly dialogue to take place among teachers and students. The ability to raise questions that are practical, relevant, and necessary to the exploration of issues and being able and willing to participate with students in discussions is an essential ingredient in educative teaching.

USING SOME OF THE MODELS TO STRUCTURE TEACHING

Lecturing

Lecturing is an excellent strategy for giving information not available in another form; for sharing unpublished materials; for providing a different viewpoint or framework for viewing material; for combining ideas, insights, and information in unique combinations and structures; and for condensing and limiting material that students would have to spend hours finding and reading. The lecture is excellent for providing inspiration and for sharing the teacher's private world of experience. It is the strategy of choice when working with large numbers of students in settings that do not lend themselves well to "buzz groups." And of course, lecture is irreplaceable for showcasing the teacher's charisma, sense of humor, showmanship, and delightful and comprehensive knowledge of the subject.

Probably one of the most important reasons for a lecture is to build connections between the content and methods of the field of study and the student's own personal experience. Meyers (1986) explains that all learning proceeds from analogy. He believes we can only understand something new by recognizing how it is similar to or different from something familiar. Abstractions that are very far removed from a student's own experience are very poorly understood. This is the reason hearts become "pumps" and blood vessels "pipes." Lectures can help make these synapses.

However, on the whole, it is not what the teacher says or does that is important; it is what the teacher has the students do that is important in the overall scheme of education. One must be aware that when reorganizing a classroom, with the teachers becoming co-learners who are experts in content and the strategies of learning, who in effect become meta strategists, the whole politics of the classroom changes.

Regardless of its strengths, lecturing is an oppressive teaching strategy. It is oppressive because, among other reasons, learners must listen to information filtered through someone else's perspective and value system. Usually content is chosen because it is accepted discipline knowledge or the instructor believes the material will at some point in the student's career have relevance. It is "faith" teaching because it is passively absorbed by students who must have faith that sometime in the future the information lectured on will be of use. This "faith" teaching enables the teacher to retain full control of the class, to call upon whomever he or she favors with recognition, and to determine what is and what is not appropriate issue for inquiry. It calls for passivity in students; it panders to immaturity and lulls the brain to sleep. Even charismatic lecturers are oppressive (see Chapter 4). Although they often "resonate" with students, inspire, and motivate them, their overpowering personal presence unintentionally propagandizes and persuades. The charismatic teacher can inspire students to seek more learning and can "hook" their interest and curiosity. At the same time, they can be so persuasive that students become infected with "guruism" and become uncritical followers.

Huebner (1966) discusses influence at length. He legitimizes influence as part of the educational process but places great ethical accountability for it in the educator. He speaks of teachers helping students develop "response-abilities" and says, "The educator does try to influence, but with the optimism and faith in knowledge as a vehicle to new response-abilities and to new conversational possibilities" (p. 22). He says, "Knowledge, used in the process of educational influence between educator and student, becomes an instrument of promise" (p. 22). He, like Freire, proposes that with knowledge, the teacher is promising "not enslavement, not diminished power, but fulfillment and possibility and response-ability" (p. 22). When Huebner speaks of influence, it is in the context of dialogue, not of lecture. Huebner states his position:

> The educational activity differs from other human encounters by this emphasis on influence, for clearly the educator is seen, and accepted, as a person who legitimately attempts to influence. However, he operates within the uniquely human endeavor of conversation, the giving and receiving of the word at the frontiers of each other's being. It is in conversation that the newness of each participant can come forth and the unconditioned can be revealed in new forms of gesture and language. (p. 20–21)

Lecture, on the other hand, may do much for influence but little for the promise of confronting each other's being. According to Meyers (1986), "the lecture tradition fosters a generally passive style of education in which critical thinking is taught only implicitly or not at all" (p. 2).

Piaget (1976) asserts that children are not passive recipients of knowledge but rather discover and construct knowledge through activities. If this is true for children, certainly it pertains to adults as well. Yet, despite the wide respect for such theories dating back to Dewey and Hopkins, Meyers (1986) maintains, "Many colleges and universities continue to emphasize the learning of information and content rather than the development of thinking abilities. Thus, lecture remains a dominant mode of instruction" (p. 2). As instruments of education, they are of little or no value and must be abandoned as an everyday methodology to be used for special occasions only. For selected "special occasions," lecturing can be the strategy of choice.

An Approach to Educative Teaching

When I was a child, my parents were forever going to college. (Well, to a child it seemed forever.) I was the "gofor" and was sent on various scholarly errands, the most frequent being to the library to return books. I loved that errand best and perhaps so acquired my love of the musty quiet of bookladen places. Over the door of the library, engraved in stone in large, gothic letters, was the phrase, "Half of knowledge is knowing where to find it." I asked my father what the other half was. His reply was, "Knowing what questions to ask." His wisdom has proven more true and alive for me than the stone words of the library door. One cannot always "find" knowledge, but one is half way home if one knows what questions to ask and how to phrase them. Teaching, in its true form, is helping students learn new ways of approaching ideas and examining things by helping them learn to ask the appropriate questions. As mentioned above, teaching as "telling" or providing information is mere instruction that holds a much less important place in the teacher's rich gifts. In clinical and classroom instruction, asking questions is often limited to asking for the rationale behind decisions. In the classroom, it is often a guessing game. Items are asked for such as, "Does anyone know who discovered insulin?" or "What accident of nature pointed the way to smallpox vaccinations?" These questions call for answers that can be memorized. They do not call for questions that make one think through a position or an idea, reflect on a thesis, examine assumptions or implications, or devise a strategy either for nursing care or for inquiry.

There are a wealth of questions begging to be asked that will set students upon new pathways, open their minds to new ideas and areas for investigation, and provide exciting new horizons.

Raising Questions and Issues

Raising questions and issues is perhaps the most useful way a teacher can interact with a student. By this I am referring to meaningful, exploratory questioning, not to the "Socratic" method. The dialogues of Plato that contain examples of Socrates' questioning devices provide a picture of questions and answers in which the questions are very leading, with the aim of persuasion. They are excellent examples of logical progression where an antagonist leads another to the answer desired through excellent reason and rhetoric. While the dialogues make good reading and good philosophy, I do not believe they make for very good teaching.

One can choose at random among any of the dialogues and perceive instantly what is occurring. The quotation here is from the dialogue entitled "Meno," in which Socrates and Meno discuss virtue (Plato, 1952, p. 189). It follows the conversation most quoted in educational literature, in which Socrates maintains that "there is not teaching but only recollection" and leads a boy attendant to Meno through a "lesson" on geometry. Socrates was maintaining that neither knowledge nor right opinion is given to man by nature nor is acquired by him.

> Socrates: Then if they are not given by nature neither are the good by nature good?
> Meno: Certainly not.
> Socrates: And nature being excluded, then came the question whether virtue is acquired by teaching?
> Meno: Yes.
> Socrates: If virtue was wisdom [or knowledge], then, as we thought, it was taught?
> Meno: Yes.
> Socrates: And if it was taught it was wisdom?
> Meno: Certainly.
> Socrates: And if there were teachers, it might be taught; and if there were no teachers, not?
> Meno: True.
> Socrates: But surely we acknowledged that there were no teachers of virtue?
> Meno: Yes.

Meno really was not a straight man to Socrates, although all of the dialogues use the same type of structure. My criticism is not that his arguments do not make one think, only that his questions are not framed to stimulate one to think enough nor to provide one room to exercise personal initiative. It would have been better pedagogy had Socrates given his students a position and asked them to determine the assumptions underlying it and create an argument refuting it.

Determining a mode of teaching that accomplishes the general goals and ends-in-view of education requires several approaches. No one formula will work because strategies must change with the intent, the content, the teacher's experiences and talents, the setting, the numbers of students, the equipment available, the time constraints, and many other variables that must be considered.

Raising questions and issues pervades all educative teaching strategies. This is not to say that the educative teacher never answers questions or gives information. The educative teacher does give information and answer questions when the students want and need to know. The educative teacher never assumes that need and "faith" teaches.

Information giving is done intermittently during student work, when they ask, when they look stumped or puzzled, or when they bog down. And then it is given in small doses.

The questions are arrived at by the teacher systematically. If the teacher asks educative questions, it follows that students will learn to ask educative questions.

Chapter 4 presents a theoretical model of learning types. This typology suggests 6 types of learning (see Chapter 4, Table 2). To recapitulate: The model does not assume that one must move from item learning through inquiry learning. That is a linear, simplistic approach to the model. However, there is some hierarchy involved. One must know items and directives before rationales make any sense. A good grounding in item, directive, and rationale makes contextual, syntactical, and inquiry easier to learn. Obviously, contextual can be, and is learned, at any point and concurrently with all other types. Syntactical and inquiry can be learned together or separately. The point that must not be missed is that to the novice learner, item, directive, and rationale learning constitutes training. Aspects of contextual can be training, depending upon what one views as professional. (The traditional nursing "professional" injunctions regarding grooming would fit into this category.) Yet, to the expert learner, items, directives, and rationales take on a different aspect. Because of their ability to get insights quickly, to note significance, to see patterns, to arrive at meanings, and other such advanced scholarly skills, and because of their knowledge of the deeper structures of the field of study, it follows that item, directive, and rationale learning are no longer training but education. This ability becomes an indicator of learning expertise.

The use of this model is fairly simple. It is simply a guide to help fashion questions. Take, for example, a student who is caring for a child with croup. Ask the student to read the charts and observe other children with croup. Ask the student to talk with other students who have children with croup. Assuming the student has come prepared with the item, directive, and rationale aspects, move into syntactical learning by asking the student to look for patterns, relationships between symptoms, the meaning of stridor, and the significance of anxiety in parents. Have the student compare symptoms and care and determine the assumptions behind certain protocols of care. Ask the student in what ways the care given differed from the "textbook" care or departs from the "rules of care." Ask the student, if the day's care were to be repeated, what might be changed based on present knowledge, understanding, and intuition. These kinds of questions help students build experiences that become what Benner (1984) refers to as "paradigm cases."

Structuring Learning Episodes

The preceding general discussions are sufficient to enable some teachers to conduct teaching trials that incorporate the suggested ideas. They need no further words about "how to" and indeed might feel that too much help was being offered to further concretize the ideas. However, for others, some guidelines and examples are helpful so that the shift in paradigm becomes more concrete. This section is written for this latter group.

There are any number of ways to structure a course or class so that emancipation, sorority/fraternity, and humanistic-education occurs. The methods described below represent various ways to do that. Some methods are stronger in acknowledging the students' abilities and rights to help organize the content than are others, and some represent the compromises made with the teacher's own growing ability to develop confidence in the students and in self.

First, one begins. Beginning is the secret. One begins with an intent to teach in an emancipatory-participatory-sororal/fraternal modality and works toward ownership of a methodology. Methodologies must have the flavor of the teacher, the unique fit that marks one's pattern of being, a song that is one's own. Following the guidelines listed here may be a start for some, but, like the work of an artist, the courses will soon bear the mark of individuality so that one teacher's courses easily can be distinguished from another's.

Learning episodes were discussed earlier in this chapter. The three aspects of learning episodes, the amount of structure, the active–passive continuum, the factors influencing complexity, the learning maps, and the examples of educational modes and heuristics were all presented to give some ideas to teachers who are choosing or structuring learning episodes for their courses.

Learning episodes can be planned or unplanned. Some of the best learning takes place spontaneously. However, if one is to plan classroom teaching around active rather than passive learning, some ideas about how to do that are in order. This will necessarily be brief.

Active learning can occur in many ways. Most of them will not be discussed here because this is not a teaching strategy book. Games are certainly good strategies, as are debates and simulations such as role play or television clips. Only small group work will be discussed here to illustrate educative learning as a search for understanding.

Classes Structured as Small Discussion Groups

Every class or educational group has a culture. That culture is developed by the unique mystery of the interactions and flavor that persons have when grouped together with purposes to achieve. Inherent in the culture are values, understandings, and meanings that are learned and shared. It expresses the friendships, respect, hopes, compromises, intensity of feelings, and commitment to the goals that exist in the group. Group cohesion, work, and social feelings keep the culture going and enable it to change.

growth in the class culture. This is a form of transmitting culture. The teacher sets the course up for group work and entices the group toward new and higher standards of being in the world together by the very way the teacher interacts with the group—in other words, by the climate created. Therefore, one of the first features of such courses is a discussion around how the course will be conducted. Some principles of procedure devised by the group to guide the process and the work are helpful. The "Principles of Unity" from Wheeler and Chinn (1989) are a good model. These principles address beliefs, values, and ways of working together. Four of their principles are given here as examples:

- We value our own friendships among one another and are committed to living our friendship with deliberate awareness, examining and creating our experience as we go.

- We will address conflicts, feelings, and issues between us openly as soon as they reach our awareness, with the understanding that early awareness may not be perfect but deserves expression.

- We will not intentionally take any action individually or collectively that exploits any individual within the group or any other women.

- We are committed to using feminist process, including making decisions through consensus and learning to provide constructive, growthful criticism for one another. (pp. 5–8)

Many other valuable principles are given by this project's position paper on the Principles of Unity. Most groups need to formulate such principles. In many groups these are called ground rules, although ground rules have a connotation of laws rather than shared values.

To operate in a mode such as this, the group work must be meaningful and fit into the context of significant problems and issues worthy of engaging the minds, hearts, and energy of the group. The class participants and teacher as co-learner participate in designing the principles of unity as well as the topics and strategies for approach. Otherwise, the group culture excludes the teacher or becomes adversarial to the teacher. The teacher gets discounted as a factor of importance in the group's cohesive being. If this happens, it curtails the evolution of values that are effective in shaping standards of scholarship that are emancipatory.

There is a further ideal that shapes the way of being in the world of teachers and students in daily activity. It is best expressed by Huebner (1966):

> For some, the encounter of man with man is seen as the essence of life, and the form that this encounter takes is the meaning of life. The encounter is not used to produce change, to enhance prestige, to identify new knowledge, or to be symbolic of something else. The encounter is. In it is the essence of life. In it life is revealed and lived. The student is not viewed as an object, an it; but as a fellow human being, another subject, a thou, who is to be lived with in the fullness of the present moment or the eternal present. From the ethical stance the educator meets the student, not as an embodied role, as a lesser category, but as a fellow human being who demands to be accepted on the basis of fraternity not simply on the basis of equality. No thing, no conceptual barrier, no purpose intrudes between educator and student when educational activity is valued ethically. The fullness of the educational activity, as students encounter each other, the world around them, and the teacher, is all there is. The educational activity is life—and life's meanings are witnessed and lived in the classroom. (p. 19)

So the classroom becomes for the group (which includes the teacher) a place of encounter—encounter with each other and the realities of nursing. It becomes an encounter with discourse and language as a primary method, and seeking a real activity that unconceals mystery—the mystery here of being a nurse—a mystery of and an activity about sorority and fraternity, equality, skill, caring, and enlightenment.

This is active learning—so active that it spiritually engages; so active that it is an ethical endeavor that captures the value of human life. This activity first must be structured—for students are unaccustomed to the relationships of fraternity and sorority, and the discourse of educational seeking. Once the modality becomes part of the fabric of daily scholarship, it assumes a life of its own, and teacher–structure diminishes. It is the structure and form of developing students who are accustomed to being lectured at, diminished as humans, oppressed of thought, and robbed of an education that we must now address. Structure and form must liberate. Just as discipline of mind and habit liberates, so does scholarly structure.

Form.   All classroom learning activities have form. The form consists of tasks that are clearly spelled out; an explanation of where this learning episode or activity fits in the overall scheme of things (sometimes called an overview); some general goals or ends-in-view so the groups know where they are headed; a situation, problem, issue, or event that serves as the focus for the activity; some agreements about how the groups are to function, what they are to do, a time limit; and a plenary session to pull things together or surface what has occurred or been learned.

The place to begin in the ultimately liberated curriculum is with the topic of the course. Students participate with the teacher in devising the course. This can be done in several ways. One common way is for the teacher to pose a problem: "Given that this course is about the common nursing needs of persons experiencing life-altering health problems, what kinds of things do you wish to study?" Defining that can be done in a variety of ways. Take the student into the clinical areas (homes, clinics, hospitals of all sorts) to visit and talk with patients who have experience with life-altering health problems. Ask them to structure an interview for these patients so they can get some information about their experiences. Have them talk with nurses who work with patients who have experienced such problems. Then ask them to analyze (see earlier part of chapter) the information and generate a list of things they think they need to know. The teacher then works with the students to establish a reasonable work load for the course. As expert learner, the teacher structures, in collaboration with students, the ways of approaching the topics chosen for study.

There are all degrees/levels of empowering students regarding content to be chosen. If the teacher chooses the content and prestructures the course outline, it is important that it be negotiable and that students

be guided through the negotiating process (if they have not been partners in such a course before). Negotiations, in this case, revolve around
whether or not to include things that are not there that students want
and eliminate things that are in the course that they do not want. This
process must not be limited to the first week or so of the course but
must go on constantly as the students become increasingly attuned to
the content and clear on what they want and need. Needless to say, this
requires a teacher who knows the content so well as not to be outline
dependent.

Throughout the whole, reality-grounding is an essential ingredient.
The use of paradigm cases is very powerful for group work. Benner
(1984) says that expert clinical teachers can best teach through presentation of paradigm cases. She says that these paradigm cases transmit
more than can be conveyed through abstract principles or guidelines.
She states, "In order for students to learn from another person's
paradigm case, they must actively rehearse or imagine the situation.
Simulations can be even more effective because they require action and
decisions from the learner" (p. 9).

For graduate students, issues, theory, research, literature, and the
deeper structures of nursing knowledge all provide subjects for the
person-to-person encounter that Huebner speaks of.

Group Size.   Classroom group size is not a very important feature
unless schools have bought into the nonpractice discipline line of reasoning that believes that the larger the lecture section, the more cost-ef-
fective the education. The consequences of this is that courses are
constituted with groups of 50 or more. Class sizes of 40–50 students can
work well with discursive teaching as long as the group is divided into
small groups (4–5 students) for the discussions. More than 50 is un-
wieldy. My personal preference is about 25–30.

Learning based on active involvement seems to occur more readily
when the course group is divided into small work groups. In a class of
40, one might have 10 such groups in one room. Discussion groups that
have four to five persons in each enable everyone to participate, and yet
there are enough minds at work to open the problems and explore the
issues with a higher probability of covering all the pertinent aspects.
The more members one has in a group, the more slowly the work goes
and the less that is accomplished in the same time. Also, less human-to-
human discourse takes place. In larger groups it is too easy for a few
people to dominate the discussion. People can get preoccupied with

how they are perceived or with observing proper rules of courtesy to each other. Larger groups see more power struggles rise to the surface, more visiting and socializing take place, silent persons tend to remain silent, and participants can more easily drift into trivial tangents. The smaller groups can change in membership as desired. They can form, dissolve, and reform, and students can seek one another's talents, continue discussions, attempt to broaden their relationships, and follow a line of thought.

As a part of small group work, it is important to bring the groups back together as a class group for plenary. Plenary helps students to compare what each group has discussed, to examine the various shapes of their ideas, to seek some common denominators and/or differences, and to examine emerging patterns. It allows time to discuss these commonalities and differences in ways that enhance the small group work. It also helps to pull together what salient ideas and features people perceive in the day's work. It provides a summary that can be a steppingstone for more discussions or contribute a sense of closure to the day, if not for the subject. It helps students to grasp the ambiguity that is often inherent in nursing and to settle with that ambiguity.

Plenary sessions can consist of the total group or subtotals that combine three to five small groups. Although one is not constrained to have a whole group plenary, it is important to bring the whole group together at times to promote a sense of unity and cohesion and to allow groups to critique or shed light on each other's work.

Time. Small groups enable the time for group discussion to be maximized. The time allotted to a topic can be a variable that adds "intensity" and therefore needs to be taken into consideration. Time can also limit the degree of latitude the group has with the subject. Time is not of unlimited quantity in courses and must be monitored. Discussions on any subject will take up the time allotted, so short time periods of 5–10 minutes can be tried and then more time given if necessary. It is better to leave the groups still hungry for more time than bored because the classroom is slowed up until the last group has finished. It does not matter that all groups finish. Almost all important points will have been covered by some group and will be surfaced in the plenary sessions.

What can be done is a series of small discussions with a general goal in mind followed by a larger group discussion geared to pulling things together. Let us take as an example a situation in which students have decided they wish to examine the issues around patients with recently diagnosed cancer who might not desire treatment. The following situation is an example paradigm case modified to make it a simulated situation.

SITUATION

You are a senior student caring for Mr. Cohen, a 76-year-old widower of 8 years who has just been diagnosed with metastatic adenocarcinoma of the lower bowel. Wide metastasis is suspected with some liver involvement probable. He has four children. One lives in Canada; one, in Israel; two, in the United States. He has several grandchildren and three great-grandchildren. He lives with his daughter, her husband, and their 16-year-old daughter in a three-room apartment. He has a mild heart condition that is under control with medication. He has suffered frequent episodes of ulcerative colitis since he was 25 and has had bouts with increasing frequency and severity since his wife died. His chronic colitis may have masked his carcinoma and delayed his diagnosis.

In reading his chart and talking with him you conclude that his general health and energy level seem good. The patient acknowledges his diagnosis and seems to have read some materials he found in the city library on his disease. It is not clear what he has read, and so far you have not had an opportunity to talk with him about it enough to be clear about what he understands.

He seems neither depressed nor deeply distressed to you. He makes easy conversation about light topics and jokes a little but offers no unsolicited personal information.

He has refused surgery and chemotherapy, although he continues to be cooperative regarding his diagnostic work-up. You found his morning medications (multivitamins, digitalis, and Bumex) in the trash can.

The head nurse is concerned, as is the physician, about his noncompliance and has instructed the staff and you to make this the number one priority and to work toward compliance with the medical regimen.

Using such a paradigm experience, you can ask the small groups to enter into a series of dialogues. Some of the topics for these sessions might be:

1. What are the significant issues the nurse needs to consider in caring for Mr. Cohen?

2. Have you encountered other patients with similar issues? If so, what are the similarities and differences and do they begin to form a pattern that provides insights regarding his care?

3. What does your intuition tell you is going on with Mr. Cohen?

4. What further investigations do you need to make and how can you go about making them? (Then you provide the needed further information or ask them to imagine it.)

5. Which issues that you have surfaced concern the politics of health care, power, ethics, loyalty, caring, and nursing culture? And what underlying assumptions about the identified issues are inherent in the situation?

6. What implications does your position on ethical issues have for your work-role relationships (assuming a position has been worked out)?

These questions could take many forms. They are constructed using the learning typology categories of syntactical, contextual, and inquiry as guide. If you wished to pursue this situation you could raise issues of theorizing, strategizing, and predicting. Criteria could be constructed that the group feels would be helpful in critiquing proposed care. The possibilities are endless, and the yield can be exciting and unforgettable. The use of others' paradigm cases in this kind of simulation can serve to give the students a vicariously broadened pool of paradigm experiences on which to base their practice.

CRITERIA FOR CRITIQUING AN EDUCATIVE LEARNING ACTIVITY

Reference has been made to Murray and Merrefield's (1989) criteria for selecting and devising learning activities. Criteria of this kind devised by faculties help to ensure that the course is proceeding along in ways that are congruent with the intent of the curriculum. The following list of criteria was devised using some ideas suggested by Murray and Merrefield while stressing the specific needs suggested by the paradigm being offered here. One can use the following short list of criteria for critiquing learning activities such as the one offered above.

CRITERIA FOR CRITIQUING
AN EDUCATIVE LEARNING ACTIVITY

1. Is it liberating and reflective of a condition of sorority and fraternity?

2. Does it have a "hook" or something to engage the students' interest?

3. Does it require students to become involved (Benner's active rehearsal or imagining themselves in the situation)?

4. Does it require students to be responsible for their own learning?

5. Does it allow for training and education as appropriate to the content and needs of the students?

6. Does it facilitate writing or discussions that require formulating, supporting, and defending of propositions, postulates, and hypothesis?

7. Does it require following logical pathways as well as enabling the use of intuitive knowing?

8. Does it require intellectual modes such as analysis, critiquing, identifying, and evaluating assumptions, inquiring into the nature of things, projecting, futuring, anticipating, predicting, hypothesizing, searching for organizing motifs and patterns, engaging in praxis, evaluating, viewing wholes, acknowledging paradigm experiences, and finding meanings in experiences and ideas?

9. Does it require that educative heuristics be used such as reflection, incubation, discussion, dialogue, debate, fantasizing, imagining, imaging, intuiting, hunching, and trials?

10. Does it provide for creativity?

11. Does it allow for differences and diversity among discussants?

12. Does it structure for syntactical, contextual, and inquiry learning?

13. Does it require good scholarship?

14. Is it written or explained in a way that clearly lets participants know what they are to do?

15. Does it allow for the use of personal, phenomenological, subjective experiences and meanings?

Such a list can be helpful in keeping the course learning episodes on the track. Both the way participants (students and teachers) interact in learning and the methods/content of the course are synergistic in exploiting the full potentials of learning.

CURRICULUM AS
TEACHING–LEARNING INTERACTIONS

The purpose of this chapter is to illuminate teaching. This chapter, along with Chapter 6, both on the subject of teaching, point to the central importance of teaching to the curriculum development model. One theme, repeated throughout this book, is that curriculum *is the interactions and transaction that occur between and among teachers and students with the intent that learning occur.* This thesis runs throughout the new literature regarding a paradigm shift in nursing education (see, e.g., Diekelmann, 1988; Moccia, 1988). It follows, as the first principle of that thesis, that any and all changes in nursing's curriculum development paradigm must in some way affect the liberation and empowering of people—both students and teachers. Power, in any movement toward liberation, becomes an important issue, and one may anticipate that some teachers will be reluctant to empower students because they believe that such empowering by necessity decreases their own power.

I raise the question: Is power of limited quantity so that when I empower others (students), I concomitantly disempower myself? Or is power, like love, of unlimited quantity, so that the more I share the more I have? Through empowering others, I also empower myself. When addressing ideas about power, I am not speaking of "having power over" but "having power to." If power is conceived as "power to," then students and teachers are both empowered by the liberating force of co-learnership.

Munhall (1988, p. 221), in what she labels "Implications for Curriculum Within the Theme of the Aquarian Conspiracy," lists fostering community and searching for meaning, self-discovery, freedom, choices, and relationships as suggested curriculum processes. The implication here is that these processes are essential to a new curriculum development model for nursing.

It seems, therefore, that the very essence of curriculum rests in the quality of interactions between and among students and faculty. These interactions rely on a changed relationship between teachers and students in which the teacher's role is one of metastrategist who establishes a climate of sorority and fraternity, of equality, of scholarly seeking; who raises questions and issues and dialogues with students so that they become partners in education, not objects of education.

In new models, clinical practice realities become the modality for study, and the approach is qualitative in methodology rather than quantitative. Phenomenology, hermeneutical analysis, poetics, and other qualitative methods form the teaching-learning modalities. Both Munhall (1988) and Watson (1985, 1988) speak of the phenomenological thrust of the "new" nursing. Watson, in speaking of the transpersonal caring relationship of the nurse, states:

> Human care can begin when the nurse enters into the life space or phenomenal field of another person, is able to detect the other person's condition of being (spirit, soul), feels this condition within him- or herself, and responds to the condition in such a way that the recipient has a release of subjective feelings and thoughts he or she had been longing to release. As such, there is an intersubjective flow between the nurse and patient. (p. 63)

Munhall (1988) states that "the social humandate for change calls us to conspire together in the transformation of behavioristic, externally driven curriculum to one that focuses on expanding consciousness and the subjective and inter-subjective experiences of being human" (p. 228).

Boyd (1988) says:

> We stand vulnerably in the wake of a spiraling system of controls on human irregularity made possible by "scientific progress." For some of us, the human condition—what it means to exist, to be alive in a world seized by technology—is an appropriate, even important focus for nursing. Existentialism and phenomenology provide a lens. (p. 66)

There is little doubt for me that both existentialism and phenomenology are the lenses through which our curricula will reach the goals of excellence in professional service. They give us a sense of essence, they give us intentionality, and they ground the curriculum in "being in the world." Additionally, unlike the scientific, they give us flexibility—the justification for looking at unconcealing . . . at coming to know . . . at exploring together. These ideas are antithetical to the common scientific positions of right and wrong answers, of categorization of humans, of human predictability, of division into parts. These two modes, existentialism and phenomenology, express wholes and explore consciousness.

Phenomenology is grounded in reality, in wholes, in reflection, in insight, in everyday events. Such, too, is hermeneutics. Hermeneutic inquiry examines the textual or language-semantic structure of everyday practical activity. It begins in the everyday, practical roles and functions of nursing—what nurses actually do. Using hermeneutics, teachers and students seek meaning through language about practice.

Clinical and classroom learning methodologies must be phenomenological in all their various manifestations and must be based on human caring-human science. In speaking of phenomenological themes and concepts, Boyd (1988) states:

> These themes provide an open framework descriptive of the nature of being human: the first distinguishing feature of the phenomenological perspective. Rather than starting with a philosophy and constructing a curriculum, phenomenology grounds us only in an understanding of the nature of being human. There are fewer linear, derived guidelines and prescriptives, more openness, and more constancy in processes of choice. (p. 67)

Benner (1984) makes the case that "the proficient clinician compares past whole situations with current whole situations" (p. 9). Wholeness is something the behaviorist-empiricist paradigms seldom examine.

Poetics, another phenomenological methodology, can be useful in teaching. Poetics is a natural outcome of phenomenology. Watson (1988) speaks to that point when she characterizes poetizing as the "true vocation of the experiential phenomenologist" (p. 92). She builds her position on Levin (1983) and maintains that poetizing is "necessary in that transcendental depth phenomenology, if focused and reflective of depth human experiences, cannot be other than poetic." If our teaching is centered on helping students find meaning, then poetics is a necessary element. Watson goes on to say, "Poetic expression has the power to touch and move us, to open and transport us. Thus, the poetic quality is related to the experiential meaning and, indeed, deepens the meaning, the felt senses, so that there is increased openness to describe and preserve the truth and depth of the experience."

So many educators, when speaking of their teaching, become poetic in their language. Huebner (1985) says that "education is only possible because the human being is a being that can transcend itself" (p. 165). This transcendence is ineffable, and to express the ineffable requires rendering it into metaphor and simile. These terms, when addressing the transcendence of insight, new understanding, creativity, struggle, conflict, new forms, and the joy of the whole of learning, is by necessity poetic. The same can be said of nursing. Poetry becomes the means of expressing that which by no other means can be said.

Nursing can be the means for transforming the human experiences around health; it can make a statement about human dignity; it can support human transition to higher wholes; it can provide a bridge to greater awareness and inner harmony. Nursing transcends politics, religion, cultures. Speaking with Huebner's (1966) words, teachers can say to students of nursing:

> Look, with this knowledge I can promise you that you can find new wonders in the world; you can find new people who can interest you; and in so finding you can discover what you are and what you can become. In so doing you can help discover what man is, has been, and can be. With this knowledge I promise you, not enslavement, not a reduction of your power, but fulfillment and possibility and response-ability. (p. 22)

We can say to students that with this knowledge you can bring healing and hope. This promise is possible only through education that frees.

REFERENCES

Benner, P. (1984). *From novice to expert: Excellence and power in clinical nursing practice.* Menlo Park, CA: Addison-Wesley.

Bevis, E. (1989). *Curriculum building in nursing: A process* (3rd ed.). New York: National League for Nursing.

Boyd, C. O. (1988). Phenomenology: A foundation for nursing curriculum. In *Curriculum revolution: Mandate for change.* New York: National League for Nursing.

Denton, D. E. (1974). That mode of being called teaching. In D. E. Denton (Ed.), *Existentialism and phenomenology in education.* New York: Teachers College Press.

Dickoff, J., James, P., & Weidenbach, E. (1968). Theory in a practice discipline. *Nursing Research, 17,* 415–435.

Diekelmann, N. (1988). Curriculum revolution: A theoretical and philosophical mandate for change. In *Curriculum revolution: Mandate for change.* New York: National League for Nursing.

Dollard, J., & Miller, N. (1960). *Personality and psychotherapy.* New York: McGraw-Hill.

Gagne, R. (1970). *The conditions of learning* (2nd ed.). New York: Holt, Rinehart and Winston.

Giorgi, A. (1970). *Psychology as a human science.* New York: Harper and Row.

Goetz, I. L. (1983). Heidegger and the art of teaching. *Educational Theory, 33* (1), 1–9.

Goulet, D. (1976). Introduction. In P. Freire (Ed.), *Education: The practice of freedom.* London: Writers and Readers Publishing Cooperative.

Huebner, D. (1966). Curricular language and classroom meanings. In *Language and meaning.* Washington, DC: The Association for Supervision and Curriculum Development.

Huebner, D. (1985). Spirituality and knowing. In E. Eisner (Ed.), *Learning and teaching the ways of knowing.* Chicago: The University of Chicago Press.

Levin, D. (1983). The poetic function in phenomenological discourse. In W. McBride and C. Schrag (Eds.), *Phenomenology in a pluralistic context.* Albany, NY: State University of New York Press.

McDonald, F. (1966). *Educational psychology.* Belmont, CA: Wadsworth.

Meyers, C. (1986). *Teaching students to think critically.* San Francisco: Jossey-Bass.

Moccia, P. (1988). Curriculum revolution: An agenda for change. In *Curriculum revolution: Mandate for change.* New York: National League for Nursing.

Munhall, P. (1988). Curriculum revolution: A social mandate for change. In *Curriculum revolution: Mandate for change.* New York: National League for Nursing.

Murray J., & Merrefield, S. (1989). Criteria for teacher–student interactions and learning experiences. In J. Murray, *Developing criteria to support new curriculum models for doctoral education in nursing.* Doctoral dissertation, University of Georgia.

Piaget, J. (1976). *Psychology of intelligence.* Totowa, NJ: Littlefield Adams. (Originally published 1974)

Plato. (1952). In R. M. Hutchins (Ed.), *Great books of the Western world.* Chicago: Encyclopaedia Brittanica.

Smuts, J. (1926). *Holism and evolution.* New York: Macmillan.

Stenhouse, L. (1975). *An introduction to curriculum research and development.* London: Heinemann Educational Books.

Watson, J. (1985, 1988). *Nursing: Human science and human care.* New York: National League for Nursing.

Wheeler, C., & Chinn, P. (1989). *Peace and power, a handbook of feminist process.* Buffalo, NY: Margaretdaughters.

Whitehead, A. N. (1929). Universities and their function. In *The aims of education and other essays* (pp. 91–101). New York: The Free Press.

Whitehead, A. N. (1969). *Process and reality.* New York: The Free Press. (Originally published in 1929)

Wissot, J. (1979, March). Teaching as an art form. *The Educational Forum,* 265–278.

BIBLIOGRAPHY

Freire, P. (1976). *Education: The practice of freedom.* London: Writers and Readers Publishing Cooperative.

9

Accessing Learning: Determining Worth or Developing Excellence—From a Behaviorist toward an Interpretive-Criticism Model

Em Olivia Bevis

Verification is the only scientific criterion of reality. That does not mean that there may not be realities that are unverifiable.

John Fowles, *The Magus*

INTRODUCTION

Evaluation is about the verification of reality. It is an *attempt* to determine what reality is in relation to or in comparison with standards or criteria that the evaluator thinks (at the evaluating moment in time) reality should be. The quandary is to determine (1) what verification methods satisfy the criterion of necessary and sufficient, (2) what or whose reality is being addressed, and (3) what criteria or standards are being used as comparisons. Answers to these three questions vary, depending upon the framework used for approaching evaluation. One cannot approach the subject of evaluating student learning without touching on these issues.

Evaluation of student learning is the way teachers and learners find a landmark or a point of reference. Evaluation provides indicators, clues, cues, signs and signals that tell both teachers and students where they are in relation to where they want to be or where they are going. It has been defined in a variety of ways and from a variety of angles. Evaluation specialists speak of formative and summative, process and product, assessment, measurement, testing and grading, and normative and criterion referenced evaluation. They provide designs, patterns, plans, maps, lists, and criteria. Additionally, except for Scriven (1972), who, in speaking of program evaluation, suggests "goal free" evaluation as a way to be more attuned to nongoal-related outcomes, most evaluation specialists are tied to the objectives model. Even Scriven ends his goal-free model with an examination of objectives. This means that specific goals, in the form of behaviorally stated objectives, are the guiding light of these models.

Some commentary on the inadequacy of these methods for use in this paradigm are required at this point: (1) Empiricist evaluation models, except for inductive ones, require goals and objectives and even inductive models derive objectives in the end. (2) Most empiricist evaluation models, inductive or deductive, are after all behaviorist and at some point require behavioral objectives. (3) If behaviorist models are used, they undermine the educative-caring paradigm. Merton (1975, p. 31) suggests that paradigms that are perceptually different can be "mutually enriching" and contends:

> The cognitive problems of coexisting paradigms call for discovering the capabilities and limitations of each. This involves identifying the kinds and range of problems each is good for (and noting those for which it is incompetent or irrelevant), thus providing for potential awareness of the respects in which they are complementary or contradictory. (p. 50)

The position taken here is that the range of problems appropriate to the behaviorist evaluation paradigm are those in the first three types of learning: item, directive, and rational. These are training types of learning. Criticism as evaluation works with the educative-caring paradigms. Therefore, if training and education are evaluated by using behaviorial objectives, it subverts the educative model.

Since nursing has a training component, that aspect can and should be evaluated using behaviorist methods. These methods have been used for more than 30 years and have proven successful at what they are designed to do: to determine the degree and extent that curriculum-specified behaviors have been achieved. The problem is that, when behavioral objectives are not specified, another means must be found. The model described here for use in evaluating educative learning is an interpretive-criticism model. Prior to exploring that model, it seems advisable to follow Merton's advice and explore the assumptions, range, and limitations of the behaviorist model, so that using a different model makes paradigmatic sense.

EVALUATION IN THE BEHAVIORIST MODEL

Evaluation is a tool: a means for determining merit or worth; a means for providing data or information; and a way to find clues and cues about progress, directions, performance, effectiveness, efficiency, achievement, or usefulness. It is a tool and a *means*. Unfortunately, when unwisely used, it becomes the *ends* instead of the means, and as the ends it surfaces as the energy system that drives the whole of education. In this event evaluation emerges as the most powerful aspect of curriculum and becomes to curriculum what money is to budgets and what budgets are to organizations: the driver, the engine. All else remains subservient. This subverts the purposes of education in a way that can undermine the very process of teaching and learning.

In the behaviorist curriculum, where the objectives are written so that they can be evaluated, it is inevitable that evaluation becomes the driver. If the behavior cannot be evaluated, if it is not observable or testable, it cannot be part of the curriculum. Then the content is chosen so that, when learned, it results in those behavioral changes described in the objectives. Then criteria are devised so that they describe what constitutes evidence of having demonstrated those behaviors (Bevis, 1988; Oliva, 1982; Morgan & Irby, 1978; Tyler, 1949). Based on this evidence, scores are established by a well-defined, quantifying formula and converted to a letter grade. Sometimes, if a student varies by as much as a half point, it can mean the difference between an A and a B (or, to be more dramatic, between a C and a D), which, when calculated as grade points, can greatly influence the student's future.

One can see how easily evaluation becomes the power in the behaviorist curriculum.

Table 1
The Traditional Steps Involved in
Evaluating Student Learning

First	Describe the desired behaviors
Second	Establish criteria for behavior
Third	Select content to cause behavior
Fourth	Observe student performance
Fifth	Interpret student performance
Sixth	Determine what constitutes evidence
Seventh	Convert evidence to numerical scores
Eighth	Convert numerical scores to letters
Ninth	Average course grades to form grade point average

Table 1 illustrates the number of levels of abstraction and manipulation the process undergoes in such an evaluation scheme. Note that each level is liable to many confounding variables and subsequent errors depending upon the tools used and the evaluation expertise of the teacher.

Were this formula limited to evaluating and grading the memorization of rules and rationale (training), it would have a greater possibility of being accurate. But when one is dealing with problems of higher-order learning, such as ways of thinking and approaching problems and values, seeing patterns and significance, and caring—it has so many limitations and confounding factors as to be suspect.

COMPARISON OF PARADIGMS

In order to provide a rationale for the creation of a different model, one must first review several points discussed in previous chapters.

Definitions

The first point of exploration is what constitutes learning. In the behaviorist paradigm learning is a change in performance. Gagne (1970) expresses the behaviorist position clearly when he states:

A learning event, then takes place when the *stimulus situation* affects the learner in such a way that *his performance* changes from a time *before* being in that situation to a time *after* being in it. The *change in performance* is what leads to the conclusion that learning has occurred. (p. 5)

He defines learning as:

a change in human disposition or capability, which can be retained, and which is not simply ascribable to the process of growth. The kind of change called learning exhibits itself as a change in behavior, and the inference of learning is made by comparing what behavior was possible before the individual was placed in a "learning situation" and what behavior can be exhibited after such treatment. (p. 3)

This definition is similar in character to most behaviorist definitions and has a beautiful consistency with the empiricist/quantitative position.

It is possible that definitions of learning vary with the type of learning being defined. For example, if one shifts ground from an empiricist position to a phenomenological/qualitative one, such as the educative-caring model proposed in this book, a different definition must be formulated. The one previously offered proposes that *educative learning be defined as a process in which an individual cultivates the disciplined scholarship and experiences necessary for expertise. This includes the following: acquiring insights, seeing patterns, finding meanings and significance, seeing balance and wholeness, making compassionate and wise judgments while acquiring foresight, generating creative flexible strategies, developing informed, skilled intentionality, identifying with the ethical and cultural traditions of the field, grasping the deeper structures of the knowledge base, enlarging the ability to think critically and creatively, and finding pathways to new knowledge.*

All of this provides a potential for behavioral change and growth. However, all learning does not result in behaviors or even in empirical clues to behaviors. Indeed, Stenhouse (1970) proposes that learning can be independent of any demonstration of its occurrence. (It is possible to detect some learning through observing a change in behavior or by contriving a situation in which changes in behavior can be manifested, but some learning is latent and surfaces at unexpected moments.) Furthermore, according to the assumptions of the paradigm suggested in this book, the only person who really knows what has been learned is the learner. Others get helpful and significant glimpses but not conclusive evidence. In the educative-caring paradigm, there is no such thing as conclusive evidence, because of the almost insurmountable difficulties in measuring intuition, insight, caring, compassion, reflection, creativity, or flexibility. Indeed, how can one be confident in his or her competence to evaluate the student's ability to see patterns, find meanings and significance, see balance and wholeness, identify with the ethical and cultural traditions of the discipline, and so on?

Positional Differences

A second dimension in exploration is one of the positional differences in evaluation models stemming from dissimilar world views. In Figure 1 contrasting positions in evaluation models are shown. This reveals how the world view influences the paradigm, which in turn dictates the type of learning to be evaluated, which indicates the methodology to be used.

Examining Figure 1 leads one to conclude that the world view is the factor that influences the choice of paradigm, the methodology used, and the types of learning to be evaluated. If that conclusion holds, then

Figure 1
Contrasting Positions Regarding Evaluation of Student Learning Models in Nursing Education

World View	
DUALISTIC/REDUCTIONISTIC	ORGANISMIC/HOLISTIC
Type Paradigm	
BEHAVIORIST/OBJECTIVES	EDUCATIVE/CARING HUMAN SCIENCE/HUMAN CARE
Type Methodology	
EMPIRICIST OBSERVATIONS OF BEHAVIOR WITH FEEDBACK	EXPERT CRITICISM THROUGH EXPERIENCE AND INTERACTIONS
Type Learning Appropriately Evaluated	
TRAINING	EDUCATION

the world view becomes the starting point for examining the issues involved.

WORLD VIEW

The differences in world-view-influencing evaluation models is essentially one of reductionism as required by behaviorism as contrasted with holism as required by human science. If educative learning involves finding meaning and significance in authentic personal experience, examining the deeper structures of the field of study, developing personal paradigm experiences and exploring ways to inquire into the nature of the field's phenomena, then learning is much more difficult to evaluate than merely establishing some behavioral standards and determining how close the student comes to meeting those behaviors. It is a contrast between evaluating the particulars, the parts and pieces, and criticizing the whole phenomenon as totality. As stated above, it is ultimately the distinction between reductionism and holism.

In reductionism the teacher, for both teaching and evaluation purposes, views the elements that must be taught and tests to determine that those parts have been learned. In holism the teacher, for both teaching and evaluation, views a gestalt, a whole, and a pattern of inter-related phenomena as a panorama that the student must find a way to learn and a way to criticize what has been learned. The shift from evaluation to criticism is a natural one. Munhall (1981), in speaking of the "scientific method" and the empiricist position (which can be equated to the behaviorist position), states:

> The scientist chooses what to study, then engages in a process of self-generated reductionism. By choosing an observable or measurable part of an individual's environment, the scientist sets limits on the problem. This is the first requisite of the scientific method. (p. 177)

She goes on to say, "Reality is reduced to the measurable and the empirical" (p. 177).

In contrast, when speaking of phenomenological approaches, which are more in keeping with the criticism model, Psathas (1973) addresses valuing enlargement rather than reduction and says that where economy is valued in quantitative methods, generosity is valued in phenomenological ones. In other words, as mentioned earlier, an enlarged world view—one of wholes, of scope, of gestalt—becomes necessary for phenomenologically based criticism.

TYPE PARADIGM

World view influences the type of paradigm to be used. If one's world view is reductionistic, one looks at individual behaviors, such as the ability to make a bed, check a blood pressure, and monitor a heart. But if the world view is holistic, one looks at those things as part of a whole—wholeness and balance in not only the *things* nurses do, but also in the way they think and feel. Wholeness also means using the nurse–patient environment as a whole. Professional nursing (as different from technical nursing) is a human science in contrast to a traditional science and therefore generates a different paradigm. Watson (1988) proposes using the term *human science*, borrowing from Giorgi (1970). Giorgi describes psychology as studying the person as a whole, contravening the psychoanalytic or behaviorist views of psychology that reduce to parts. The position taken here, as stated earlier, is that nursing can continue to use the behaviorist/objectives model for evaluating student learning of the technical aspects of nursing, just as it can profitably continue to use it for guiding student learning in that model. However, because of the difference in world view, a different model must be developed for an educative paradigm based on human science/human care.

TYPE LEARNING APPROPRIATELY EVALUATED AND THE SUBSEQUENT TYPE METHODOLOGY

There is a natural grouping of related positions illustrated in the two contrasting stances shown in Figure 1. This sequence of positions makes it apparent that the type of learning to be evaluated mandates the methodology to be used. Working backward from there, the type of paradigm arises from the world view and suggests the type of learning to be appropriately evaluated.

This means that if one is to evaluate a student's ability to give an injection, measure a dosage of medicine, or turn a patient with spinal surgery safely and painlessly, one can use behaviorist methods because these are learnings that result from training. They are mechanistic techniques for which there are prescribed specifications and checklists.

But if one is to evaluate a student's ability to deal with an irritable and screaming child, or to care for an anxious, preoperative person, or to exercise judgment in dealing with family members quarreling in the intensive care unit, or to use compassion and concern in working with a 28-year-old mother of four who has just learned she has metastatic cancer, or to handle any of thousands of daily nursing situations that do not lend themselves to rule-driven behavior, then one must have an alternative. The alternative must address education (contrasted with training) as the outcome of learning and choose or develop an evaluation methodology model that is consistent with education.

EVALUATION IN AN EDUCATIVE-CARING MODEL

The model offered here is the interpretive-criticism model. This model is not complete, nor is it the only feasible way to do *educational* evaluation. It is simply an offering, an attempt to help the teacher garner ideas from several sources, and an attempt to devise some means to determine student progress and learning. It is not expected that all problems of evaluating students will be solved, only a beginning examination of one of the ways that can be uncovered as educators once begin to explore the possibilities.

Some Issues and Problems

The issue of evaluation becoming the driver of the curriculum referred to earlier in this chapter is one of primary importance. Evaluation in the behaviorist/empirical model represents very real power and begins to occupy the time and energy of both teachers and students— teachers to make sure they are being "fair," and students to make sure they are not being too harshly judged. However, it is not the time and energy that are of most concern, for any good model is labor intensive; the energy will just be focused on a different modality. The significant issue is that in the presently sanctioned model, educational decisions about content and teaching methods are made around whether or not the content or processes to be taught or included in the curriculum can be evaluated with behavioral objectives and criteria, not around the worthiness of the principles or processes to be taught. For instance, orthodox behaviorist literature (Mager, 1977) expressly forbids the writing of objectives that cannot be behaviorally demonstrated, for example, words like *understanding, appreciation, insights,* and *feelings* are banned from the lexicon. Nursing approval and accreditation agencies have until recently had de facto rules that enforce Mager's injunctions. Most state boards of nursing have educational regulations that still do. Since much educative learning, as described in Chapter 4, is usually not expressed in behaviors, empiricist observations of behavior are inadequate to the task. A second important consideration that gets lost is that students do not learn to judge nursing care, or their own reasoning, scholarship, and growth using the behaviorist paradigm; they depend upon others to do it, primarily teachers. Since this places them in hierarchal relationships in teaching and learning, one of the aspects that gets reinforced in students is the anticipatory-compliant position on the learner maturity scale (see Chapter 4). Students attempt to find out what is going to be on a test and study for it; they learn what the criteria are by which they will be judged and how to meet those criteria regardless of how sound they may think the requisite behavior is. This supports students in the anticipatory-compliant position on the maturity continuum and ensures that they stay there, because if they do not, they fail.

Compliance is, of course, a two-way street. The student cannot assume the role of anticipatory-compliance without teachers who support that role. The role has a payoff for both teachers and students because teachers often take their sense of success from how well their students perform on tests. This encourages "teaching to the test." Teaching to the test is reasonable and paradigmatically correct for teachers using the behaviorist model, and the popular folkway in teaching culture that condemns it as "bad" is inconsistent with the framework of behavioral objectives. It seems incontrovertible that if one has specified objectives, and the evaluation must be geared to those objectives, and the content is chosen to insure the objectives are met, then it would be irresponsible *not* to teach to the test. This track ensures that learning is tunneled, it makes irrelevancies of engrossing side issues and areas or subjects of interest to students, and it therefore has no place for unintended outcomes.

Another problem inherent in the system is that in the traditional evaluation models, evaluation is made primarily for the purpose of determining merit or worth and is not used as a teaching opportunity. It is sometimes used to gather information for use in teaching or program improvement. Scriven (1967), in his classic article, coined the term *formative evaluation* (p. 43) for this interim process. The term was chosen by Scriven to describe the evaluation mentioned by Chronbach (1966) as "evaluation, used to improve the course while it is still fluid" (p. 236). It is also discussed by Saylor and Alexander (1974) and is usually used in reference to program evaluation. However, its common usage in evaluating learning in nursing education indicates evaluation performed during a course or learning activity, and the *information from the evaluation is then used to improve teaching in order to help students reach goals* (Bevis, 1988, p. 248).

The difference in what is being suggested here and in formative evaluation is that formative evaluation occurs during the process but is usually kept separate from the teaching itself, and the findings are used as after-the-fact feedback for teaching purposes. In the criticism model to be discussed later in this chapter, students are *engaged in* the process of criticism with teachers as one means of helping them learn to use knowledge and experience to make comparisons and to be critics. In other words, participatory criticism becomes a teaching–learning tool. The very activity of criticism helps students grow towards meeting standards and improving their expertise. Figures 2 and 3 illustrate this.

In this collaborative activity, criticism becomes a teaching–learning activity as well as an evaluative one. If one desires to use the term "formative evaluation" for this, it must be defined as including *evaluation as teaching opportunity.* This is consistent with the curriculum development model in that the position of teachers is that of expert learners—and co-learners—and evaluation is no longer a "test." Therefore, separation of evaluation and teaching no longer becomes necessary. The common practice in nursing education, especially clinical teaching, of attempting to keep a strict separation of teaching and evaluation springs from a research tradition as well as from the character of the behaviorist paradigm and is part of the mores of evaluators.

Under the behaviorist paradigm, one should not evaluate and teach at the same time. The reason lies in the nature of the relationship between teacher and learner. The threat of evaluation is natural to the relationship of teacher as the authority figure evaluating students who are the trainee-receivers of knowledge. Under these conditions, every

Figure 2
Traditional Model of Formative Evaluation

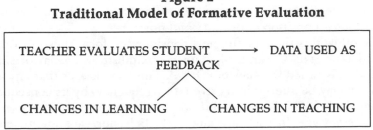

Figure 3
Model of Formative Criticism

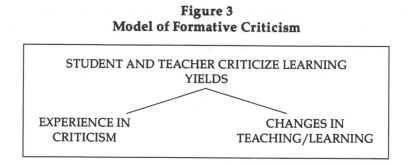

question the teacher poses becomes not an issue for discussion and exploration but a "test" question. The student feels that if he or she is not forthcoming with a "correct" answer, there will be a reckoning at final evaluation time. This may not be the intent of the teacher but is an inevitability because of the nature of the evaluation process under the behaviorist mode. It is very possible, even probable, that such separations and threatening "testing" interactions are not merely opportunities lost but are antithetical to the real process of education, which should involve becoming a discriminating connoisseur-critic (as later defined in this chapter) of good nursing care and a self-motivating colleague-learner.

Another similar chain of logic goes this way: If learning is defined as a change in behavior (the de facto definition in the behaviorist curriculum), and if the acceptable changes in behavior have been preselected and carefully described in behavioral terms, then, ipso facto, no learning has taken place unless those behaviors have been demonstrated. No learning is not quite accurate; actually one should say no learning that is deemed important to behaviorist evaluation or no learning that is visible has occurred. It follows that determining whether or not those specified behaviors are being attained becomes of primary importance both to teaching and to the curriculum. Since in the behaviorist model teaching's legitimate goal is to *mediate* the changes of behavior, evaluation assumes a position of primacy and power.

To follow this thought further, consider the focal thesis of operant conditioning. This keystone of all instrumentalism and behaviorism contains what is called the "law of effect." This "law" states that any act or behavior may be altered in its strength (frequency) by its consequences (Keller, 1969). This works well if one is intent upon students' *acquiring specific behaviors*. In such a framework, behaviors are identified and described, content is selected by its potential to bring about those behaviors, and written and performance tests are constructed to determine if the behavior is properly displayed. The traditional Tyler model lends itself well to a rigidly formulated evaluation scheme so that one evaluates to ascertain whether or not the student has achieved the specified outcomes.

If, on the other hand, learning is defined differently as proposed earlier in this chapter, then the issues in evaluating student learning change. Empiricism by nature is materialistic, and without material indicators one enters a different realm, one in which it is assumed that learning is independent of any demonstration of its occurrence (Stenhouse, 1970, p. 482). Furthermore, in the educative-caring model, unintended learnings assume great importance. Under these conditions, the rules change, and the evaluation decision scheme is laced with more than the usual uncertainty and ambiguity.

It is not my intent to condemn statistical inquiry and evaluation in itself, only to question its universal pervasiveness. Its uniform application to all forms of research and evaluation to the neglect of all other models is ultimately to discount other types as lacking rigor and being unscientific and invalid. To assert that statistical/empirical or objectives models provide the only fitting form of evidence limits the scope of our vision and prejudices our perception and criticism of the world of nursing. For nursing, like education, is a human science and as such differs substantively from other sciences in that it is less amenable to the certainties that are operative in the more concrete fields. This leads to the following posit: The more concrete the nursing content and processes being learned, the more appropriate are empiricist observations of behavior. The corollary is that the less concrete the content and processes being learned, the more appropriate is a criticism/connoisseurship model.

Assumptions Influencing the Model

Munhall (1981), in her classic article, "Nursing Philosophy and Nursing Research: In Apposition or Opposition," proposes that nursing identifies itself as humanistic and focuses on individuality and the belief that the actions of persons are to a large part free, in that humans act upon their experience and are therefore free to choose. In this way humans are active and self-determined. Furthermore, each human is integrated in such a way as to prevent "analysis by breaking him down into reducible parts and appending him back together again" (p. 176). She goes on to say that nursing philosophy further proposes that humans are an open system with unlimited capacity for growth and are autonomous. As such, the assumptions that underlie the study of humans must be different from those underlying the study of things. In other words, humans cannot be objects; they must be subjects, and when they are studied as objects, grave errors are made. The same may be said to apply to evaluation as well as to research. Watson (1988) articulated the basis for a human science context for nursing. Even though they are quoted elsewhere in this book, her remarks are worth reviewing. She is in agreement with Munhall when she says that a human-science context is based upon:

> A philosophy of human freedom, choice responsibility.
>
> A biology and psychology of holism (nonreducible persons interconnected with others and nature).
>
> An epistemology that allows not only for empirics, but for advancement of esthetics, ethical values, intuition, and process discovery.
>
> An ontology of time and space.
>
> A context of interhuman events, processes, and relationships.
>
> A scientific world view that is open. (p. 16)

Watson further states that

> if we view nursing as a human science, we can combine and integrate the science with beauty, art, ethics, and esthetics of the human-to-human care process in nursing. Human science is based upon an epistemology that can include metaphysics as well as esthetics, the humanities, art, and empirics. (p. 17)

She goes on to comment:

> As a human rather than a traditional science, nursing can view human life as a gift to be cherished—a process of wonder, awe, and mystery. Nurses can choose methods that allow for the subjective, inner world of personal meanings of the nurse and the other person. We can choose to study the inner world of experiences rather than the outer world of observation. We can choose to be a part of our method and involved in the clinical research process rather than be distant, objectively remote, and primarily concerned with the product of science. We can choose to pursue more of the

> private, intimate world of human care and inner subjective human experiences, rather than to concentrate on the public world of non-human cure techniques and outer behavior. (pp. 17–18)

Watson's words are as applicable to the evaluation of student learning as to research, for behavioral objectives as the guides to evaluation support a philosophy of evaluation that is reductionistic, mechanistic, control and predictive oriented, empirical, and manipulative. This framework seeks to manipulate subjects into behaving in predetermined ways. This is accomplished through using evaluation as feedback designed to cause changes in the organism (person) that conform or adapt to the behaviors assigned as desirable or necessary. If *adaptation* to a norm or to a pattern (as contrasted to integration, as discussed in Chapter 6) is the goal of education, then behaviorist forms of evaluation are exquisitely designed to that end and, as such, are tools of student training, not education. Furthermore, according to Freire (1976), they are oppressive.

What is being proposed here is that evaluation as known and practiced both in classrooms and clinically is consistent with training, and in training (e.g., item, directive, and rationale learning) the assumptions of empiricist philosophy hold. It is probably not the best model, but for the time being it is a workable one.

Munhall (1981) makes some further assumptions regarding empirical research that are applicable to evaluation. She states that empiricism assumes that:

1. Limits can be set on the problem of evaluation by choosing to evaluate only that which is observable and measurable.
2. Individuals are alike according to categories.
3. Experience is quantifiable.
4. Human and environmental constancy and passivity can be produced.
5. Reality can be reduced to the measurable and empirical.

The objectives model further assumes that:

1. Given the same or similar experiences, all students learn the same or similar things.
2. Learning always manifests itself in behavioral changes.
3. What the teacher identifies as desirable behaviors are the only ones worth evaluating and assigning grades to.

4. Students will take on faith that the prescribed behaviors are the desirable ones and strive to attain them.

5. Everything worth learning is in the legitimate curriculum and is reflected in the behavioral objectives.

Some of these assumptions, when placed in a comparative format, markedly demonstrate the differences (see Table 2).

These are only a few of the comparisons of assumptions that could be made, but they should be sufficient to illustrate the point. The curriculum models proposed by the behaviorist educators and those proposed by human science educators are different, not only in their perception and recommendations about how curriculum should be constructed and how students should be taught, but also in how learning should be assessed. The differences are so great that they can only be explained by the incompatible divergence in the assumptions that underlie the paradigms.

TOWARD A NEW EVALUATION MODEL

The theoretical model proposed in this section is a model for connoisseurship and interpretive-criticism to be used in evaluation of educative learning. It is a synthesis of ideas from Benner (1984), Eisner (1985), and Stenhouse (1975), mixed with a sauce of my own imagination and experience.

Since nursing is a caring, interactive, practice field with social responsibility, evaluation must be handled with great care. This is true because evaluators must first of all feel comfortable in the abilities of graduates to be safe. The problem is that safety may not be as behavioristically simplistic as it seems. Safety is more than performing the technical task without error and harm to the patient. Safety also resides in being able to depart rule-driven behavior quickly, to cut through distractors to the heart of a problem and to solve it creatively. In this way knowledge, understanding, insights, and intuition wisely used also determine safety. The attention of the evaluator must turn to those factors that provide clues to student learning and growth as an element of safety. Going beyond the objectives model requires grappling with the complex task of finding ways to assess or to find indicators of growth and learning. Therefore, the attempt here is not to reconcile the two philosophically antithetical paradigms, the empiricist/behaviorist and the educative-caring, but to develop a model for

Table 2
Comparison of Assumptions Underlying Evaluating Students

Technical Model	Professional Model
The only learning worth evaluating can be seen as behavioral changes	Worthwhile learning is often personal, obscure, and private. Only some learning appears as behavioral changes
Everything that exists, exists in some quantity and therefore can be counted and measured	Many things that exist are not empirically verifiable
The teacher-selected goals are the important, therefore the evaluated, ones	Both teacher- and student-selected goals are important, as is learning attained without goals
Every learner learns approximately the same things from the same or similar learning episode	Every learner learns something different from the same or similar learning episode
How well something is learned can be determined by comparing behaviors to objectively held criteria or comparing to the progress of other students	Educative learning cannot be rated on a scale; most learning cannot be compared either to some "objectively" conceived criteria or to the progress of other students
The teacher–student relationship is hierarchal and the teacher assigns grades to students by assigning value to what and how well they have met specific objectives	The teacher–student relationship is egalitarian; learning requires a process of trusting exploration among expert and novice learners and thrives on criticism, not grades
The quality or rigor of a course can be determined by how well it helps students meet the discipline requirements as reflected by test scores, attainment of behavioral objectives, NCLEX pass rates, and accreditation requirements, since these things reflect the agreed-upon discipline content	The quality or rigor of a course can be determined by how well it helps students collect paradigm experiences, develop insights, see patterns, find meaning in ideas and experiences, explore creative modes of inquiry, examine assumptions, form values and ethics in keeping with the moral ideal of the caring scholar-clinician, respond to societal needs, live fully, and advance the profession

educational interpretive-criticism as suggested by Stenhouse (1970, 1975), Raths (1971), Benner (1984), and Eisner (1985).

The First Step: A Change of Alliance

The evaluation problems emerge quite plainly when one diagrams the teaching–learning process from both the empiricist/behaviorist/ training point of view and the human–science/educational one. It is worthwhile therefore to review briefly the section on this from Chapter 6 ("Teaching and Learning"). In the behaviorist paradigm, the teaching–learning process (see Fig. 4) shows that the student stands alone, and the teacher is aligned with the content.

Since, in the behaviorist curriculum, the teacher is aligned with the content, the teacher is directed by the dictates of the content and is thereby content responsible. The learning activity is part of the teacher/content aspect and is created by the teacher in support of the attainment of specified behaviors that are eligible to be evaluated as learning. The teacher is the content priest, mediating between the content and the student. The teacher cannot reasonably move outside the dogma of the content for either legitimate teaching or legitimate evaluation (and, therefore, the hidden curricula, the illegitimate curricula, and the null curricula cannot be recognized). This sets up what obviously exists in traditional teaching–learning situations: an adversarial relationship between the student and the teacher/content. The students "do battle" with the content, and the teacher tries to *help the content* to be learned. This is the reason the relationships reflected in these figures are called "alliances."

View, on the other hand, Figure 5, in which the alliance shifts for the educative-caring paradigm.

In the educative paradigm, the student is liberated from contention with the content as represented by teacher-formulated behavioral objectives. This is not to decrease the importance of nursing content but to increase the importance of the students' role in their own lives. The teacher as co-learner creates an alliance between student and teacher in

Figure 4
The Teaching–Learning Process Alliance Diagram: Behaviorist

STUDENT	>	TEACHER/CONTENT	>	LEARNING

Figure 5
The Teaching–Learning Process Alliance Diagram:
Educative-Caring

STUDENT–TEACHER	>	CONTENT	>	LEARNING

which they tackle the subject matter together. They also may legitimately follow any other scholarly problems that emerge and that seem
of interest or importance.

The impact this has on the evaluation of learning is tremendous.
Evaluation in this case becomes a shared teacher–student activity. As
such, it shifts from empiricist-type evaluation to criticism in the classical
sense. To do this, evaluation must depart from the traditional mode of
examining student behaviors in isolation.

What can be put in its place? What is offered here is not a definitive
solution. It is an attempt to add a dimension that is consistent with the
new posture of nursing as a human science. For it to work, the teacher
as co-learner must rely more heavily on a trusting relationship with
students, one in which students are taught to be connoisseur-critics, as
later discussed. Teachers must find ways to have discourse with students that provide clues to learning. Discussions must be held that get at
what meanings students invest in experiences, what patterns they see
emerging in their nursing care, how they "know," and what type of
knowing they experience. Only then can teachers begin to help students critique their work and learning progress and determine a numer-
ical or letter grade.

As with any paradigm that seeks to evaluate human learning,
whether the behaviorist or the educative, there is much uncertainty and
ambiguity in the process. This is nothing new to the nurse-educator, to
whom unresolved issues are a part of daily experience; evaluation simply adds another portion of ambiguity and irresolution. But, whereas
common perception assumes that the greatest possible rigor lies in empirical evaluation, in fact all evaluation of educative learning is laced
with inaccuracy and uncertainty. However, the probability of achieving
greater clarity and accuracy is increased by the educative paradigm's
inclusion of learners in dialogue about their own learning. Teachers
who are willing to forego the false security of numbers and to accept
the inevitability of some uncertainty can use the positive aspects of the

involvement of learners in interpretation and criticism to achieve the goals of both teaching and evaluation.

The Second Step: Creating a New Model

A "new model" is never new. Three thousand years ago, Solomon wisely said that there is nothing new under the sun. New models come from a synthesis of ideas and procedures developed and tested by others. As stated earlier, the model proposed here melds the work of Benner (1984), Stenhouse (1975), and Eisner (1972, 1975a, b, 1985). The model is new only in the respect that it has not been devised in this form before. The model is only appropriate for use in curricula in which teachers perceive of themselves as expert co-learners with students and in which active learning is the primary teaching–learning modality.

Benner's research on excellence in clinical expertise, entitled *From Novice to Expert* (1984), can, if we allow it, make a remarkable impact on teaching and evaluation. In her preface she suggests that:

> Perceptual awareness is central to good nursing judgment and . . . this begins with vague hunches and global assessments that initially bypass critical analysis; conceptual clarity follows more often than it precedes. Expert nurses often describe their perceptual abilities using phrases such as "gut feeling," a "sense of uneasiness," or "feeling that things are not quite right." This kind of talk makes educators and clinicians uncomfortable, because the assessment must move from these perceptual beginnings to conclusive evidence. Expert nurses know that in all cases definitive evaluation of a patient's condition requires more than vague hunches, but through experience they have learned to allow their perceptions to lead to confirming evidence. (p. xviii–xix)

Benner's assertions could, without alteration, be said of evaluating students' clinical work when working in the educative/humanistic/ human–science paradigm. Even when using behavioral objectives as starting points for criteria for clinical evaluations, expert teachers use their perceptual awareness and educational judgment to perceive a gestalt, to attend to a "gut feeling," and then to seek evidence to substantiate what they know to be true. This is much more important to the teacher who depends upon criticism as the major form of evaluation.

Confirming evidence is often difficult to find and lies hidden beneath layers of preconceived notions about what the data must be, for example, that the student may be able to succeed in spite of the teacher's "gut feeling" that the student is not learning the aspects of nursing that are ultimately the mark of a professional nurse. Yet the evidence is hard to find, because one is looking for a failure to produce the correct "rationale" or the inability to produce the correct response. Confirming evidence often comes more easily once one moves beyond item, directive, and rationale learning. This evidence would be found in the criticism of learning in the categories of syntax, context, and inquiry. What might be uncovered in critical dialogue is a lack of insight, compassion, ethical awareness, flexibility, or the simple ability to perceive patterns. But unless teachers have conviction that these elements of nursing mark the educated professional, there will be no consideration of them as significant for determining worth or merit in the process of progressing from lay person to novice nurse.

Benner's (1984) proposal is a radical departure from traditional ways of viewing nursing practice, and, when used as a component of an evaluation paradigm, it becomes revolutionary. However, to be consistent with the basic assumptions and tenets of the paradigm, a departure from behaviorist evaluation is needed. Benner's work is based upon that of Heidegger (1962), Polanyi (1962), and Dreyfus and Dreyfus (1980), among others. Her work, essential as a component to any new consideration of a paradigm shift in nursing, provides some rich material appropriate to a model for interpreting and criticizing learning. The following ideas are gleaned from Benner's (1984) book:

- Students are taught context-free rules as guides to action, yet these rules are inflexible and limited. Following the rules decreases the chances for successful performance because rules cannot divulge what is relevant in an actual situation.[1]

- Paradigm experiences (called "cases" by Benner) form a rich tapestry of experience that enables comparing and contrasting circumstances, situations, conditions, and nursing care. This helps the nurse to describe and interpret behavior or care and to understand it.

- Students have limited experiences and therefore lack the richness necessary to a multifaceted interpretation of new situations. Yet, even with this limitation experiences have meanings.

---

[1] This creates a bind, at least in the mind of the student and sometimes in the mind of the instructor. If they follow the rules and the rules are inappropriate in the present contextual reality, they lack judgment; if they fail to follow the rules, then they lack a theoretical basis for practice. The bind diminishes as students gain paradigm experiences on which to base nursing care.

- To understand and interpret behavior, one must look at the larger context—practical knowledge must be studied holistically.

- The interpretive approach inevitably relies on the context of the unique situation, that is, the timing, meanings, and intentions. These must be richly described.

- The possible interpretations of a nursing act or situation are limited, usually to one or two "best" interpretations, because in rich descriptions the meaning of the "situation is maintained rather than stripped away to objectified, context-free traits or behaviors" (p. 40).

- Connoisseurship has as aspects descriptive and interpretive recording of recognitional abilities, context, meanings, characteristics, and outcomes.

- Connoisseurship is the natural outcome of comparisons of judgments of qualitative distinctions in actual nursing care situations.

- Connoisseurship enables nurses to refine their skills and demonstrate qualitative distinctions that they have learned to recognize. (p. 40)

Benner offers some interesting insights into the necessity of rich descriptions, the development of connoisseurship, and interpretation. If we are to develop connoisseurship in students, we must alter the substance and form of the teacher–student relationship so that the teacher is allied with the student and not with the content (see Fig. 5).

Stenhouse (1975) is in accord with this position and proposes that the teacher who shifts from authority person to co-learner ("expert learner," as he calls it) must simultaneously shift from evaluation and grading to "criticism." He says criticism rests on trust, and trust is the basis of the co-learner position as teacher. As a basis for criticism, Stenhouse supports Raths' (1971) concepts of standards or principles of procedure, as discussed in Chapter 7. He suggests that these principles of procedure could be used as standards for judging teaching. If so, is there not also an implication that they could be used to critique learning by the dynamic duo that is now the alliance of teacher–expert learner and student–novice learner? I think it possible that some ideas for criticism could be derived from these criteria.[2]

Stenhouse credits Mann (1969) with initially influencing his ideas about criteria. Mann, in the same paper in which he addresses the nature of criteria, speaks of the function of criticism as being *to disclose*

---

[2]Used here are Murray and Merrefield's (1988) criteria for teacher–student interactions and for selecting or devising learning activities.

meanings and illuminate answers (p. 29). The ideas offered by Stenhouse and Mann are consistent with Eisner's ideas, except that Eisner makes a clear distinction between connoisseurship and criticism. Benner and Eisner call connoisseurship what Stenhouse and Mann include in the idea of criticism.

Thus, we move easily into Eisner's connoisseurship and criticism as a possible model for evaluating learning. It is consistent with Benner's "expertise" that rests on experience and moves from "gut feelings" to confirmation. The marriage of these works with other ideas may make a beginning for a new model for nursing evaluation.

CONNOISSEURSHIP

The process of criticism, as this section will reveal, revolves around *connoisseurship*. To be a connoisseur, one must be an expert, an expert in both nursing content and in the processes of the educated mind, in learning. This means that in order to be a good critic/connoisseur, the teacher must have an expert's grasp of the following:

1. The meaning of experience in the field.
2. The deeper structures of the subject.
3. The history and historically significant issues of the field.
4. Both the classical and the current literature of the field.
5. The characteristics of the educated expert nurse.
6. The educative processes that shapes the expert professional nurse.
7. The modes of inquiry appropriate to the field.

This expertise is important because the judgments made by the expert—the teacher—are the criticism that must stand accountable for the rigor and for the quality care that must be provided the public. In the "best of all possible worlds," this accountability would be a shared one. Even in this not-so-best of worlds, every attempt must be made to make it a shared one—both for "formative" and "summative" criticisms. However, in the final analysis, the teacher is accountable to society and to the college or university for decisions regarding the merit of student learning.

One difficult issue that all nursing teachers must face is that although most merit decisions can be collaborative with students, it is usually the student with the least ability, the most immaturities, and the greatest deficits who also has little insight into the merit of his work. These students have great difficulty in learning the art of criticism and often have equal difficulty in all educative learning categories. It then falls to the teacher to exercise the accountability role necessary to the present academic system.

EXPERTISE AND EXPERIENCE

As mentioned, the descriptions, interpretations, comparisons, and judgments that mark the connoisseur require an expert. Only experts have the experiences that form the basis for connoisseurship. This means that in order to be a nursing educational connoisseur, the teacher must be an expert both in learning-education and in nursing practice. Herein lies the secret to all aspects of a new professional educational paradigm for nursing, because without this expert teacher-practitioner, the keystone is missing, and the paradigm collapses. Of course this is also true of the behaviorist paradigm. But behavioral objectives act as a crutch and obscure the key role of teacher-practitioner expert and give the appearance of a "teacher-proof" curriculum. In the professional educational paradigm, the teacher must be a connoisseur of both the scholarly processes and good nursing care. Connoisseurship itself is a complex level of expertise, and the model requires not only expertise but also some effort in learning how to use criticism as an evaluative tool and in teaching that process to the co-learners who are the students. There is a certain degree of humility inherent in the shared process of educational criticism that is absent when the teacher, using behavioral criteria as an absolute standard, *measures* a student's performance against that standard. By contrast, humility comes in the act of seeking together to find ways to see, describe, render, interpret, and judge nursing care. The object is not whether or not something is "right" or "wrong," but seeking ways to improve. It is a process of the teacher who, having the experiences in teaching, learning, and nursing necessary to comparisons, helps the student build up experiences and tune the senses to perceive the elements that constitute good care. This is the reason that it is both an evaluative and a learning process.

It is the very lack of experience on the part of students that handicaps them in developing "taste" and sophistication in perceiving and interpreting events of care. It is this deficit that supports the position that perhaps training should precede education in the nursing curriculum. If matters of technique and procedure can be learned during the first year of a professional program, and if the item and rule learning can be focused upon early, then perhaps the art of criticism can be taught concurrently with rationale, syntax, context, and inquiry learning. It seems evident that the practice of nursing skills will begin to provide an experience tapestry against which connoisseurship can be developed.

In support of this, it might be profitable to review what was said in Chapter 4. Peters (1966) distinguishes between "knowing how" and "knowing that." He contends that "knowing how" (skills) does not have a wide-ranging cognitive content and requires a knack rather than understanding. But the important distinction he makes is that what there is to know about a skill throws very little light on much else. In other words, it is not very widely generalizable. By contrast, in any field "knowing that" requires one to know an immense amount, and if that knowing is properly assimilated, it constantly illuminates countless other fields, experiences, and things (it is widely generalizable). This seems to be a sound rationale for placing emphasis upon critiquing those aspects of a field that are categorized as "knowing *that*" while allowing the aspects of learning categorized as "knowing *how*" to be treated as skills and behaviorally evaluated. It is easy to equate "knowing *how*" with the three training types of learning in the learning typology and "knowing *that*" with educative types of learning (see Fig. 6).

There are dangers in teachers attempting to switch from a behaviorist framework with teacher as authority-evaluator to an interpretive-criticism model with teacher as co-learner/co-critic. It is an almost impossible switch, since the two roles arise from such disparate philosophical positions. The behaviorist-evaluator role is one that places the teacher in a power position. The teacher has totalitarian power over students' grades and, therefore, can make or break a career choice. It is such power that often undermines the trust relationship. For the critic relationship to be successful, power must be shared.

Figure 6
"Knowing How" as Training and "Knowing That" as Education

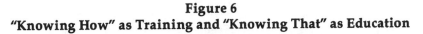
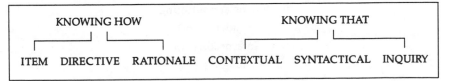

INTERPRETIVE-CRITICISM: EDUCATIONAL CONNOISSEURSHIP—A WAY TO CRITIQUE STUDENT LEARNING

This is a modified version of the Eisner model of educational connoisseurship. The interpretive-criticism model is a student–teacher collaborative model composed of six parts: looking, seeing, perceiving and intuiting, rendering, interpreting, and judging (see Table 3). These parts must not be conceived as a linear process in that each aspect must proceed in a specific sequence. No one thinks in linear fashion, and of course no critical scheme can possibly be that unidirectional. Furthermore, in a liberated, caring, and educational model, the process is shared among students and teachers so that not only does the flow go back and forth among the aspects of the model, but it also swirls around the scholars in rich discussions that enhance the perceptions and comparisons and help to check out intuition's quiet but persistent voice.

Eisner believes that there is a vital difference between connoisseurship and criticism. According to Eisner (1985), connoisseurship is the art of appreciation. It is more than knowing how to look; it is how to see. And in what one sees, it is to be able to distinguish the significant and important from the trivial. Moreover, it recognizes the qualities of the unique and particular. It is not that the connoisseur does not generalize by classifying, but that he or she goes beyond those generalizations and is not misled or blocked by the pre-sets that generalizations often beget. A connoisseur goes further than the generalizations or classifications by perceiving the unique attributes of phenomena that distinguish one thing from another even within a category. This requires a knowledge of how to look and see and further to appreciate what are subtle, important qualities and characteristics.

Table 3
Interpretive-Criticism Model

Looking

Seeing

Perceiving and intuiting

Rendering

Interpreting

Judging

Eisner believes connoisseurship to be a private act. He maintains that, unlike criticism, it does not require a public judgment or public description of those qualities that have been perceived. He maintains that criticism is the public rendering of the connoisseur's insights and that connoisseurship is private and requires an experienced sensory memory that has the flavor of expertise: a sensory memory that enables comparing and contrasting to a backdrop of imagined perfection based on a composite experientially based picture. Eisner (1985) calls this "knowledgeable perception" (p. 219) and proposes that one can be a connoisseur without being a critic, but one cannot be a critic without being a connoisseur.

This position misses the mark. The issue is that criticism and connoisseurship are publicly acquired skills. These skills exist as an activity that goes on in the world, not only in the privacy of one's inner self. As a public practice, they become one flowing activity: the connoisseurship of experience and taste linked with criticism, which implies the use of criteria, models, and guiding principles (such as internal consistency, consistency with examples, relevance, etc.).

It would be misleading students to suggest that they can, while being students, have enough experience to become connoisseurs. What they can do is begin an apprenticeship in the art of perception, appreciation, and comparing that will become connoisseurship as they become more experienced. This connoisseurship has in it all the elements of criticism, and, although it may not be publicly acclaimed, it is put to public use because it alters the way the nurse proceeds with care. Both connoisseurship and criticism can be invaluable in the live world of nursing work in that the nurse becomes a finely tuned gourmet of nursing care, always using that exquisite palate to improve quality.

In the interest of illuminating the model, each aspect will be discussed separately.

Looking

Looking is different from seeing. Looking is simply viewing. Eisner (1985) calls it a "task one undertakes" primarily to classify; it is seeing that it is an achievement (p. 220). Looking is not demanding nor does it require attending to. It is a simple physical act. One can put a parcel of trash by the door to be taken out expecting the spouse to *see* it and take it on the way out. But the spouse may *look* at the trash for several days and not *see* it. The spouse may even step over or around the trash to get out of the door and still not be aware of its presence.

Seeing

Seeing is looking with attention and focus. Seeing is attending to the details, the context, the situation, the environment, the parts, and the whole. It is an interesting experience to take several students into the room of an ill person either in a home or in a hospital, then, once outside the room, ask them separately, out of each other's hearing, what they saw. Seeing is centered, highlighted, and directed. It is *recognition* of what one is looking at. The students will have recognized different elements in the ill person's room.

Perceiving and Intuiting

Perceiving and intuiting are sensing and interpreting on a personal level. By that is meant interpreting the stimuli of seeing, not interpreting in a larger sense of what meaning is in what is perceived. Perception is a step beyond recognition. According to Eisner (1985), "Perception based on recognition alone stops with assigning the particular to the class to which it belongs" (p. 220). It does not go on to do what is necessary to connoisseurship: explore the specific, subtle differences and similarities of this unique and particular with its general class. Looking, focusing on classification, or use of a specific framework can prejudice and mislead in a human science because human beings are not so easily classified without losing the unique attributes of the difference that is the special emphasis of freedom. Intuitive perception must go beyond categorical limitations. This is not to imply that categories are useless—far from it—but we must not be limited by them.

For example, the whole concept of *caring* implies appreciating the individuality of each person and event. Caring is the moral imperative of both nursing and teaching, and the very definition of caring implies caring for the *unique* and *distinctive* needs of each human and caring about a person's special qualities because, like Mt. Everest, they are there. It becomes a part of the ethical system of nursing, then, to teach attending to the unique and particular attributes both of persons and of situations.

Perception translates looking and seeing into experience. If we are helping students learn the art of criticism, the words of Eisner (1985) are worth remembering: "Criticism can be only as rich as the critic's perceptions" (p. 237). Perception, to be useful, must be intuitive and imaginative. Perception without intuition makes it difficult to grasp wholes or at least to relate the parts in ways that make it easy to quickly and easily assimilate an organismic sense of meanings in situations. This involves the ability to perceive what is significant and what is trivial in a situation, a judgment that can only be made in the light of experience. Once a nursing aide was told to take the blood pressure and pulse every 15 minutes of a woman postdelivery of twins and to report any significant changes. When the nurse returned 2 hours later, the woman was in deep irreversible shock. The aide had dutifully taken the blood pressure and pulse and recorded it on the appropriate record. She did not know that it was significant that the blood pressure was constantly dropping and the pulse concomitantly rising. This is an extreme example from a true event where the aide, a new trainee, had insufficient experience to recognize significance. One reason that the Eisner model is so excellent is that it enriches the opportunities for engaging students in examining the significance of what they see, that is, educating their perception.

Benner (1984) says that experts often start perceiving a situation with a "gut feeling" or intuition. Arieh Issar, the Israeli hydrogeologist who discovered the Nubian Sandstone Aquifer in the Negev Desert with no hard evidence of its existence, said:

> Somewhere along the line you jump a few steps and come to a conclusion. It's dangerous; you always have to calculate the steps back. But you must make that leap into the dark. If scientists become technologists, they'll degenerate. They must be philosophers too. (Hazelton, 1979, p. 19)

Issar, being a scientist, may call it philosophy, but no euphemism can mask the fact that it was intuition that led him to the idea of a sandstone aquifer, and Israel expended millions of dollars on water exploration on the educated intuitive guess of an expert. Intuition is not merely a guess based on facts. It goes beyond facts into metaphysics. Some call it an educated guess; probably this is because experts in a field develop a sort of "sixth" sense about things in their field. Expert nurses can walk onto a unit with which they are familiar and almost instantly sense that something is wrong. Similarly, mothers and fathers can often exercise keen intuition when dealing with their children. Intuition can be based on facts/data but goes so far beyond the data as to defy logical explanation.

Teaching students to attend to their "guts," their intuition, has long been anathema to nursing. In our search for recognition and status through "science," nursing faculty in academia have discounted intuitive knowing and adjured students not only to avoid relying on it, but to refuse to admit using it at all. One of the worst evaluation statements a teacher could make about an aspiring student in the 1950s through the 1970s was that the student relied on intuition rather than scientific rationale for making nursing care decisions. The goal should not be the substitution of one for the other but the development of many ways of knowing without limiting the legitimate ways to the empirical (see Chapter 5). To develop apprentice connoisseurs, teachers must help students enhance their perceptive powers and attend to their intuition. Then, in the words of Issar, teachers should attempt to help them "calculate the steps back." In this way the perceptions become amenable to descriptions.

Rendering

Rendering is a way of describing the ineffable. According to Kozloff (1969, p. 10), who coined this term for describing the indescribable, *rendering* is an account of the interaction between a work of art and the response of the viewer. A response is a feeling, and feelings are not amenable to descriptions that aspire to be accurate accounts of *actual* events or experiences. A rendering has *virtual* rather than actual meaning and depends upon symbolic language.

Connoisseurship and criticism demand elucidation. In education, critics must render a situation in language that is not language to begin with but experience and reactions to experience. The language used for this must be the qualitative language of metaphor, simile, analogy, and allegory. It is not evaluative but evocative and, therefore, is powerful in its ability to communicate in thick, rich imagery.

It is one thing to say simply, "When I arrived the room was a mess and smelled bad. The patient felt alone and neglected." It is quite another to say:

> When I arrived everything seemed out of place, it seemed that a dump truck had backed up to the room junking it with all the old used equipment and linen from a week's collecting of the hospital's hampers and bins. The place smelled of ammonia like a neglected cat litter box; the blinds were closed, as was the door, and though the day was not dark the room was oppressive and heavy, like before a storm. The patient lay staring unfocused at the images in her own world, withdrawn and unavailable as if she were an abandoned house with a vacancy sign on the lawn. She whimpered with the neglect of a stray dog. I felt enraged: at the family, at the system, at

the selfish brutality of our treatment of the aged. It is as if we owe them no fealty, no recognition for their contribution to the present.

This is a rendering, laced with metaphor, simile and imagery, pregnant with meaning, and ready for interpretation.

Rendering of this type is antithetical to the behaviorist paradigm in which evaluators are taught to stay to the facts that are observable and to avoid any feelings or subjectivity at all. Benner (1984), in discussing her "interpretive" approach, has the following to say:

> Thus to understand specific meaning of any behavior (or nursing care measure), one must know the specific context, and knowing the context inherently limits the possible meanings of behavior into manageable and relevant wholes. With an interpretive approach, the intentions and understanding of the participants are taken into consideration and seen as dependent on a shared world of meanings. For example, intentions and empathy are a personal expression of the participants in a situation. Once described, however, they are clear to those who share the same background meanings. That is, the participants can talk about them, and the interpreter who shares their knowledge and experience base can understand them. (p. 40)

In this way the "meaning of the situation is maintained rather than stripped away to objective, context-free traits or behaviors" (Benner, 1984, p. 40). The criticism model is similar in many respects to Benner's interpretive model.

The criticism model, therefore, relies on situation-based, rich descriptions that are context rooted, that expand rather than reduce, show feelings and interactions rather than deleting them, enrich information with subjectivity, present a whole, and are laced with metaphor and poetics. This would not be possible in an empiricist/behaviorist model, but the criticism model allows interpretations that are more accurate because they are context and content laden.

Good rendering is often poetic and at the very least excellent and attractive prose. Poetics is becoming increasingly recognized as a phenomenological method. Heidegger (1975) speaks of poetizing as the voice of the experiential phenomenologist. Watson (1988) says it beautifully: "Indeed, when a phenomenologist is true to the depths of the moving human experience, he or she almost naturally poetizes" (p. 92). She goes on to say:

If we are to consider this deep level of phenomenology, that is beyond pure descriptions, and allow for the transcendental experience as both felt and expressed through poetic language, then we have to give up the correspondence theory of truth and adapt the aletheia theory of truth which is associated with discovery of the unknown, or unconcealment. We also have to abandon the notion of "descriptive" as well as "factual," "quantitative" truth that simply corresponds to facts and figures. The human science and art of nursing and human care, which is indeed transpersonal, must incorporate feeling, depth of experience, and transcendental processes that result in poetic expression; that moves us toward authentic experiential expression and helps us maintain openness with our humanism and our potential for growth. Finally, transcendental phenomenology also reminds us that as nurses, in either practice or research efforts, we are first of all human beings, capable of transcending the moment, capable of engaging in a truly felt experience, emerging from that experience with a desire for self-expression while still being capable of maintaining contact with the original, spontaneous thrust of the experience. (pp. 92–93)

Watson's advocacy of poetic language in phenomenological discourse and research strikes the right note for its use in rendering the marriage of experience and response. There is sufficient similarity in the poetics of transcendental phenomenology and the "renderings" of criticism to apply her words to this topic.

Krall (1981) presents an understated case for poetizing as inquiry in his article "Navajo Tapestry: A Curriculum for Ethno-ecological Perspectives." The article itself is narrative taken from his journal made during a class he gave on the interrelationships between the Navajo and their reservation environment. His journal excerpts are rich, thick, renderings of lived experience. He uses as theoretical support for his methods Pinar and Grumet (1976), Eisner (1975a, b), McCutchen (1979), and Spradley and McCurdy (1972). He says that his "efforts toward interpretation and appraisal (if, indeed rendering can be considered appraisal as McCutchen suggests) are offered with full realization of the personal and subjective orientation of my view." His aim is "to make that view, rooted in my personal biography, passion, values, and justifications as clear as possible to the reader and to myself." His article is rife with disclosure and the metaphor, simile, and rhythm of poetry.

Pinar and Grumet (1976), whom Krall uses as theoretical support, speak of a strategy of existential experiential disclosure that enables one to view an experience more clearly. McCutchen (1979) addresses educational criticism as a process of inquiry between the critic and the educational phenomenon and says it must include appraisal and interpretation as well as illuminative descriptions. She also discusses the use of comparisons. Comparisons by experts are the basis of both Benner's (1984) and Eisner's (1985) concepts of criticism.

When rendering an experience and one's response to that experience, one need not be logical or objective (unbiased). In fact, such renderings are often illogical and biased. When one leaves the world of empirical evaluation, one may abandon, in at least this aspect of criticism, the need for reductionistic objectivity. The subjectivity of lived experience is inescapable.

Polanyi and Prosch (1975) say it well:

> Thus the ideal of pure objectivity in knowing and in science has been shown to be a myth. It is perhaps a harmless myth if most of its implications are not followed out, but it is certainly a poisonous one if they are. For the implication that the truth about human behavior demands an amoral standpoint is, as we have seen, part of what our moral inversions have been made of. (p. 63)

In this same vein Eisner (1985) says, "The essence of perception is that it is selective; there is no value-free mode of seeing. In seeking renderings, subjectivity is not only unavoidable, it is desirable for it must make public the private world of perception" (p. 222).

Interpreting Meaning

Polanyi and Prosch (1975) state, "Man lives in the meanings he is able to discern. He extends himself into that which he finds coherent and is at home there" (p. 66). They speak of "meaning" being sought through explanation and explanation being a means to get relief from puzzlement. They further offer the consideration that, given an experience that finds no coherence in the belief system of the individual, the explanations may deny the objective clues and find expression as an explanation that imaginatively fits the belief system.

An example is the official denial of the existence of unidentified flying objects. I once stood in the street with two neighbors and viewed such an object. A ball with comet tail of energy-simmering light fairly close to earth hovered for a while and then took off at about a 45-degree angle, going out into the distant, clear California summer sky. I said, "Wow, a UFO!" They, a father and son, said, "That's not a UFO, they don't exist!" I then asked what they thought it was. They started on an imaginative search for other explanations: explanations that denied the behavior and appearance of the object. It was an interesting experience that verified Polanyi and Prosch's claims that people live in and with meanings they are able to discern and seek for coherence. The UFO did not fit—it was not coherent with the belief systems my neighbors held, and so other meanings were sought. This kind of selective perception is reminiscent of Brilliant's (1979) poem "Seeing is Believing":

> I wouldn't
> have seen it
> if I hadn't
> believed it.

Meanings are individual and personal, and they must have congruence with the person's experience, belief system, rationality, expectations, and the context of the event.

Context assumes great significance in uncovering meaning. Eisner and Benner agree on this point: "To discern what an event means requires an understanding of the context in which it occurs; that context requires not only some knowledge of the people involved and the circumstances within which the event occurs, but in many situations also something about the past, against which the particulars of the present can be placed. Again, memory is indispensable" (Eisner, 1985, p. 222).

Benner's (1984) research on the levels of competency in clinical nursing practice uses an interpretive approach. She maintains that in the interpretive approach, synthesis, not analysis, is used. She maintains that one can only understand a part as it is an aspect of a whole, and the interpretations of meaning are from the context in which the part is found. She contends, as does Eisner, that to "understand behavior, therefore, one must look at it in its larger context." The interpretation of an event includes the intentions, timing, and understandings of the participants (p. 40). She goes on to say, "once the context of the actual situation is described, the number of possible interpretations or meanings is limited" (p. 40). She believes this is due to the rich descriptions required (what are called "renderings" here). In rendering one does not strive for objectivity, which would rob the interpretation of the contextual traits of the situation.

Interpretation and meaning are part of the syntactical category of learning. In syntax one looks at wholes, broad relationships, insights, and patterns, and finds or seeks the meanings. Only until some meaning is found can an experience become a paradigm experience. Meaningless experiences are seldom retained to form a tapestry for future reference.

Erickson (1986), in speaking of interpretive social research, makes reference to the influence of culture on interpreting meaning. He states that a shared culture often makes humans seem to have similar meaning interpretations. But, he says, "these surface similarities mask an underlying diversity; in a given situation of action one cannot assume that the behaviors of two individuals, physical acts with similar form, have the same meaning to the two individuals" (p. 126). He suggests that when possibility and probability are present meaning interpretations of similar behavior-action will differ. He places great importance on meaning interpretation because, in his view, people take action on the basis of their interpretations of the actions of others. If this is true, then meaning interpretation is causal (p. 127). This adds an important component to interpretive criticism.

Therefore, in examining meaning for criticism, two kinds of meanings must be uncovered. The first is the meaning of events or experiences or their interpretation for reasons of critiquing care. The second is the personal meanings they import for the learner. The meaning for nursing care is dependent upon exposing the personal meanings, for unlike behaviorist evaluation where only the processes and products bear examining for evaluation purposes, in the interpretive-criticism model, the motives, intentions, and events are interpreted from the renderings. Meanings emerge against a backdrop of other experiences, and the more experiences acquired, the more complex become the pathways to meaning.

Meanings are also a product of expertise. Understanding an event from thick descriptions or renderings must be sought from a point of knowledge, not ignorance. Comparisons are made by experts using an abundant library of similar or relevant experiences and an understanding of the theory of their discipline. Interpretations are as dependent upon the knowledge and expertise of the critics as upon the renderings of the participants. It is this that underlines the importance of the teacher as *expert* learner and, as such, as guide to novice learners in interpretations.

Judging

Judging is the evaluation aspect of the interpretive-criticism approach. In this aspect, the critic attempts to determine the value or importance of the episode or experience to education, its significance within the overall scheme. This requires the application of criteria so that judgments are "grounded in some view of what counts within an educational perspective" (Eisner, 1985, p. 238). To make good judgments requires two things: experience in learning and nursing so that one may have a context for the comparisons necessary to judgment, and knowledge about the theories and content of the fields of teaching and nursing so that the judgments are grounded in the reality of nursing and learning. Even if one has criteria, the way the criteria are used and the judgments are made must rest on comparisons and knowledge. Were it not so, any observer could make judgments on the prima facie evidence of objective behavior and expect to be fair in those judgments. It would be naive to ignore the absolute necessity of teachers who are expert learners and expert nurses participating in the process so that students may become critics of their own scholarship and their own nursing care.

What then of objectives? As previously discussed, objectives as specified behaviors are not used in the educative aspects of the curriculum paradigm and therefore do not exist for use in evaluation. Goals or ends-in-view exist and are useful. General goals or ends-in-view of the course or learning activities being evaluated act as part of the material used as criteria for evaluation. However, much may have been learned that was not chosen or anticipated by the teacher as important or possible. Scriven (1972) addresses "goal free evaluation" in discussing program evaluation. His point that unintended achievements can be just as important as intended ones is well made. Therefore, evaluation must not be limited by the goals but can be guided by them in part.

The problem immediately arises of other standards or criteria. From where are they obtained, and who is responsible for compiling them? To answer those questions, we must reconsider the basic theme of this proposal for a new paradigm for professional nursing curriculum development. That theme is this: Curriculum basically is what transpires between students and teachers and among students with the intention that learning occurs. What transpires is governed by two things: (1) the character and quality of the teacher–student interactions and (2) the type of learning activities that engage students. If that is so, then the basic task of the faculty in developing curriculum is to devise a list of criteria for guiding teacher–student interactions or transactions and a second list of criteria for selecting or generating learning activities. These two lists, then, become some of the criteria used in the judgment phase of the interpretive-criticism model. The list for teacher–student interactions is most useful for evaluating teaching and for ascertaining how students respond to teachers. The list of criteria for learning episodes or experiences is helpful in judging nursing and learning. The content of the course can form the basis for a third set of criteria or standards.

One must remember that the criteria are not used to judge the *behavior* of the student from teacher observations. Judgments, in this model, are made conjointly with students and are based on the process of the looking, seeing, perceiving, intuiting, rendering, and interpreting that must precede judging. Judging that takes place before the teacher–student dialogue succeeds in building thick renderings based on perceptions and interpreted for meanings inevitably reverts to behaviorism and insidiously sabotages the whole paradigm. As long as one continues to make evaluative judgments based upon "changes" of behavior, the paradigm remains behaviorist no matter what else has altered in it.

The criteria themselves, created as guides for selecting and devising learning experiences, do not address directly the issue of student performance, but they provide clues about what kinds of learning are valued in the curriculum. So, the criteria for critiquing student learning is implied in these criteria. For example, the Murray and Merrefield criteria (1989) provided in Appendix I supply the following examples. The numbers reference the numbers in the appendix. Only three are used as examples.

CRITERIA FOR LEARNING EXPERIENCES

6. Makes clear that the critique of the student's work is the valued part of the learning process.
7. Creates a cognitive dissonance that requires the student to engage in educative heuristics such as reflection, incubation, dialogue, debate, imagining, hypothesizing to approach the resolution of the dissonance.
8. Requires the student to practice creative approaches to the subject matter.

If one were to use criteria 6–8, a judgment discussion might follow that would involve the teacher and student in examining the rendered descriptions together in an attempt to determine what cognitive dissonance was experienced, what educational heuristics were used and how well they worked, what other heuristics might have been used and what might have been gained by their use, and what other experiences in criticizing care they have had that might be useful here as comparison and guide. The dialogue can continue until both student and teacher think the subject is exhausted for its worth in learning.

In speaking of using the criteria of our example, it was stated that critical dialogue continues until it is exhausted for its *worth in learning*. Criticism exists for the purpose of supporting improvements, not for marking. The educative-caring paradigm rests on criticism, not on grading. Stenhouse (1975), in commenting about his "process" model of curriculum states, "The process model is essentially a critical model, not a marking model. It can never be directed towards an examination as an objective without loss of quality, since the standards of the examination then override the standards immanent in the subject" (p. 95).

He also proposes that there is a conflict of demand between appraisal as teaching and appraisal as grading. His process model, an attempt to offer a better alternative to teachers than the behaviorist model, is similar in some respects to the humanist educative model, especially in the role of evaluation in the paradigm. In commenting about objective examinations, he says, "The more objective an examination, the more it fails to reveal the quality of good teaching and good learning."

Criteria, or standards, need not all arise from the two lists discussed above. Using the types of teaching and learning supported by the two groups of criteria and the scholarly processes involved, one can formulate other criteria—derivative criteria. These criteria or standards must have the quality of congruency with the faculty-developed lists and must be useful for helping students critique their own work. Teacher criticism used alone has limited usefulness in that it might accomplish helping a student develop insights into the experience itself, but it does little to help the student develop his critical powers.

Another useful source of help for criteria are the elements of criticism itself, which are explained in Chapter 8.

A note of caution here: Earlier in the chapter, it was suggested that in connoisseurship and criticism, one looks at the whole. But that does not mean that the parts are not to be criticized insofar as they affect the whole. For example, when one views a face, a nose might be thought too long or a mouth too wide when they are examined individually. But when they are considered with the whole face, they may be just right and very effective in making the face distinctive and beautiful or very attractive. If one took all the "perfect" features and put them together on the same face—eyes, mouth, nose, forehead, cheeks, and chin—the face may give an overall appearance of blandness.

What is being offered here as a criticism model has as requisite a lot of student writing as well as the teacher–student and student–student discussions previously considered. The reason is simple. In the act of writing, thinking is improved; in the act of rendering, the events are carefully thought about, memory is enhanced, and a paradigm experience is much more likely to have meaning in the ultimate practice of nursing in the student's life. Additionally, the educated must, verbally and in writing, be able to articulate their thoughts; to express their feelings, to take a position and defend it; and to explore a subject, problem, or issue with scholarly thoroughness, with clarity, with succinctness and with some degree of eloquence. Without this ability, it is doubtful that education has taken place. As Cousins (1985) says, "The area in which a poor education shows up first is in self-expression, whether it be oral or written. It makes little difference how many university courses or degrees a person may own. If he cannot use words to move an idea from one point to another, his education is incomplete" (p. 4).

GRADING

Grading is a difficult problem. Academic settings demand that grades be submitted. These grades are supposed to reflect or at least be symbolic of student achievement, although how a teacher is supposed to place an accurate value on another's learning is anyone's guess. Grades are powerful. They evoke a sense of worthiness, achievement, and pride—or, on the other end of the spectrum, unworthiness, stupidity, or shame. They are also powerful for prestige and for career progress. Graduate schools and jobs often are grade-related opportunities. When grades are marginal, they can actually make a difference in whether or not a student may pursue a chosen field.

Another issue that emerges in any field such as nursing is the trust the public places in teachers to keep incompetents from practice. In an attempt to do this, teachers often develop absolute standards based on the assumption that their materials are valid. While grades are a mechanism useful for this purpose, this is not the problem in postgeneric nursing education. The problem is the school's reputation for graduating scholars.

There are no good solutions for these dilemmas. There are a few ideas that should be considered when a faculty makes decisions about grading. These ideas are assumptions upon which this criticism-interpretive model is based.

1. Learning activities are devised for the purpose of facilitating learning, not for evaluating "competency" or "performance" and grading its worth.

2. Some learning is latent and surfaces at unexpected moments. (It is possible to detect learning in some instances through a change in behavior or by contriving a situation in which changes in behavior can be manifested, but often learning lies incubating for years only to emerge at some later time.)

3. The learner is the only person who really knows what has been learned and how valuable it is.

4. What a student has learned from an activity may not be what the teacher intended but may be just as valuable to society, to the profession, and/or to the learner.

5. Grading by a teacher is the placing of value on learning by one unqualified to know the value that learning has for another individual. In other words, when the teacher grades, he or she places value using his or her own system of values, which may or may not coincide with the student's value system.

6. Except for the issue of safety, the value of learning is personal, private, and often secret both from the learner and from the teacher. It often does not emerge as valuable until something triggers it, and then it pops into awareness.

As mentioned earlier, there are no good answers to the problem of grading. The system seems entrenched in the United States, and, at present, teachers must seek creative ways to live with it. To survive in academia, teachers must find responsible ways to place value upon learning by grading. A workable compromise is collaboration between learners and teachers in seeking to assess learning and placing a value on it. Teachers could request students to reveal as much as possible of their inner life as scholars for a semester. This is done using the interpretive-critical approach, that is, through a process of intuitive perception, rendering, interpreting and judging, and using criteria that are consistent with the criteria for teacher–student interactions and learning activities. Then the students assign themselves a grade, supporting this grade with the data from their criticism. Teachers then critique the paper using criteria developed specifically for that purpose.

LOOKING TO THE FUTURE

What we need is some way to enlarge our vision instead of reduce it, to see wholes instead of parts, to see the complexity of human learning and growth and not attempt to simplify it to mere behaviors. Somewhere in the evaluation process, one must catch a vision that although a student may not have memorized the desired answer and may not know the expected responses, perhaps that student has caught a glimpse of other equally valuable things and perhaps has developed insights and aware-nesses that transport him or her beyond the answers into the patterns and meanings. Perhaps the test answers can be looked up when needed, but insights and meanings are personal and are arrived at through the hard work of reflection, examining assumptions, comparing, reading, discussing, and raising issues and questions. Perhaps, instead of mea-surement by behaviorist criteria and objective tests, teachers will en-gage their students in conversations that are critical in nature and that teach students to criticize. Perhaps then we will not objectify persons but will respect them as subjects. Perhaps then we will liberate and not oppress. Perhaps then we will enable instead of facilitate. Perhaps then we will teach rather than instruct.

Someday, perhaps.

REFERENCES

Benner, P. (1984). *From novice to expert: Excellence and power in clinical nursing practice.* Menlo Park, CA: Addison-Wesley.

Bevis, E. (1988). *Curriculum building in nursing.* New York: National League for Nursing.

Chronbach, L. J. (1966). The logic of experiments on discovery. In L. M. Shul-man and E. Keislar (Eds.), *Learning by discovery.* Chicago: Rand McNally.

Cousins, N. (1985). The options of learning. *Creative Living, The Magazine of Life, 14*(4), 1–4.

Dreyfus, S. E., & Dreyfus, H. L. (1980). *A five-stage model of the mental activities involved in directed skill acquisition.* Unpublished report supported by the Air Force Office of Scientific Research (AFSC), USAF (Contract F49620-79-C-0063), University of California at Berkeley.

Eisner, E. (1972, August). Emerging models for educational evaluation. *School Review,* 573–589.

Eisner, E. (1975a). *The perspective eye.* Washington, DC: Address at Annual Meeting of the American Educational Research Association.

Eisner, E. (1975b, April). Toward a more adequate conception of evaluation in the arts. *Peabody Journal of Education,* 172–179.

Eisner, E. (1985). *The educational imagination* (2nd ed.). New York: Macmillan.

Erickson, F. (1986). Qualitative methods in research on teaching. In M. C. Whittrock (Ed.), *Handbook of research on teaching* (3rd ed). A project of the American Educational Research Association. New York: Macmillan.

Freire, P. (1976). *Education: The practice of freedom.* London: Writers and Readers Publishing Cooperative.

Gagne, R. (1970). *The conditions of learning* (2nd ed.). New York: Holt, Rinehart and Winston.

Giorgi, A. (1970). *Psychology as a human science.* New York: Harper and Row.

Hazelton, L. (1979). Water from rock, tomatoes from sand. *Quest, 3*(5), 19.

Heidegger, M. (1962). *Being and time.* New York: Harper and Row.

Heidegger, M. (1975). *Poetry, language and thought.* New York: Harper and Row.

Keller, F. (1969). *Learning: Reinforcement theory* (2nd ed). New York: Random House.

Kozloff, M. (1969). *Renderings: Critical essays on a century of modern art.* New York: Simon and Schuster.

Krall, F. R. (1981). Navajo tapestry: A curriculum for ethno-ecological perspectives. *The Journal of Curriculum Theorizing, 3 (2),* 165–208.

Mager, R. (1977). *Preparing instructional objectives.* Belmont, CA: Feron Publishers.

Mann, J. S. (1969). Curriculum criticism. *Teachers' College Record, 71,* 27–40.

McCutchen, G. (1979, summer). Educational curriculum: Methods and applications. *The Journal of Curriculum Theorizing, 1*(2).

Merton, R. K. (1975). Structural analysis in sociology. In P. Blau (Ed.), *Approaches to the study of social structure.* New York: The Free Press.

Morgan, M., & Irby, D. (1978). *Evaluating clinical competence in the health professions.* St. Louis: C. V. Mosby.

Munhall, P. (1981). Nursing philosophy and nursing research: In apposition or opposition? *Nursing Research, 31*(3), 176–181.

Murray, J., & Merrefield, S. (1989). Criteria for student–teacher interactions end learning experiences. In J. Murray, *Developing criteria to support new curriculum models for doctoral education in nursing.* Doctoral dissertation, University of Georgia.

Oliva, P. (1982). *Developing the curriculum.* Boston: Little, Brown.

Peters, R. S. (1966). *Ethics and education.* London: Allen and Unwin.

Pinar, W., & Grumet, M. (1976). *Toward a poor curriculum.* Dubuque, IA: Kendull-Hunt Publishing.

Polanyi, M. (1962). *Personal knowledge.* London: Routledge and Kegan Paul.

Polanyi, M., & Prosch, H. (1975). *Meaning.* Chicago: University of Chicago Press.

Psathas, G. (1973). *Phemonenological sociology: Issues and applications.* New York: John Wiley & Sons.

Raths, J. (1971). Teaching without specific objectives. *Educational Leadership,* 714–720.

Saylor, J., & Alexander, W. (1974). *Planning curriculum for schools* New York: Holt, Rinehart and Winston.

Scriven, M. (1967). The methodology of evaluation. *AERA Monograph Series on Curriculum Evaluation, No. 1. Perspectives of Curriculum Evaluation* (pp. 39–83). Chicago: Rand McNally.

Scriven, M. (1972, December). Pros and cons about goal-free evaluation. *Evaluation Comment. The Journal of Educational Evaluation.* Center for the Study of Evaluation, University of California.

Spradley, J., & McCurdy, D. (1972). *The cultural experience: Ethnography in complex society.* Chicago: Science Research Associates.

Stenhouse, L. (1970). *The humanities project: An introduction.* London: Heinemann Educational Books.

Stenhouse, L. (1975). *An introduction to curriculum research and development.* London: Heinemann Educational Books.

Tyler, R. (1949). *Basic principles of curriculum and instruction.* Chicago: The University of Chicago Press.

Watson, J. (1988). *Nursing: Human science and human care.* Norwalk, CT: Appleton-Century-Crofts.

BIBLIOGRAPHY

Peters, R. S. (1973). Must an educator have an aim? In R. S. Peters (Ed.), *Authority, responsibility and education* (pp. 83–95). London: Allen and Unwin.

Saylor, J., & Alexander, W. (1954). *Curriculum planning for better teaching and learning.* New York: Holt, Rinehart and Winston.

Part III

Toward a New Destiny:
The Elegance of Liberation
—A Conclusion

The dominant view of knowledge in the Western tradition emphasizes abstract, general, theoretical knowledge while overlooking and devaluing local, specific, practical knowledge and expert skillful clinical judgments about particular clinical situations. The way involvement is central to expert knowledge is overlooked, reinforcing the myth that the expert must stand outside the situation, aloof and detached, in order to pronounce expert judgment.

Nursing and other caring practices have become paradoxical in a highly technical culture that seeks sweeping technological breakthroughs to provide liberation and disburdenment. For example, American health care emphasizes the heroics of trauma centers, while overlooking and under-funding programs for nutrition and prenatal care. Heart transplants receive tremendous funding and attention while preventive measures are less exciting and fundable because they are less culturally appealing. In the case of heart transplantation, people typically focus on the dramatic stitching in of a transplanted heart as the "breakthrough." Few notice that the intensive medical and nursing followup—solving the day-to-day problems of living with a transplanted organ, treating sores in the mouth due to immunosuppression, coping with a new hormonal milieu, promptly recognizing and responding to infection and rejection—were all caring "breakthroughs" that led to the eventual success of heart transplantation. These essential day-to-day nursing-care issues had to be solved in order to make heart transplantation a viable therapy. Yet they are all but overlooked in the scientific and popular media coverage of the transplant story.

Pat Benner and Judith Wrubel,
The Primacy of Caring, 1989, p. XV.

INTRODUCTION

The central day to day issues that had to be solved for successful heart transplants are only part of the story. There are many remaining issues to be solved—issues that can only be solved by nurses who are substantively different from the traditional prototype of the "good" woman, "good" nurse; the technological expert; the emerging professional. This substantive difference can only occur under a different system of education married to a different system of health care.

There is a basic requirement: liberating education for nurses. This is a redundancy, for real education is liberating, it is empowering, it provides the tools for maturity in judgment and compassion that are translated into action, and a reality view of the world that combines power with control, ability and skill with composure, and caring with firmness and resolution.

This is the elegance of liberation: It frees both the teacher and student in the educational system, and it empowers the graduate. Elegance has a meaning all its own. It is simplicity expressed as style, elan, and grace. Elegance is clean, with a focused purpose, a lack of trivia, and a timeless appropriateness that is understated vigor.

Liberation requires an openness that refutes dogma, that refuses unreasonable restraints, that respects tradition while moving beyond it, that changes and shapes the future without destroying the past. This section is about emancipation in nursing curriculum and the ideals that it is designed to realize. Toward that end, there are three chapters: Chapter 10 examines the behaviorist paradigm that has driven nursing curriculum for almost 40 years. It makes an attempt to help curriculum developers sort out and choose which of the traditional components of the Tylerian model to retain, use, and change and which to discard entirely. Chapter 11 examines impact—it tries to answer the question: so what? It examines what the potential impact for society and for nursing will be if this, or another alternative educative paradigm, were to become pervasively used in nursing education. Chapter 12 examines nursing's future, its destiny, its dreams made manifest.

10

From Dogma to Emancipation: An Examination of Traditional Behaviorist Curriculum Development

Em Olivia Bevis

When a man announces himself a high priest of the new education, he thereby brands those who do not fall down before the god of his pedagogical method as old fogies. Since this is easily satisfying to the high priest and doesn't worry the old fogies, the new education becomes a phrase for summoning spirits from the vasty deep. . . . It is suspected that the leaders of the cult themselves do not understand what it is; certainly they do not agree as to its true inwardness; which leads many to suppose that it is entirely composed of out-wardness. . . .

Once upon a time three archbishops of the creed [high priests of the new education] gave addresses at a certain educational gather-ing on the new education. After the ambulances had cleared away the audience, the three speakers were gathered by a reporter around a secluded table at the hotel. It was in the room where the lights dance merrily through the many-colored glasses, and all men are reduced to a common denominator. The three speakers, by the way, were really good fellows and quite sane upon all subjects but their pedagogical fad.

After the reporter had set up several rounds of the grateful fluids mentioned slightingly by the prohibition physiologies, he remarked,

"We go to press in an hour, and I've been listening to you fellows since eight o'clock. Now please tell me, as man to man, what is this new education anyway?"

As he looked from one to another, the answers were respectively:

a. "Damfino."
b. "Search me."
c. "Nother o' shame, pleash."

Welland Hendrick, *A Joysome History of Education*, 1909, pp. 39–40

INTRODUCTION

One could change the gender and replay this scene in several hotels in the past few years and not be in error. So, in an attempt to clarify the "new education," the paradigm shift in nursing education now occurring, this chapter will look at behaviorist curriculum in the light of educative-caring suggestions and examine how the curriculum development products of the behaviorist might be affected or altered by the new paradigm. To give perspective, let's review a little history.

Behaviorist-curriculum paradigms did not begin with Tyler (1949). However, Tyler's *Syllabus for Education 360*, since its publication in 1949 at the University of Chicago, has influenced the structure and direction of world education. It was Tyler who established the ends–means model as a force in education; it was he who gave structure to deliberate curriculum planning along coherent, logical, step-by-step lines; and it was he who pointed out the central focus of the curriculum as behavioral objectives (p. 1). In his introduction, he calls his book a "rationale for viewing, analyzing and interpreting the curriculum and instructional program of an educational institution" (p. 1). Nowhere does he call it a theory, for it is not; nor did he call it a paradigm or model, although it may be that. In honor of his perception of it, three generations of educators have called it the "Tyler Rationale" and used it as touchstone for creating and revising curriculum. Subsequent to Tyler, almost all educational writers have created rationales, models, and paradigms that have in some way modified or been derived from his work (Beauchamp, 1981; Leyton Soto & Tyler, 1969; Oliva, 1982; Saylor & Alexander, 1974; Taba, 1962). Not all these models are classified as ends–means models, as is Tyler's, but all have the same or similar Tyler-type curriculum-development products, for example, philosophy, objectives (all levels), program of study, and evaluation based upon the objectives. Some have a conceptual framework, some not. They differ in detail, in how to proceed from one element to another, and are the same in product if not always in the success of the outcome.

The works of many different educators constitute behaviorist doctrine. Some of this work complements, supplements, or augments Tyler. Some of the work would have existed whether or not Tyler had ever written his treatise on curriculum, and often these writers and researchers differed from Tyler on what they thought were major issues. But to those of us who are curriculum practitioners, the work is a whole—each writer/researcher giving scope and depth to the other and contradicting each other on points that are often important but sometimes inconsequential to curriculum practitioners.

Gagne (1970), in listing the conditions of learning, gave direction for building objectives and learning activities so that they fulfilled his conditions for learning and unerringly led the student to the achievement of the objectives. Bloom and his coworkers, in providing taxonomies on the domains of learning, provided guides for writing behavioral objectives (carrying reductionism to its Cartesian dualistic, inevitable end). Caroll and Bloom, in proposing mastery learning, provided a way to enable most students to meet the specified objectives. Taba (1962) and Beauchamp (through four editions, 1961–1981), in suggesting theories or conceptual frameworks, simplified Tyler's "screens." Mager (1972) and Gronlund (1970) gave detailed instruction on the framing and use of behavioral objectives. Scriven (1967); Popham (1971); Stake (1967); Provus (1971); Bloom, Hastings, and Madaus (1981); and others devised program evaluation models, each based on an assumption of behavioral objectives. And so together, despite their differences and their embroglios, the behaviorists held education in thrall for more than 40 years.

Out of the body of work and research called behaviorism came such epochs as the programed instruction movement, initiated in 1954 by Skinner's *The Science of Learning and the Art of Teaching* (1968). This opened the flood gates to "auto-tutorial packages," "self-paced learning," "individualized instruction," "learning modules," and early "computer assisted instruction." Throughout it all, the Tyler Rationale continued to influence educational practice. Many educators modified parts of the process to adapt the Tyler model to a specific problem or to put their own individual stamps upon it.

In nursing the behaviorists were revered, written about, used, and institutionalized—institutionalized in ways that made it impossible to become approved by state boards of nursing or to gain National League for Nursing accreditation without having curriculum materials that reflected behaviorist theory. As a result, nursing curriculum prospered. It became uniform in the products of curriculum development, it became relatively easy to evaluate, and it improved in quality because of standards that reflected behaviorist theory. It brought us to the shores of professionalism. But used alone, it can take nursing no further. Behaviorism is a learning theory for training and is good for skills as described in the maintenance learning of Botkin, Elmandjra, and Malitza (1979). Professions demand educated practitioners whose imagination and creativity take them beyond behaviorist parameters.

Behaviorism in nursing has spawned other notions that are in keeping with its philosophy and assumptions. Two of these are "nursing process" and "nursing diagnosis." These two popular tools of nursing have the same problems and limitations as behaviorism and will be discussed later.

The Tyler Rationale and its subsequent modifications have standardized the curriculum-development products in nursing education (see Fig. 1). Four of these products, those most influential in nursing education, will be taken in turn and discussed for their impact on and potential for use in a humanistic-educative nursing curriculum.

The aspects of this model that will be explored in this chapter are philosophy, conceptual frameworks, program goals, and behavioral objectives. Content, learning activities, and evaluation are covered elsewhere.

PHILOSOPHY

In the National League for Nursing (NLN) Council of Baccalaureate and Higher Degree Programs' *Criteria for the Evaluation of Baccalaureate and Higher Degree Programs in Nursing* (1983), criterion number one reads, "The program's philosophy and goals are consistent with the mission(s) of the parent institution" (p. 3). Both criteria 29 and 35, under first and second professional degree, respectively, read, "The instructional processes support the philosophy and goals of the program and the objectives of the curriculum" (p. 8). The fact that program philosophy is mentioned before all the others in the criteria and that it is mentioned three times among 36 criteria for both baccalaureate and master's programs communicates something regarding the nature of its importance in the national

Figure 1
Modified Tyler-Type Ends–Means Model

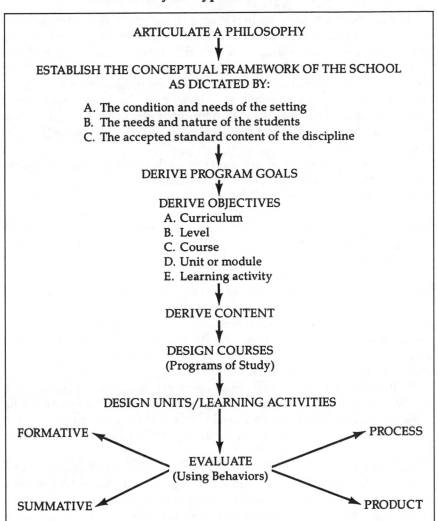

ARTICULATE A PHILOSOPHY

ESTABLISH THE CONCEPTUAL FRAMEWORK OF THE SCHOOL
AS DICTATED BY:

    A. The condition and needs of the setting
    B. The needs and nature of the students
    C. The accepted standard content of the discipline

DERIVE PROGRAM GOALS

DERIVE OBJECTIVES
    A. Curriculum
    B. Level
    C. Course
    D. Unit or module
    E. Learning activity

DERIVE CONTENT

DESIGN COURSES
(Programs of Study)

DESIGN UNITS/LEARNING ACTIVITIES

FORMATIVE   PROCESS

EVALUATE
(Using Behaviors)

SUMMATIVE   PRODUCT

accrediting process. No one seems to have questioned the premier place of philosophy in nursing education nor the amount of time and energy faculties spend in writing them.

The influence of philosophies is seen in historical documents. Stewart (1947), nursing education's classical historian, describes the period from Florence Nightingale's first interest in nursing and the need for reforms until her accomplishments in the Crimean war as a time when "Miss Nightingale was working out her philosophy of nursing and nursing education." She describes this philosophy as a "synthesis of ancient, medieval, and modern ideas and viewpoints" (p. 43). So we have a legacy of philosophy in modern nursing from its founder.

In discussing some basic principles of philosophy for nursing, Stewart (1947) speaks of two aspects: "the development of the individual and the progressive enrichment of his life experience, on the one hand, and the reconstruction and improvement of society on the other" (p. 319). What Stewart describes is a philosophy that encompasses both an individual educational and a social philosophy. Some other philosophical principles she addresses follow.

1. Mutual respect for personality, on the part of teachers and learners (her first axiom): She writes that individuals are to be regarded as ends in themselves, never as means to ends, and that basic democratic rights such as freedom of speech and opinion, freedom from fear, etc., are for learners as well as teachers, for nurses as well as patients. She says, "No one has the right to starve or stereotype or dominate the individuality of another" (p. 320).

2. Equality of opportunity and of cooperation or shared responsibility: She says that "democracy teaches that obeying orders and doing what one is told is not enough. Individuals should share in proportion to capacity in shaping the plans and policies of the groups to which they belong" (p. 320).

3. The greatest possible opportunity to think and act freely and naturally: She asserts, "when human beings have a chance to use their own ideas, direct their own activities, make their own decisions, and be responsible for their own conduct they are likely to show the most satisfactory growth" (pp. 320–321).

4. Learner accountability: She offers the opinion that "learners should be helped to recognize and solve their own problems as far as possible, instead of having ready-made problems and solutions handed out to them" (p. 321).

5. Evaluation: Stewart's counsel is that learners "should learn to

expect and welcome criticism as an essential part of the learning process, but criticism should be constructive and individuals should learn as far as possible to check and evaluate their own work, criticize themselves, and correct their mistakes" (p. 321).

Stewart's 1947 summary of her philosophy of education is, surprisingly, a historical anomaly; it could well form the philosophy for this book. It is surprising only until one realizes that the Tyler Rationale did not come into being until 1949 and did not take nursing by storm until the mid-1950s. The behaviorist movement, however, was underway long before Tyler and Miss Stewart, a well-educated woman, maintained her influence in nursing education and her reputation and position at Columbia University by being well read in educational theory. It must be assumed that she was knowledgeable about Bobbitt, Dewey, Hutchins, Hopkins, Thorndike, and other educational writers popular in the early part of this century. Her writings do reflect some behaviorist positions.

Since Stewart spoke about philosophy of nursing education as a historical issue, it is obvious that Tyler did not initiate educational philosophy in schools of nursing. Many nurse-educators, desiring to excel in teaching and to help mould nursing education, sought degrees in education. Teachers' colleges were common and were widely available to women. In fact they were one of the educational institutions designed with women in mind.

The rise of women in education is reflective of the whole of the history of women. Until the 1830s, teaching was thought to be for men only. The notion existed that women were inadequate to control students and to take care of disciplinary problems. However, since teaching was historically a low-paying job, it was soon discovered that one could pay a woman one-third to one-half as much as a man. That economic factor was persuasive enough to open teaching to women. Normal schools began to be opened around the country, beginning, of course, with the successful Mann effort in 1839 in Lexington, Massachusetts (Cohen, 1971, pp. 20–21). The availability of these normal schools, and the fact that they were organized primarily for women, made it easy for nurse educators to matriculate. For this reason, we find that educational precepts rapidly found their way into nursing schools. Philosophy, then, as an integral part of curriculum efforts, existed in nursing schools far earlier than the advent of Tyler.

Supporting this notion is Stewart (1947), who mentions the influence of Counts on nursing educational philosophy. Counts (1934) speaks of the administrator's responsibility:

embodying in his theories and programs some interpretation of history in the making, some general outlook upon the world, some frame of reference with respect to society, some conception of things deemed necessary, of things deemed possible, of things deemed desirable in the proximate future. (p. 3)

He clearly places the need for a philosophy to guide the theories and programs on the administrator's shoulders.

Nursing not only incorporated philosophy as part of the necessary products of curriculum development but eventually, as we shall see later, took it to the level of prescribing exactly what must be included in the philosophy of every school.

Tyler (1949) also speaks of an educational and social philosophy. He lists four democratic values as important to effective and satisfying personal and social life:

(1) The recognition of the importance of every individual human being as a human being regardless of his race, national, social, or economic status; (2) opportunity for wide participation in all phases of activities in the social groups in the society; (3) encouragement of variability rather than demanding a single type of personality; (4) faith in intelligence as a method of dealing with important problems rather than depending upon the authority of an autocratic or aristocratic group. (p. 34)

Tyler suggests, "When a school accepts these values as basic the implication is that these are values to be aimed at in the educational program of the school" (p. 34).

The problem arises when one progresses to his discussion on the form of objectives—for then he contradicts himself by saying,

It can safely be concluded that a statement of objectives clear enough to be used in guiding the selection of learning experiences and in planning instruction will indicate both the kind of behavior to be developed in the student and the area of content or of life in which the behavior is to be applied. (p. 47)

This is obviously at variance with "encouragement of variability" and "faith in intelligence as a method of dealing with important problems rather than depending upon the authority."

Initiating the era of a prescribed list of topics to be included in a school's philosophy, Tyler (pp. 35–37) lists several other topics that faculties must include in their educational philosophy. These are:

- Whether or not the school accepts the contemporary emphasis on materialism.
- Whether or not financial, personal, or social success is a desired educational value.
- Whether the educated person should accept the social order by adjusting to it or whether education should fit persons to seek to improve society.
- Whether there "should be a different education for different classes in society."
- Whether democracy is to "be defined solely in political terms, or does democracy imply a way of life at home, in the school, and in economic matters as well."

Tyler advises faculties not to limit their philosophical statements to these but to explore all philosophical issues they think relevant.

In 1973, Bevis suggested that:

> Topically, it [the philosophy] should contain the following elements:
>
> 1. Statements about the values upon which the nursing education is based.
>   a. The future of nursing practice as viewed by the faculty.
>   b. The moral, ethical, or religious context of the school, if appropriate.
>   c. The scope and limits of the education provided.
>   d. The characteristics of people in a democratic society and the implications of these beliefs in the practice of nursing as well as in curriculum.
> 2. Statements about the nature of nursing, its origins, its processes, and its practice roles. (p. 195)

National League for Nursing literature soon began to suggest a prescription for nursing school philosophies. Even though the appraisal criteria for accrediting and approval bodies seldom give the prescription, there exists other literature that prescribes the content and categories for nursing educational program philosophies. One early evidence of the beginnings of this occurs in the literature generated by regional workshops. In 1974 the NLN conducted a series of regional curriculum workshops designed for faculty in baccalaureate nursing programs. In these workshops, they stressed the systematic development of curriculum. Torres, a key speaker at these meetings and an employee of the Department of Baccalaureate and Higher Degree Programs of the NLN, stated, "Generally, baccalaureate nursing programs speak to society, health, nursing, and learning, as well as man, in their written philosophies" (p. 16). This comment was rapidly picked up and used to prescribe the contents of a philosophy for each school of nursing and became de facto regulations.

In keeping with the de facto regulations of the accrediting and approval bodies, Bevis (1978), departing from her more general ideas of the earlier edition, prescribes a list of topics that "almost all schools of nursing address in their statement of philosophy: (1) What is the nature of the client? (2) What is the nature of Nursing? (3) What is health? (4) What are the basic commitments of the nursing educational enterprise." Then almost as if by afterthought, Bevis comments, "In addition to these, the National League for Nursing suggests that each school should discuss the nature of society" (p. 43).

Each teacher has a philosophy and acts upon it. The philosophy may not be articulated, but it exists. So too does each school have values that guide its curriculum development, its interactive practices, and its selection of content. That is inescapable. In that vein, Kneller (1971) specifies philosophy as both natural and necessary to man.

> Philosophy attempts to establish conceptual coherence throughout the whole domain of experience. . . . Just as formal philosophy attempts to understand reality as a whole by explaining it in the most general and systematic way, so educational philosophy seeks to comprehend education in its entirety, interpreting it by means of general concepts that will guide our choice of educational ends and policies. (p. 201)

These philosophies that guide educational ends and policies have given rise to the "perennialist," the "idealist," the "realist," the "pragmatist," the "reconstructionist," the "existentialist," the "disciplined" centered curriculum, the "progressives," the "academist," the "rationalist," and the "reconceptualist," to name a few. Philosophy does without doubt direct educational thought, support educational paradigms, influence teaching practices, and motivate evaluation methods. There is no dispute over that, nor is there dispute that philosophy is an integral part of the curriculum-planning process.

The problem that arises is that, according to traditional theory, the first task of the curriculum-planning group is to come to grips with, and to set forth, a philosophy that represents the thinking of the faculty of the school of nursing. First, the school of nursing exists through the faculty and students and, therefore, in reality reflects their individual philosophies, whether or not they are recorded. Second, the faculty and students are unique individuals whose philosophies differ. As a consequence of these differences, any statements of philosophy are arrived at through negotiation and are altered to be more collectively agreeable. They are thereby so compromised that they are watered down to the point of reflecting no one's belief and too often are meaningless.

Bevis (1988), with uncharacteristic understatement, defines this situation: "faculties often have difficulty arriving at consensus in a statement of philosophy" (p. 43). Indeed, with very few exceptions, the philosophy of every school of nursing could be put into a pot, mixed up, redistributed to altogether different schools, and the only persons who would recognize the difference would be members of the committee who were appointed to do the final editing. Even they might have some difficulty. I have been expecting to see an advertisement by some enterprising nurse-educator offering to boiler-plate philosophies for requesting schools of nursing at $200 each (cheap at the price considering how much time and energy is spent doing it).

In fact, Munhall (1981) finds that certain common denominators in nursing philosophy do exist. In statements of philosophy in schools of nursing throughout the country and in nursing literature, they hold the same place for nurse educators as "mom" and "apple pie" for the indigenous American. Munhall summarizes them as humanistic, focusing on individuality, believing that humans have free will and are self-determined, autonomous, and active, that people are holistic and holism does not allow reductionistic methods, and that people have unlimited capacity for growth, and are evolving and emerging in mutual interaction with the environment (p. 176).

Bevis (1988, pp. 43–44) also lists five philosophical points of general agreement found in nursing literature. These are:

1. The individual has intrinsic value, and there is worth inherent in human life.
2. Nursing is a rational activity.
3. Nursing's uniqueness is in the way the basic social and biological sciences are synthesized in functions that promote health.
4. The individual nurse-citizen has some control over and responsibility for the political and social milieu.

5. Nursing is a process with a central subjective purpose, an inherent organization or system, and dynamic creativity.

Point 2 above, that "nursing is a rational activity," was derived from the amount of space given to "nursing process" or problem solving and decision making, quantitative research, and nursing diagnosis. Were the trends found in current literature searched there would be more emphasis on nursing as a human science. However, at any rate, there is some unity reflected in the literature regarding philosophical thought . . . if not unity, at least it reflects the styles that come and go in education.

These statements do have curriculum implications that are inescapable but are not always found to be consistent with the actual curriculum materials. For instance, these statements can be found in the philosophies of schools that still teach in the medical model; that only teach research methods that are reductionistic, instrumental, and empiricist; that talk about "bio-psycho-social" as if hyphenating the word would hide its reductionism; and that continue to operate in behaviorist paradigms for teaching and evaluating. One conclusion that can be reached from these observations is that the words are so commonplace that faculty, although they believe them, allow other assumptions to dictate their actual curricula, that is, what actually goes on between and among students and teachers. In order to restructure the curriculum paradigm, the gap between what faculty say they believe and what they actually do must be dealt with in direct and unavoidable means.

The position taken here is that statements of philosophy, meant to guide the curriculum development of a school of nursing, are practically useless for that purpose. They are shaped by tradition into statements about the nature of man,[1] education, nursing, society, the teaching–learning process, baccalaureate (or whatever level) nursing, professional nursing practice, and the nature of the "product we would produce"[2] (Lewis, 1974, p. 62).

---

[1] It is interesting to note that in this paper, and in NLN materials, "man" is stressed—sexist language was perpetuated in a predominantly women's field.
[2] "Producing" a "product" is common language used in curriculum circles. It is the traditional industrial metaphor educators use to discuss their field and transforms students who are the subjects and coparticipants in curriculum endeavors to objects. This is not done through any intent to objectify, but it is the result of informal enculturation into nursing education.

A problem that intrudes itself and makes obvious the discontinuity between the philosophy and the actual curriculum plans and implementation is that nursing philosophy has moved more rapidly to acknowledge the kinds of positions that nurses must take to be true to their societal mission and to acknowledge their own feminist roots. Nursing curriculum, on the other hand, is still entangled with the behaviorist model, which contradicts that philosophy at every turn. The resolution of this conflict must be a task of highest priority to nursing educators.

One fruitful consequence of the long weeks of faculty debate that usually go into the making of a philosophy is that faculty learn a little more about these areas and what their colleagues think about each of them. It has some beneficial uses for faculty development.

In order to solve the conflict evident between nursing philosophy and educational practices, we might depart from the prescriptive categories that are usually addressed by nursing school philosophies. If we must have a philosophy at the beginning of our curriculum materials (and I am not convinced we need one in the current form), we might explore the educational rewards of discussing the traditional six major divisions of philosophy: metaphysics, the nature of reality; ontology, the nature of being; epistemology, the nature of knowledge; axiology, the nature of values; ethics, the nature of human conduct; and aesthetics, the nature of beauty. Scholarly exploration of these areas and how they are related to each other might yield at least some assumptions of educational value and direct use in curriculum development. However, no gains will be seen unless sincere efforts are made to teach by the values inherent in the philosophy.

Assumptions might be more useful than high-flown language for the school's philosophy and might provide an alternative to the problem of the sound-alike, look-alike philosophies. Assumptions, too, would be outgrowths of faculty discussions but would be placed differently in order to make them more powerful. For instance, when a course is described in the curriculum-planning documents, place the assumptions about teaching methods with the teaching methods, about evaluation and grading methods with the evaluation and grading section, and the assumptions about students with the policy about student responsibilities and rights. In that manner, the philosophy comes alive in the actual materials used in the curriculum. The philosophy then would not be some cold document, tucked away in the files and trotted out for inspectors, visitors, accreditors, and catalog copy. The philosophy then could be individual—reflecting the values of the teacher(s) who are actually involved in the course(s). There would be an obvious and direct connection between the philosophical discussions of metaphysics, ontology, epistemology, axiology, ethics, and aesthetics reflected in the nursing school's curriculum, as represented by the assumptions and the curriculum materials actually in use in the school. Additionally, the congruence between the assumptions and the curriculum matters they influence would be more obvious so that discrepancies would be more easily detected and remedied.

CONCEPTUAL FRAMEWORKS

Tyler (1949) does not mention conceptual frameworks. He speaks instead about the educational purposes the school should seek to attain, in one paragraph calling them purposes, aims, goals, and objectives (p. 3). He asks how the objectives are to be obtained and answers that there are three sources: the student or learner, studies of contemporary life outside the school (society), and the subject matter. These three "S's"—student, society, and subject—evolved through Taba (1962) and Beauchamp into conceptual frameworks that have influenced nursing education for the last 20 years.

Taba (1962) was largely responsible for the emergence of conceptual frameworks as a force in curriculum. She writes:

> [It] spells out the crucial elements of curriculum and their relationship to each other. The central problems of a curriculum design are to determine the scope of expected learning, to establish a continuity of learning and proper sequence of content, and to unify ideas from diverse areas. (p. 13)

She says further that:

> A conceptual system for the curriculum or a theory of curriculum is a way of organizing thinking about all matters that are important to curriculum development: what the curriculum consists of, what its important elements are, how these are chosen and organized, what the sources of curriculum decisions are, and how the information and criteria from these sources are translated into curriculum decisions. (p. 420)

Taba traces the term to Herrick (Herrick & Tyler, 1950), who used the term *curriculum theory,* and to Goodlad (1958), who used the term *conceptual system.* She says such frameworks/theories are "a way of asking and answering questions about important issues in curriculum development, and of asking them systematically" (p. 421).

In Bevis' first edition (1973) of *Curriculum Building in Nursing*, this aspect of curriculum is called a "theoretical framework." It is defined as "the decision-making guide for the curriculum-building process" (p. 6). She says it is variously called a curriculum framework, a framework for curriculum development, the conceptual system, the curriculum theory, a theory of education, and the conceptual framework (p. 18). In the next two editions (1978, 1988), Bevis began to call it a "conceptual framework." She described it (1978) as:

> the conceptualization and articulation of concepts, facts, propositions, postulates, theories, phenomena, and variables relevant to a specific nursing educational system. It comprises concepts, facts, hypotheses, theories, and/or other crucial elements or ideas on which a nursing curriculum is based and the relationship these concepts have to each other and to the nursing curriculum in a specific educational situation. The frame of reference, or a conceptual framework, is the structure that provides the map for all curriculum matters. It is like the framing of a house in that it furnishes the specifications and decision-making guidelines for the walls, rooms, form, and function of the house. The conceptual framework provides the perimeters (limits and constraints) and parameters (values) for curriculum development, giving consistency and integrity to the learning plan. (p. 25)

Chater (1975), adding a dimension, participated in helping nursing understand the importance of conceptual frameworks. Taking a cue from Tyler, she divided the influences on the curriculum into three areas: students, setting, and knowledge base. These movements highlighted a requirement, growing out of the Tyler (1949) model, that horizontal and vertical strands, threads, or concepts be identified and used throughout the curriculum. In addressing the organization of content, Tyler had spoken about continuity, sequence, and integration. Continuity, he said, "refers to the vertical reiteration of major curriculum elements" (p. 84). Integration "refers to the horizontal relationship of curriculum experiences" (p. 85). From these statements issued the preoccupation of nursing with horizontal and vertical threads/strands/concepts that eventually became "conceptual frameworks."

Meanwhile, at the National League for Nursing, the criteria for the appraisal of programs were changing to reflect the new trends. The criteria had never mentioned horizontal and vertical threads, strands, or concepts—they were part of the very powerful nonofficial criteria. This was reflected in the writings of Torres (1974), which suggested:

> After the development of the philosophy, the characteristics of the graduate, and the conceptual framework, it is most helpful for a faculty to identify the horizontal and vertical strands so that the essence of the philosophy can be incorporated more easily into the behavioral objectives. These strands reflect the essence of the nursing curriculum. (p. 19)

In this article, Torres managed to preserve the horizontal and vertical strands and add a conceptual framework to the materials required as faculty curriculum development products. Horizontal and vertical threads continued to be part of de facto regulations in nursing. Peterson (1978) describes "threads" as themes addressed in the conceptual framework that are "emphasized throughout the curriculum with increasing expectations of the student's skill" (p. 8).

This was written 6 years after conceptual frameworks became part of the official NLN requirements. Conceptual frameworks were written into the criteria, first appearing in 1972. The criterion in question stated, "The curriculum plan is based on a conceptual framework(s) consistent with the stated philosophy, purposes, and objectives of the program(s)" (NLN, 1972, p. 8).

That very statement makes it seem apparent that the conceptual framework was an afterthought to the objectives, where in reality it was conceived as guiding the selection of objectives and content much like Tyler's "screens." Having picked up this problem, the next edition of the criteria, the first to carry an edition number (4th ed.), altered the criteria to read: "The curriculum implements the philosophy, purposes, and objectives of the program and is developed within a conceptual framework" (NLN, 1978, p. 13).

That was its last official appearance in the criteria, the fifth edition (1983) merely stating as its 21st and 29th criteria:

> The curriculum is logically organized and internally consistent.
>   The instructional processes support the philosophy and goals of the program and objectives of the curriculum. (NLN, 1983, p. 8)

Mention of conceptual frameworks did not, however, disappear from the "Guidelines for Interpretation" listed in the NLN *Self-Study Manual, Guidelines for Preparation of the Self-Study Report* (1984). As instructions to schools preparing for accreditation, this manual gives information about how to write a self-study. It is divided into four parts: The first states the criterion, the second the "Guidelines for Interpretation," the third "Evidence for Self-Study Report," and the last "Evidence for Visitors." Under "Guidelines for Interpretation," paragraph 21.2 of the manual prescribes, "Organizing framework(s) is/are used for the selection and sequencing of content" (p. 39). Under "Evidence for Self-Study Report," paragraph 4 of the manual reads, "Describe how the program content is derived and organized from the philosophy, purposes, objectives and organizing framework" (p. 39).

So conceptual framework language, although disappearing from the criteria, stayed in the guidelines and remained part of the de facto criteria governing accreditation of baccalaureate and higher degree programs. These de facto criteria were used by both the Board of Review and the site visitors representing the Board of Review. Evidence was required for both organizing "frameworks" and concepts and threads.

There was departure from educational thinking represented in the NLN-sponsored workshops and meetings as interpreted by non-nursing educators. Instead of viewing it, as Taba (1962, p. 420) does, as a "theory of curriculum" and "a way of organizing thinking about all matters that are important to curriculum development," Torres (1974, p. 18) says that a conceptual framework "represents the faculty's notions about nursing and nursing education and gives structure to the curriculum." She elaborates by saying that the outcome is to produce "core" concepts about nursing and suggesting that these "core" concepts speak about man, society, health, nursing, and their interrelatedness. That idea was reiterated and elaborated in Torres and Yura (1974). This changes the intent of a conceptual framework from shaping the curriculum to shaping and choosing content. However, in the discussions about society, no mention is made of the importance of society as the context for nursing, its needs, characteristics, problems, trends, and probable future, and how they influence curricular decisions.

It is easy to see the drift toward viewing conceptual frameworks as a theory of nursing. Nations (1978) reflects this trend by using "theme" and "framework" interchangeably. She speaks of the "selection of a conceptual framework" (p. 25) and lists some possible "frameworks" that can be used. She then goes into "theoretical formulations" concerning "man," "nursing," and "health." So, when the accreditation criteria and guidelines refer to a framework for organizing content, it is perceived by most as simply that—a content-related curriculum factor—not, as Taba originally intended, a way of thinking about everything having to do with curriculum development.

Concomitant with the increase in popularity of conceptual frameworks as a *required* part of the curriculum plans, and in seeing theories either as *the* conceptual framework or as part of it, came a rich increase in nursing theories. This became important to curriculum planners because of the trend and because Bevis (1973) and Chater (1975) were calling for concepts and theories of nursing as part of the framework. Nursing was short on theoretical constructs that gave conceptual organization to its content and therefore welcomed theories that helped them see the content in ways that were in keeping with nursing's unique societal mission. In earlier years, these were hard to find.

Historically, the first real departure from the medical model to a nursing one was Abdullah, Martin, Beland, and Matheny (1960), who wrote *Patient-Centered Approaches to Nursing Care.* This book offered 21 nursing problems as categories for nurses' unique role with clients. Its historical significance was that, for the first time, a convincing case was made that there was a way to perceive and teach nursing that was not based on medical diagnosis but on patient needs and was nursing care oriented.[3] As nursing research and reflection regarding nursing's unique role developed, models and theories exploded. Roy (1970), King (1971), Johnson (Grubbs, 1980), Neuman (1980), Orem (1971), and Rogers (1970) are but a few of the more popular theorists.

What occurred was that nurse educators began to think of these theories as conceptual frameworks. They were used in curricula as part of the whole of the school's official version of what nursing was and how it should be practiced. When adopted by faculty, these theories were used to guide teaching and student practice and became *the* conceptual framework. The other components of frameworks that guide curriculum development were either not considered at all or were relegated to things that influenced content selection only. Mistakenly, they were not seen as factors that influence all aspects of curriculum planning and implementation.

Gradually nursing educators came to realize that when one of these theories was chosen and all other theories eliminated, it was more constraining than liberating. Each theory has something to give, some insight to offer, some dimension the others do not have. Some theories

---

[3] An interesting historical note is that with the efforts of Matheny and others like her, it was Associate of Arts programs that first successfully worked with integrated curricula based on nursing instead of medical models.

work better with some patient problems than others, and some faculty simply have a preference for one or the other. As the limitations of choosing one as the exclusive framework for nursing became more evident, "frameworks"—or in reality single theories—became less and less popular.

The question arises, is the conceptual framework, or even concepts and threads, necessary to guide the teaching and practice of nursing? Would it be better to take some type of structure for examining the sources of content and devising a way to organize the curriculum so that there is some assurance of continuity, increasing complexity (sequence), and integration (Tyler, 1949)? Or would curriculum planners do better simply to look, again as Tyler suggests, to students, subject, and setting or society as the sources of content and let the organization fall as it may?

The answers to these, and questions like them, might best be left to faculty. There are many factors that faculties who struggle with this problem will need to consider. One that is important is the factor of exclusiveness. Nursing theories influence the way nurses practice. They provide structure and maps for creative nursing care. They help steer the nurse scholar-clinician toward ways and means to help clients. As such, they are invaluable tools for nursing. When only one is chosen, and it is used to the exclusion of all other theories, that exclusiveness limits the options, the flexibility of care, the ways nurses have of examining the multifaceted, complex way humans experience their health problems and deal with health issues. Theories are necessary and very useful to teachers, for they influence the way we think, the way we organize our care for patients, and the way we give care. Theories are tools that nurses use in approaching care; the more tools we have in our toolbox, the more likely we can select the best/most appropriate tool to do the job. It seems obvious that using only one theory to guide nursing teaching and practice would limit perceptions of the nature of the problems as well as the possibilities for their solution. Creativity requires options.

That factors in the environment, setting, or society influence nursing curriculum is indisputable (Bevis, 1988); that the type of students and the needs of the students influence the content and how it is taught is also beyond question; and obviously the state of the field of study, the concepts, facts, theories, and postulates that comprise the knowledge base and influence the selection of content. These things need not be too restrictive an influence and can actually be an aide for flexibility.

GOALS

In the melodrama of curriculum, goals are the good guys, the white hats, the pathfinders that help students and teachers toward some end-in-view. Traditional curriculum books make a distinction between purposes, goals, and objectives. And those committed to behaviorist doctrine think of them all as some terminal point. Zais (1976) fits this stereotype:

> Whether we use the word "ends," "purposes," "aims," "goals," or "objective," we understand that reference is being made to some terminal point toward which we are moving, working, or traveling. Having created a terminal point in our minds, we ordinarily set about identifying the process or processes of getting there, employing the word "means" to name the way(s) by which we reach this terminal point. (p. 297)

As mentioned before, this model does very well if the "terminal point" is some behavior that is the result of training. *Terminal,* however, is a word that means finale, as in "ring down the curtain, the melodrama is over"; it means end, as in terminal disease. (One must admit that much instructing done in the frontal-lecture format is dull enough to kill one with boredom.) It would be more appropriate to educative learning if, in place of "terminal behaviors," we were to change the metaphor and think of goals, aims, and ends-in-view as being *directions* instead of destinations. For instance, "Go West, young man"[4] provides a goal, a direction, but not a destination. "Go to Utah" might give a clearer picture of the general area in the West, and "Go to Salt Lake City" might have given an even more specific picture. It would not, however, have allowed the young man to have the freedom to find his own place in the western sun. He might find the climate and the culture of Utah or Salt Lake City less suited to his personal needs than, say, Nevada or Carson City.

Goals, regardless of paradigm, whether behaviorist or educative-caring, work better if they are general, giving a sense of direction—not specificity—to the educational enterprise.

---

[4] An interesting bit of trivia: This familiar quotation, which is usually attributed to Horace Greeley, who used it in an editorial in the *New York Tribune* and often gave this pungent advice to young acquaintances, was in fact first employed by John B. L. Soule in an article in the Terre Haute *Express* in 1851.

In the educative-caring paradigm, goals become all that educators and students have to guide their teaching and learning endeavors. Whereas, in the behaviorist models, goals are usually an outcome of committee work and are spelled out in some detail so that objectives can flow from them with obvious congruity, goals in the educative-caring model are inherent in the topic that gives the name of the course and in whatever general outline of content may or may not be provided by curriculum committee plans. For instance, if the course is to address home care of the chronically ill, there is a direction in the title. Other goals or ends-in-view can be developed by the students as they tackle the nursing and client problems imbedded in the area in home care. If that structure is too loose for some teachers, other general goals can be chosen. If, however, a goal becomes too detailed and content oriented, it serves to contain and restrain rather than to liberate.

Often the solution is found in a scholarly approach to determining goals. Students, as a first task in a course, can survey the literature and venture into homes and interview families, patients, friends, and/or health care providers in order to get a reality-based idea of what the problems are that face the chronically ill at home. This way, students, in collaboration with teacher/co-learners, can weed out redundancy, busy work, and trivia.

Such loose structure can be frightening to those of us who for so long have followed the "happy trails" into behaviorist country. The loose structure suggested here has little or no research to support it—it has little except the deep-seated faith that human beings who really do want to learn can be effective partners with teachers. There are models in the form of master teachers who teach this way. Their work lays a path the rest of us can follow—it also provides rich ground for research. It may not be superior to lecture in aiding in the memorization of content so often tested in such research—there are other methods for that—but once students finish their grieving for hand feeding, I think it might be most effective for educating.

BEHAVIORAL OBJECTIVES

Objectives are the crux of the matter. It is the objectives, hammered into prescriptions of behaviors to be evaluated, that constrict curriculum. It is behavioral objectives that, in the final analysis, have cramped educative teaching. It is not the philosophy, the conceptual framework, or the goals.

These may have wasted time, frustrated or helped teachers, advanced or curtailed nursing education, depending upon one's point of view. But it is objectives that are the central issue for educators looking for paradigms that liberate teachers and students, that support a philosophy of human science, and that educate in addition to train. Except for the types of learning that are training (see Chapter 3), there is no place for objectives in the educative-caring paradigm, only for goals.

Charting the course of how goals and aims evolved into behavioral objectives and the influence this evolution has had on curriculum brings insights about how objectives progressed in structure and importance so that they currently pervade most of nursing education. There is historical significance in what is said and not said in the literature about nursing educational goals, aims, and objectives. To point up the evolution in perception of nursing education's use of behavioral objectives, three significant sources have been chosen. These books have been selected because they were, during their respective span of years, foundational sources for nursing curriculum and the chief influences upon the substance and direction of nursing education.

The Curriculum Guide (1917–1937)

A Curriculum Guide for Schools of Nursing (The Committee on Curriculum of the National League of Nursing Education, 1937) was the last in a series of three editions of a volume dating from 1917 to 1937. It was the sole reference on nursing curriculum for those years, all else being adjunct to or commentary on this source. Designed as a guide, it was misused as dogma just as the Tyler model was later to be.

In speaking of how the aims of nursing education were determined, the following was said:

> The first step was to consider the present aims of nursing education as far as they could be determined and to decide whether or not they are adequate in view of modern conditions of life and the demands that nurses are meeting and are likely to meet in the immediate future. [This is still considered by most persons to be the first step.] The traditional aims of discipline, self-sacrificing service, practical utility, and technical efficiency will be found in many statements. Obviously there is much value in these aims but in their interpretation too much emphasis has been placed on the subordination of the individual nurse and too little on her growth and self-realization. (pp. 15–16)

The words *subordination of the individual, growth,* and *self-realization* sound like a much-later era of nursing education. The book goes on to elucidate the discontinuity of the "military ideals and methods of training in nursing schools" with the ideals and accepted principles of democracy. The section concludes with an attempt to reconcile the two: "There is nothing incompatible in this ideal with the idea of discipline and self-sacrificing service providing the discipline is self-imposed and the self-sacrifice does not cripple but rather stimulates the growth of the individual" (p. 16). No matter how much the rhetoric of martyrdom is clothed in the raiment of self-realization, what comes through is the value of self-sacrifice.

There is in the same section the origins of a later era in nursing: that of clamoring after the methods of science. This section (p. 16) holds nurses up to be "members of the larger family of medicine," wherein nurses should be in "harmony with" and have an appreciation for the methods of science that "are needed in order to co-operate with physicians and others who are carrying on medical research." Then the committee nicely slips into the "adjustment aim" (which still affects nursing education) by saying:

> Nurses must be able to adjust to these rapidly changing conditions, and this means that they require a different type of preparation. . . . The kind of training that puts emphasis on unquestioning obedience to orders and drill in fixed habits of behavior and standardized procedures will not prepare the nurse to meet new and constantly changing situations where intelligence, initiative, and self-direction are needed. (p. 17)

Had this gone but a bit further, it might have spoken of contextual and acontextual rules and guidelines, thereby anticipating Benner (1984) by 47 years.[5]

---

[5] A side issue note is appropriate here. This ability to trace the roots of an idea that is a current force in nursing to its beginnings in the literature and, therefore, to its early formative stages and to understand its origins and the forces that shaped it through the decades is what I mean when I refer to one of the goals of doctoral education in nursing as enabling one to understand the deeper structures of the field. These deeper structures—tracing the classical ideas and persistent issues to their roots—have another necessary element, that of tying those ideas together into three-dimensional imaginary structures, so that one has a mental picture of how one group of ideas came to influence and be related to another group of ideas.

The adjustment aim is described as to "set right," to "bring to a true relative position," "to bring into right relationship" (p. 18). It takes the position that education is the means by which individuals learn to adjust. It goes further by saying that "the whole study and practice of education are for the purpose of securing a better understanding of the principles involved and a better mastery of the processes by which human beings adjust themselves to the world in which they live and work" (p. 18). It sounds much like the "adaptation" concept that became popular for patient care following the success of Selye's (1956) *The Stress of Life* and Roy's (1970) adaptation model.

The adjustment aim reflects the era of education wherein the overall goal was to "produce" a "good" work force. This, of course means, tractable, obedient, and meeting middle-class standards of industry, punctuality, and honesty. The adjustment aim arose from social trends to which United States education responded. According to Cohen (1971, pp. 26–29), one of the greatest waves of immigration to America occurred between 1880 and 1914, bringing some 22 million immigrants. These immigrants constituted about 40 percent of the population of the 12 largest cities in the United States. A public education system was needed that would solve the problems of health, hygiene, vocation, congestion, and assimilation. The task of transforming this mass of highly heterogeneous population into a homogeneous work-oriented labor force fell to the public schools. This traditional role of education underlies the "adjustment aim." By 1937, when the third edition of nursing's *Curriculum Guide* was published, the adjustment aim was a tried and true concept in educational circles.

The adjustment aim was fashioned to mean "not only changes in behavior, but changes that make for better living, better relationships, and a better contribution to society" (National League of Nursing Education, 1937, p. 18). So, in 1937, behaviorism was already omnipresent in education and could be treated as a "not only." One paragraph sums up the aims of nursing programs in the late 1930s and early 1940s. It states:

> The function of nursing schools is to select students who show particular aptitude for nursing, to provide suitable opportunities for them to learn how to make these adjustments, also to guide their learning in such a way that they will be able to give efficient service to society as professional nurses, enjoy the satisfactions that come from such service, and attain the fullest growth of which they are capable. (p. 19)

The "Guide" recommends providing practical objectives that are written in terms of nursing functions and proceeds with a list of the "duties and responsibilities" under "Practical Objectives." They are classified under types of activities, with 64 main types included in the list with a number of subdivisions. The guide says the list represents a condensed form, and it recommends that the list be made more detailed. As it stands, the list represents nine small-print pages and is, as described, a list of functions—quite an expansion from Nightingale's mere 13 duties and responsibilities quoted in Chapter 1 of this book.

The University of Washington, 1955

By the time the University of Washington Curriculum research study was published in 1955 (Sand, 1955), objectives had assumed a much more behaviorist orientation. With Tyler as consultant, it is no surprise to find him quoted in statements such as:

> The changes in behavior which teaching is expected to produce in students are the objectives of teaching. . . . Each group of students, each teaching situation, must, to a considerable degree, be treated as a problem of how to achieve certain desirable results under particular conditions. The solution of these teaching problems requires on the part of the teacher a clear idea of the objectives sought. (p. 19)

This was quoted by Sand from Tyler's article, "How Can We Improve High School Teaching?" (1948, pp. 387–399).

After this quote follows a detailed list of tasks to be accomplished in formulating objectives and the kinds of data used to do this. Next, five broad general goals statements are given, each with a list of the implied behaviors stated in such a manner that it foretells Mager[6] (1972) by 20 years. However, the list of functions has disappeared in favor of more modern-sounding objectives. The program objectives given in this book could be mixed in with some from a modern school of nursing, and little difference would emerge. To illustrate, one section of Sand

---

[6] Mager goes to extreme lengths, undreamed of by Tyler, even when Tyler offered what Kliebard (1970) called the "simplistic notion that evaluation is a process of matching objectives with outcome." Mager offers a prescription for writing behavioral objectives that can run into pages of criteria and that can confine the learner even to the reference that must be used as the source for a "correct" answer. Tyler avoids the obvious pitfalls of such an idea.

(1955), which pertains to technical and professional competence, will be quoted.

> The School of Nursing endeavors to develop a nurse who is professionally and technically a competent person possessing an understanding of the physical, biological, and social sciences and the humanities essential to effective nursing practice, and who is skillful in meeting the nursing needs of the individual and community for care during illness and in the conservation of health.
>
> The implied behavior is that she:
>
> 1. Gives skillful patient care.
> 2. Participates with effectiveness as a member of the health team.
> 3. Possesses essential basic and related cultural and scientific knowledge.
> 4. Practices to a high degree those skills necessary to meet the fundamental health needs of the individual and the community:
>   a. Skill in communication.
>   b. Skill in applying knowledge to specific situations and solving health problems.
>   c. Skill in carrying out, with understanding and appreciation of implications for the patient, technical procedures.
>   d. Skill in organizing and directing the work of others.
>   e. Skill in social techniques essential for effective working relationships with patients and all levels of health workers.
>   f. Skill in recognizing and understanding essential health needs.
> 5. Understands the principles of learning and possesses some ability in the application of these.
> 6. Evaluates the effectiveness of her own work. (pp. 26–27)

The program objectives alone run to four and one-half printed pages and cover responsibility and accountability for self and one's own actions (which indicates the roots of current existential philosophy in nursing), professional and technical competence, membership on the health team with effective interpersonal and professional relationships, responsible citizenship, and creativity in making a contribution to improve nursing and meeting one's own established goals (pp. 25–29).

The beginnings of the objectives age and the Tylerian influence on nursing education can be seen clearly in this book. It made an indelible imprint on nursing education and launched the behaviorist movement. That movement came to full bloom in Bevis' *Curriculum Building in Nursing*.

Curriculum Building in Nursing, 1973–1988

The written page is very unforgiving. It carves on paper as permanent ideas that only reflect a temporal place in a thinking person's progress. Through three editions and 15 years, this book has been used by faculty working to improve curricula and by graduate students as a text in curriculum courses. Through three editions and 9 years, this book revealed my thinking about curriculum. What it does not reveal is the increasing concern I have had that it could continue to help nursing grow in ways that are in the best interest of the public based upon my discomfort with the limitations of behaviorist models.

In *Curriculum Building in Nursing* I speak with certainty about the role of objectives in curriculum. Two points become clear. The book shows that there was, and probably still is, a deep-seated belief in nursing that behavioral objectives were crucial. "In a practice discipline the objectives do not reflect so much what the graduate will know as what the graduate will be able to do, since what the graduate will be able to do is the ultimate test of any practice-oriented curriculum" (1982, p. 181). This section of the book discusses critical thinking and the educated mind and suggests that these goals can be made into objectives by asking (p. 181) "what are the behaviors of the person who thinks critically?" Another remark worth quoting that reflects the thinking of the day is, "The problem in specifying purposes and objectives becomes one of identifying those behaviors that the faculty thinks necessary to the functions of nursing as defined in the conceptual framework" (p. 182). At this point in history (1982), conceptual frameworks were as important as philosophies. I go on to say:

> Since the emphasis of nursing curricula is on practice and practice "doing," it behooves nurse educators to spell out objectives behaviorally on all levels. Program aims, goals, or purposes tell where one is going; program objectives tell what one can do when one has arrived. Program objectives are, in effect, end-product[7] criteria. (p. 182)

---

[7] I cannot resist pointing out once again how commonly the behaviorist metaphor of industry colors our language. Behaviorists speak of "end-product," which can mean either students or student behaviors. In this metaphor, content becomes "input," and unintended learning is called, as undeserving of a major role, "by-products." It must not be lost that "products" are objects and students are subjects. The depersonalization of students, although unintended, contributes to blinding us to the oppressive tendency inherent in behaviorism.

Extensive space is given to the process of writing objectives. The suggested topics for program objectives are also listed (p. 248). The similarities in these and the earlier one of the University of Washington are notable, although the language is different. The areas that are suggested to be covered are the following: learning how to learn or independence in learning; being instrumental in the process of change; continuing education or continuous learning; being responsive to the needs of society; being creative in giving care; being expert decision-makers, teaching others; planning, giving and, evaluating nursing care; and collaborating with others.

It is interesting to note that there have never been written criteria for evaluating nursing educational programs that spelled out the rules for writing behavioral objectives. From the first published list (National Nursing Accrediting Service, 1949) until the current ones, the word "behavioral" is not mentioned. The word "specific" is sometimes used. Yet, since the late 1960s, there has been criticism of programs that had in their self-study materials any objectives that used words such as *understand, attitude,* and other words that were deemed "unevaluatable." It has been common knowledge that this is *not to be done* (to be spoken in flat, measured tones).

The basic assumption of the behaviorist model is that it is possible to predict, fairly accurately, the outcomes of instruction. Most critics of this model believe that in classrooms where teacher–student interactions are egalitarian and interactive or in which dialogue is used as the primary teaching mode, the outcomes of teaching are only in small part predictable. Since these two positions are based upon different assumptions, there is an irreconcilable difference in their world view and, hence, their ability to agree upon other points that are contingent upon this fundamental difference. The following summary of differences is an attempt to underline the points of argument arising from these two divergent belief systems.

1. According to Stenhouse (1975, p. 83), "It is the business of education to make us freer and more creative." He goes on to say, "The most important characteristic of the knowledge mode is that one can think with it. This is the nature of knowledge—as distinct from information—that it is a structure to sustain creative thought and provide frameworks for judgment" (p. 82).

In commenting about the problems with the objectives model, Kliebard (1968) questions the morality of placing emphasis on behavioral goals, saying that the goals border on indoctrination or brainwashing rather than education, since they begin with a notion of how one wants a person to *behave* and manipulate that person and the environment until he or she behaves as prescribed (p. 246). The question, unanswered by research, is whether a system, so ordered, controlled, and prescribed, can provide a structure to sustain creative thought and frameworks for judgment as Kliebard suggests is the role of education? It would be an anomaly if it were able to do so, and experience tells us it cannot. While discussing this point, Eisner (1978) comments:

> In subject matters where, for example, novel or creative responses are desired, the particular behaviors to be developed cannot easily be identified. Here curriculum and instruction should yield behaviors and products which are unpredictable. The end achieved ought to be something of a surprise to both teacher and pupil. (p. 362)

2. Stenhouse offers the position that knowledge is primarily concerned with synthesis, and the objectives model is an analytic approach (1975, p. 83). One establishes an objective, analyzes it to determine the content and behaviors that will signal achievement of it, and instructs students in the content and behaviors. This makes knowledge instrumental. Regarding this instrumentalism, Stenhouse refers to "intrinsically worthwhile content" and warns against allowing "the use of methods to distort content in order to meet objectives" (1970, p. 76). He suggests that making knowledge merely instrumental trivializes it (1975, p. 83).

There is a case for knowledge as instrument in nursing in that nursing rests on practice. And, of course, knowledge and wisdom, critical thinking, caring, and compassion all help to shape practice. However, the direct connection between a specific bit of knowledge (non-skill-related) and a specific behavior is a tenuous trail to follow—and although that link might be traceable by a capable behaviorist researcher, it is doubtful that it could be with any confidence, for it requires a cause-and-effect connection that, with the multiple sources of learning for any individual, would be difficult or impossible to track. Eisner (1978) warns that one limitation of the objectives model is its failure "to recognize the constraints various subject matters place upon objectives" (p. 361). For instance, a knowledge of classical literature gives students vicarious experiences that enrich their understanding of tragedy, joy, the fickle nature of luck and fate, a sense of the moral struggle of humans to gain, release, and express their higher selves, a tolerance for difference, a love of beauty and the ability to see it in their work, and other lessons that are manifested in many ways in their contacts with clients—all difficult or impossible to trace in a cause-effect paradigm such as behaviorism.

Popham, in his article "Probing the Validity of Arguments against Behavioral Goals" (1968), listed several of the classical criticisms of the behaviorist model and wove classical behaviorist arguments defending against these criticisms. Whether he was successful or not certainly depends upon where one stands to cheer or boo. His work is laced with "shoulds" and "oughts," which are, to say the least, heavy parenting words that substitute authoritarian responses for acknowledging that the issues are legitimate and that behaviorism has, at least, some shortcomings. He does a good job, however, of listing some of the classical objections to the behaviorist paradigm. Among those are some of the following:

3. Objectives that can be defined behaviorally are those most readily assessed and are therefore the ones emphasized where the really important outcomes of education, being more difficult to evaluate, are underemphasized.

4. Specifying explicit behavioral objectives prevents or at least inhibits teachers from taking advantage of the unexpected opportunities for teaching things not designated in the objectives. This is an important objection for nursing in that nursing curricula tend to be so content laden that teachers fear that the objective-specified content will not be covered if they take time for what they see as a "side issue."

One can take the issue of unexpected opportunities for teaching a step further into evaluation. This gives rise to the next objection:

5. Sometimes when one is evaluating the worth of instruction, it is the unanticipated results that are really important. But, since evaluators concentrate on the objectives for evaluation, the unexpected most often gets ignored.

Eisner (1978) makes a further objection regarding the belief that behaviorally stated objectives can be used as criteria to measure the outcomes of curriculum and instruction:

> The assumption that objectives can be used as standards by which to measure achievement fails, I think, to distinguish adequately between the application of a standard and the making of a judgment. Not all—perhaps not even most—outcomes of curriculum and instruction are amenable to measurement. (p. 362)

He goes on to speak specifically of fields of activity that are qualitative in character and have few, if any, rules by which objectives can be applied as standards to measure achievement.

Stenhouse (1975) makes two objections to the behaviorist model that get to the essence of the matter:

6. The objectives model mistakes the nature of knowledge (p. 79).

7. The objectives model mistakes the process of improving practice (p. 79).

Regarding the mistaken nature of knowledge and the process of improving practice, Stenhouse says that schools have the responsibility to educate and education comprises at least four different processes: training, instruction, initiation, and induction. Training is skill acquisition and results in performance; instruction is information oriented and results in retention; initiation is concerned with social values and norms and results in the ability to interpret the social environment and to react appropriately to it; and induction is concerned with introduction into the thought systems of the knowledge or field and results in understanding, for example, the ability to make relationships and judgments. He holds that the first three are amenable to behaviorism, but the fourth is not, and it is an important aspect of education. I question that even number three, initiation, can be competently evaluated from a behavioral standpoint and suggest that it would be more amenable to a criticism model.

It was partially from Stenhouse's suggestions about the educational task of schools discussed above that I derived the types of learning given in Chapter 4. What Stenhouse (1975, p. 80) does successfully is to provide a rationale for the use of the behaviorist model in some types of instructional endeavors, pointing out the kinds of schooling responsibilities the behaviorist model addresses and making it legitimate to use more than one learning theory and educational paradigm.

CONCLUSION

There are few if any rules for making decisions when one is using the humanist-educative paradigm, but some modicum of consistency is called for in order that the paradigm not be invalidated by contradiction. For instance, one could choose to have or not to have a traditional nursing educational philosophy; one could also choose to identify or not to identify some conceptual systems that integrate content; but one could not choose to have behavioral objectives for any except training aspects of the curriculum (in Chapter 4, see learning types 1, 2, and 3). To be consistent, one also would need to support and structure for participation and freedom students as colleagues in the educational enterprise. However, this still leaves little structure and relies greatly on the teacher's good offices. The fact is that the humanist-educative paradigm, though it offers some mini-models and some advice, still offers very little structure and leaves those who are accustomed to the more detailed and stricter guidelines feeling somewhat abandoned. However, Stenhouse (1975) is correct when he says:

> Now it is one of the problems of theorizing that our minds are beguiled by systematic tidiness and by comprehensive breadth. Hence, many people believe that the more systematic a theory is, the more likely it is to be correct. In curriculum studies—though perhaps not in the physical sciences—the reverse is likely to be the case. Our firm knowledge of the educational process is very limited. Large-scale theories have great utility as staging points in the advancement of knowledge, but the more logically satisfying they are, the less likely they are to be adequate. They can easily become the lotus isles of our scientific journey. (p. 71)

REFERENCES

Abdullah, F., Martin, A., Beland, I., & Matheny, R. (1960). *Patient-centered approaches to nursing care.* New York: MacMillan.

Beauchamp, G. (1981). *Curriculum theory* (4th ed.). Itasca, IL: F. E. Peacock.

Benner, P. (1984). *From novice to expert: Excellence and power in clinical nursing practice.* Menlo Park, CA: Addison-Wesley.

Bevis, E. (1973). *Curriculum building in nursing: A process.* St. Louis: C. V. Mosby.

Bevis, E. (1978). *Curriculum building in nursing: A process.* St. Louis: C. V. Mosby.

Bevis, E. (1982). *Curriculum building in nursing: A process.* St. Louis: C. V. Mosby.

Bevis, E. (1988). *Curriculum building in nursing: A process*. New York: National League for Nursing.

Bloom, B. (1968, May). Learning for mastery. *Evaluation Comment, 1–11.*

Bloom, B., Hastings, J., & Madaus, G. (1981). *Evaluate to improve learning.* New York: McGraw-Hill.

Botkin, J. W., Elmandjra, M., & Malitza, M. (1979). *No limits to learning: Bridging the human gap.* New York: Pergamon.

Chater, S. (1975). A conceptual framework for curriculum development. *Nursing Outlook, 23,* 428–433.

Cohen, S. (1971). The forming of the common school. In G. Kneller (Ed.), *Foundations of education* (pp. 3–24). New York: John Wiley and Sons.

Committee of the Six National Nursing Organizations on Unification of Accrediting Activities. (1949). *Manual of accrediting educational programs in nursing.* New York: National Nursing Accrediting Service.

Counts, G. (1934). *Social foundations for education.* New York: Scribner.

Eisner, E. (1978). Educational objectives: Help or hindrance? In J. Gress & D. Purpel (Eds.), *Curriculum, an introduction to the field* (pp. 358–366). Berkeley, CA: McCutchan.

Gagne, R. (1970). *The conditions of learning* (2nd ed.). New York: Holt, Rinehart and Winston.

Goodlad, J. (1958). Toward a conceptual system for curriculum problems. *School Review, 66,* 391–396.

Gronlund, N. E. (1970). *Stating behavioral objectives for classroom instruction.* New York: Macmillan.

Grubbs, J. (1980). The Johnson behavioral system model. In J. Riehl & S. C. Roy (Eds.), *Conceptual models of nursing: Analysis and application* (pp. 160–196). New York: Appleton-Century-Crofts.

Hendrick, W. (1909). *A joysome history of education for use in schools and small families.* Nyack, NY: The Point of View.

Herrick, V., & Tyler, R. (1950). *Toward improved curriculum theory* (supplementary educational monograph no. 71). Chicago: The University of Chicago Press.

Kliebard, H. (1968). Curricular objectives and evaluation: A reassessment. *The High School Journal,* 241–247.

Kliebard, H. (1970). The Tyler rationale. *School Review, 78*(2), 259–272.

King, I. (1971). *Toward a theory for nursing.* New York: John Wiley and Sons.

Kneller, G. (1971). Knowledge and value. In G. Kneller (Ed.), *Foundations of education* (pp. 212–230). New York: John Wiley and Sons.

Leyton Soto, M., & Tyler, R. (1969). *Planeamiento educacional.* Santiago, Chile: Editorial Universitaria.

Lewis, E. R. (1974). Initiating a new baccalaureate program in nursing. In *Developing nursing programs in institutions of higher education* (pp. 56–66). New York: National League for Nursing.

Mager, R. (1972). *Preparing instructional objectives.* Belmont, CA: Feron.

Munhall, P. (1981). Nursing philosophy and nursing research: In apposition or opposition? *Nursing Research, 31*(3), 176–181.

National League of Nursing Education, Committee on Curriculum. (1917, 1927, 1937). *A curriculum guide for schools of nursing.* New York: National League of Nursing Education.

National League for Nursing Department of Baccalaureate and Higher Degree Programs. (1972). *Criteria for the appraisal of baccalaureate and higher degree programs in nursing* (Publication no. 15-1251). (3rd ed.). New York: National League for Nursing.

National League for Nursing Department of Baccalaureate and Higher Degree Programs. (1978). *Criteria for the appraisal of baccalaureate and higher degree programs in nursing* (Publication no. 15-1251) (4th ed.). New York: National League for Nursing.

National League for Nursing Department of Baccalaureate and Higher Degree Programs. (1983). *Criteria for the evaluation of baccalaureate and higher dgree programs in nursing* (Publication no. 15-1251) (5th ed.). New York: National League for Nursing.

National League for Nursing Department of Baccalaureate and Higher Degree Programs. (1984). *Self-study manual, guidelines for preparation of the self-study report* (Publication no. 15-1255). New York: National League for Nursing.

Nations, L. (1978). Conceptual framework: Who and why? In *Curriculum development and its implementation through a conceptual framework*. New York: National League for Nursing.

Neuman, B. (1980). The Betty Neuman health-care systems model: A total person approach to patient problems. In J. Riehl & S. C. Roy (Eds.), *Conceptual models of nursing: Analysis and application* (pp. 99–114). New York: Appleton-Century-Crofts.

Oliva, P. (1982). *Developing the curriculum*. Boston: Little, Brown.

Orem, D. (1971). *Nursing: Concepts of practice*. New York: McGraw-Hill.

Peterson, C. (1978). Blueprint for curriculum development: A comprehensive view. In *Curriculum development and its implementation through a conceptual framework*. New York: National League for Nursing.

Popham, W. (1968). Probing the validity of arguments against behavioral goals. A symposium presentation at the Annual American Educational Research Association meeting, Chicago, 7–10 February. In R. Kibler, L. Barker, & D. Miles (Eds.) (1970), *Behavioral objectives and instruction*. Boston: Allyn and Bacon.

Popham, W. (1971). *Criterion-referenced measurement*. Englewood Cliffs, NJ: Prentice-Hall.

Provus, M. (1971). *Discrepancy evaluation for educational program improvement and assessment*. Berkeley, CA: McCutchan.

Roy, S. C. (1970). Adaptation: A conceptual framework for nursing. *Nursing Outlook, 18*(3), 42.

Rogers, M. (1970). *The theoretical basis of nursing*. Philadelphia: Saunders.

Sand, O. (1955). *Curriculum study in basic nursing education*. New York: G. P. Putnam & Sons.

Saylor, J., & Alexander, W. (1974). *Planning curriculum for schools.* New York: Holt, Rinehart and Winston.

Scriven, M. (1967). The methodology of evaluation. In R. Tyler, R. Gagen, & M. Scriven (Eds.), *Perspectives of curriculum evaluation. AERA Monograph Series of Curriculum Evaluation no. 1* (pp. 39–83). Chicago: Rand McNally.

Selye, H. (1956). *The stress of life.* New York: McGraw-Hill.

Skinner, B. F. (1968). The science of learning and the art of teaching. In B. F. Skinner (Ed.), *The technology of teaching.* New York: Appleton-Century-Crofts.

Stake, R. (1967). The countenance of educational evaluation. *Teachers College Record,* (68), 523–540.

Stenhouse, L. (1970). *The humanities project: An introduction.* London: Heinemann Educational Books.

Stenhouse, L. (1975). *An introduction to curriculum research and development.* London: Heinemann Educational Books.

Stewart, I. (1947). *The education of nurses, historical foundations and modern trends.* New York: MacMillan.

Taba, H. (1962). *Curriculum development: Theory and practice.* New York: Harcourt, Brace, Jovanovich.

Torres, G., & Yura, H. (1974). *Today's conceptual framework: Its relationship to the curriculum development process.* New York: National League for Nursing, Department of Baccalaureate and Higher Degree Programs.

Torres, G. (1974). Curriculum process and the integrated curriculum. In *Department of baccalaureate and higher degree programs. Faculty-curriculum development part IV, unifying the curriculum—the integrated approach* (pp. 15–31). New York: National League for Nursing.

Tyler, R. (1948). How can we improve high school teaching? *The School Review, LVI*(7), 387–399.

Tyler, R. (1949). *Basic principles of curriculum and instruction.* Chicago: University of Chicago Press.

Zais, R. (1976). *Curriculum principles and foundations.* New York: Harper & Row.

BIBLIOGRAPHY

Bloom, B. S., Englehart, M. D., Furst, E. J., Hill, W. H., & Drathwohl, D. R. (Eds.) (1956). *Taxonomy of educational objectives* New York: Longmans, Green.

Kliebard, H. (1975). Reappraisal: The Tyler rationale. In W. Pinar (Ed.), *Curriculum theorizing, the reconceptualists* (pp. 70–83). Berkeley, CA: McCutchan.

Popham, W. (1973). *Evaluating instruction.* Englewood Cliffs, NJ: Prentice-Hall.

Popham, W. (1975). *Educational evaluation.* Englewood Cliffs, NJ: Prentice-Hall.

Roy, S. C. (1980). The Roy adaptation model. In J. Riehl & S. C. Roy (Eds.), *Conceptual models of nursing: Analysis and application* (pp. 135–143). New York: Appleton-Century-Crofts.

Stufflebeam, D., Foley, W., Gephart, W., Guba, E., Hammond, R., Merriman, H., & Provus, M. (1971). *Educational evaluation and decision-making.* Bloomington, IN: Phi Delta Kappa National Study Committee on Education.

11

Making a Difference

Em Olivia Bevis

The dominant model of health care, in a word, doesn't address health and human caring, so vital to surviving as a society and a health care system. Nor does the contemporary system accommodate violence, abuse, women's and infant's health, prenatal care, child development, chronically ill, terminally ill, homeless, elderly, AIDS patients, pregnant women, basic preventative health care and so on.

Jean Watson, *Human Caring: A Human Agenda,* 1989, p. 5

The dominant view of knowledge in the Western tradition emphasizes abstract, general, theoretical knowledge while overlooking and devaluing local, specific, practical knowledge and expert skillful clinical judgments about particular clinical situations. The way involvement is central to expert knowledge is overlooked, reinforcing the myth that the expert must stand outside the situation, aloof and detached, in order to pronounce expert judgment.

Nursing and other caring practices have become paradoxical in a highly technical culture that seeks sweeping technological breakthroughs to provide liberation and disburdenment. For example, American health care emphasizes the heroics of trauma centers, while overlooking and under-funding programs for nutrition and prenatal care. Heart transplants receive tremendous funding and attention while preventive measures are less exciting and fundable because they are less culturally appealing. In the case of heart transplantation, people typically focus on the dramatic stitching in of a transplanted heart as the "breakthrough." Few notice that the intensive medical and nursing followup—solving the day-to-day problems of living with a transplanted organ, treating sores in the mouth due to immunosuppression, coping with a new hormonal milieu, promptly recognizing and responding to infection and rejection—were all caring "breakthroughs" that led to the eventual success of heart transplantation. These essential day-to-day nursing-care issues had to be solved in order to make heart transplantation a viable therapy. Yet they are all but overlooked in the scientific and popular media coverage of the transplant story.

Pat Benner and Judith Wrubel,
The Primacy of Caring, 1989, p. XV

Nurses, as do others who perform what our society defines as "women's work," have always contended with the dichotomy between the duty and desire to care for others and the right to control and define this activity. The balance between this duty and the right has shifted over time as the circumstances of nursing have changed, but the obligation to care has been at nursing's definitional core. When we become ill or injured, we expect to be cared for as we hope for a cure. . . . Nursing as work is thus based on our expectation and need for someone to take up the obligation to care.

Susan Reverby, *Ordered to Care*, 1987, p. 1

These quotations highlight the predicament of nursing today. It is a work that is out of step with the social health care paradigm. Watson (1989) says that the current model ignores or inadequately addresses such significant issues as family violence, prenatal care, elder care, chronically ill, women's health, and prevention (p. 5). It has only now begun to address AIDS. It values cure in a time crying for care and prevention. According to an article in *American Nurse* (Selby & Cizmek, 1989, p. 1), the demand for nurses is higher than ever before, and, although there are more nurses than at any other time in history, women have more career opportunities that are less restrictive, so fewer of them are entering nursing. Because of these factors, there is a critical shortage of those prepared to do that work.

It is a work of caring. It is a work in high demand, where there is a critical shortage of those prepared to do that work; it is a work of caring in an age that thrills to technology and waits breathlessly for each new technological breakthrough—breakthroughs that enable people to survive formerly devastating illnesses. It is an age that ignores the societal repercussions of such survival. These repercussions—such things as pain, helplessness, isolation, loneliness, disability, and decreases in life quality—are all problems that require caring . . . the ingredient nurses have as primary focus. Yet the very people—the experts in caring, the ones responsible for the real statistics of survival in the miracles of today's science—are denied the right to control their own practice. Although they comprise 55 percent of the health care providers and are among the best educated of health care providers, they have little impact on the policies of health care.

Things are changing. Nursing is an awakening giant. It is a group of well over 2 million, 97 percent of whom are women, late in coming to the women's movement, and late in joining together in ways that strengthen their ability to be a force on behalf of the health vulnerable. This predominantly women's group is late in learning politics, how to compete for funds, attract media attention, and centralize its concentration on its unique social mission, which is (according to Reverby [1987]) "the order to care in a society that refuses to value caring" (p. 1).

This is not a failure of nursing so much as a failure of society to create the conditions where care, essential to human survival, is valued and acknowledged as worthy of priority attention. Therefore, conditions in employing agencies have been allowed to exist that are inimical to the freedom, creativity, autonomy, and humane concern that must be the mark of a career worthy of the educated individual—a career that makes an obligation of caring and a necessity of educated expertise. All problems in nursing today cannot therefore be laid at the door of education . . . in fact, few of these problems can. However, while society must do much, nursing education can do some things that will evoke repercussions in the lived world of both students and patients. It is to these areas of potential impact that this chapter is addressed.

RECAPITULATION OF THE EXPECTED IMPACT OF THE EDUCATIVE-CARING PARADIGM

Purposes

The purposes of this book, as listed in the Introduction, are to offer an alternative nursing educational paradigm that would:

- Enable nursing graduates to be more responsive to societal needs.
- Be better able to bring scholarly approaches to client problems and issues—more capable of critical thinking.
- Be more successful in humanizing the highly technological milieus of health care—more caring and compassionate.
- Be more insightful about ethical and moral issues and better able to advocate ethical positions on behalf of clients.

These purposes become the goals of a paradigm shift in nursing and will be examined in the light of expected impact were this paradigm to be adopted in nursing education.

Responsiveness to Societal Needs

For a country that is self perceived as an advanced Western nation, a leader in technology, a leader in world human rights, and a leader among democracies with high standards of living, we tolerate, or rather ignore, some crucial health issues—bizarre for such an advanced nation. These issues continue to accumulate and will eventually either cause us to completely alter our health care paradigm or cause our economy to collapse. Here are some of the problems:

1. The United States has the highest infant mortality rate in the postindustrialized world. Its ranking for infant survival, among all industrialized nations, was last place in 1988. The infant mortality rate is generally conceded to be the most accurate indicator of a nation's health status because of the high priority placed by civilized nations on the comprehensive care of pregnant women and young children. Poverty and its accompanying lack of prenatal care is one of the major causes of infant mortality (Maraldo, 1989).

2. By 1991, the projection is for Acquired Immunodeficiency Syndrome to have infected 270,000 persons, 179,000 of whom will be dead. The others will rely primarily on home nursing care, care that is understaffed and underfunded both by private and government insurance (Maraldo, 1989).

3. Drugs are rampant. Every month brings worse statistics on drug use, and Americans continue to double and triple the amount of federal dollars expended in law enforcement to solve the problem despite continued demonstration that the law enforcement approach has failed. Creative possibilities that might have a potential for success are

blocked at every turn by legislatures unwilling to take the political risk of relinquishing a failed approach to try a different one. Therefore, escalation of addiction and drug abuse continues.

4. Thirty-seven million Americans are uninsured and have no access to health care in a nation that spends 12 percent of its gross national product on health care. This is 40 percent more per capita than any other developed nation. Additionally, we are the only developed country other than South Africa that does not have some kind of comprehensive national health insurance coverage program (Maraldo, 1989).

5. Physician outlays under Medicare have been rising 18–20 percent per year compared to 3–4 percent in other sectors of health care. This in spite of the fact that physician fees have been frozen under Medicare since 1986. This is due to the fact that physicians have been increasing their per person services by 18 percent a year for the past 10 years (Maraldo, 1989). Yet lawmaker solutions propose that employers provide health care insurance coverage for the 37 million who are uncovered, a solution that ignores the basic problem.

6. Home care is the fastest growing industry in the nation. Yet nurses—those who give that care—are at the worst point of shortage in our history. Programs to tackle that shortage are too often aimed at recruitment and retention of nurses and too seldom at the root causes of the problem.

7. Nonwhite health statistics are worsening, while those for whites are improving. This is a reflection of the widening income gap between the poor (usually nonwhite) and the rich (usually white) (Mesce, 1989).

These conditions do not even address the lack of quality in the care that is given, the number of lawsuits involving health care, the outmoded turf-protecting laws, and the cynicism that loads federal committees to study the problems of health care for the poor with experts[1] who are usually wealthy or at least from the upper middle classes. A

---

[1] A friend of mine was recently appointed to a large, federally sponsored committee comprised primarily of male "experts" to study health care of the poor. In discussing the site for the second meeting of the committee, the men were discussing the merits of various luxury resorts where they could meet and play golf. One of the few women on the committee, a social worker from Mississippi, rose to the occasion with a statement shaming the cynicism of a committee constituted to study the health plight of the poorest poor in arranging a meeting based on a site's ability to be a luxury playground. "Come to the back country of Mississippi," she said. "Let me show you what we are here for, let me

moral voice is needed, and nurses must be better prepared to be the moral voice of U.S. health care. Only a new approach to teaching nursing can so prepare such voices to speak of the social needs and problems that are so readily swept under the rug.

According to the executive director of the National League for Nursing, "The time is past when nursing can rely on others to solve its problems, or other problems in heath care" (Maraldo, 1989, p. 1).

Nursing has a unique societal mission: to care for the vulnerable and to provide caring services in prevention, cure, and maintenance. Nursing forms a partnership with people that extends their ability to maintain themselves and not be set apart in institutions; it concerns itself with lived experiences of people who have to face health problems. It provides services of the most intimate nature to people whose independence, life, and family unity are threatened. Nurses find themselves involved in the struggles faced by family units (of all possible types) in trying to cope with the problems rooted in society's bungling of its health care responsibilities.

Therefore, the social mandate is clear: to give compassionate, humane care by helping people with their lived experiences within an ineffective health care system that continually denies the individual's personhood both during and in the aftermath of medical "miracle" technology. Furthermore, this new trend in curricula paradigms is designed to help nurses learn to be politically effective in shaping health policy so that the needs of all the people can be met. Nurses will be unable to meet the challenge without an education that frees the imagination, that brings confidence in one's personal power, that teaches social consciousness and commitment to advocacy for those who cannot effectively advocate for themselves, and that provides insights into the needs of the silent 37 million Americans without insurance. This curriculum-development model is designed to build on the lived interactions of students, nurses, and clients in ways that bring these insights and skills. Furthermore, by the use of paradigm experiences of students and other nurses, it is designed to provoke in a new generation of nurses those imaginative strategies that can shape health policy and improve the quality of care.

---

take you around to talk to the people we are talking about, let me give you a real life view of those whom you cannot even imagine and for whom we are to make recommendations." After the silence that follows shame, they voted to meet in rural Mississippi. There needs to be more and louder voices to spur conscience of the health care system.

Critical Thinking

Much time was spent in Chapters 6 and 8 discussing critical thinking. The question remains, what benefits can nurses bring to clients and to society through a scholarly approach to client and societal problems and issues? Some of the benefits were referred to in the former section, in that well-educated graduates will be better able to be politically active and make a difference in shaping national and local health policy matters. There are, of course, other things that require nurses with scholarly approaches to client problems. Answers to this question require a reexamination of the reason for nursing education's move to higher education.

One of the goals of higher education for nurses was not only to identify nursing more with the academic fields, improve its research and theory base, and advance it as a profession, but also to require courses that give a broad general education. The increased numbers of nurses with master's and doctorate degrees have contributed greatly to what is known about human needs for care and how to provide it. But an additional factor motivated nursing's move into higher education: to give nursing a liberal arts base. Consequently, educators in institutions of higher learning require college courses of two types: The first and most frequent type is that deemed prerequisite to nursing; second, and much less frequently, courses in humanities are required. However, the benefits of humanities courses have been diminished because educators have not built into the nursing-patient-care curriculum those processes necessary to help nurses use the humanities' knowledge and understanding in their work with clients. This is not to say that some university schools have not found ways to increase the level of knowledge of liberal arts and ways to help students use this knowledge in nursing care—and when it has occurred, it has been largely a part of the hidden curriculum and not of the legitimate curriculum. This omission is in part due to the curriculum model currently in use: Behavioral objectives do not allow for the intangibles of caring, creativity, critical thinking, political sophistication, seeking for meaning, facilitation of growth in clients, and other important phenomena central to professional nursing. The paradigm presented by this book is shaped to help us harken to the very reason for nursing's move to institutions of higher learning: the full use of the human potential for a creative vision of the interrelatedness of the art and science of human life and the imagination, excitement, enthusiasm, and energy to translate that vision into nursing care.

Watson (1987), addressing this, says, "It is therefore incumbent on the profession and the academic community to adhere to the purpose of a university education" (p. 3).

This paradigm rests on the postulate that the purposes of a university education have been subverted by the behaviorist model, and this paradigm is designed to halt that subversion. Along these lines, Botkin, Elmandjra, and Malitza (1979) present a definition of "maintenance learning" and one of "innovative learning." Regarding maintenance learning, they write:

> Life encompasses innumerable routines—reading and writing, using tools and crafts, riding a bicycle and driving a car, harnessing animals and handling electronic devices, applying basic norms of individual conduct and social behavior and so on. All are guided by rules, all of which must be learned where needed. This type of learning consists in assimilating as quickly as possible time-honored procedures developed slowly but surely for given and recurrent "problems." The response to any such problem starts by making simplifications—the process is to define, select, and isolate a situation from a larger maze of interrelationships. This is the classical approach of science. It is also a description of maintenance learning, which is a process of problem solving based on bounded plans and agreed-upon procedures, with well-defined goals and tasks. (pp. 42–43)

If, as Botkin et al. assert, "maintenance learning is the acquisition of fixed outlooks, methods, and rules for dealing with known and recurring situations" (p. 10), then this applies to the way nursing schools currently teach nursing. Rule-driven learning is necessary for some levels of nursing, but it will not enable graduates to approach and solve the myriad of problems they must face with their clients in the complex, lived world of today's health care. Rule-driven theory is not only the result of behaviorism in nursing schools, but it is also due to the erroneous assumption that theory shapes practice. Indeed, in a practice field, theory and practice must each shape the other. Benner and Wrubel (1989) offer the goal that:

> A theory [of nursing] is needed that describes, interprets, and explains not an imagined ideal of nursing, but actual expert nursing as it is practiced day to day. This type of theory could be used to develop curricula in which practice informs nursing education in a way that nursing education has always influenced practice. (p. 5)

This might lead to the same kind of imbalance currently seen, in that we could move from the current situation in which too little attention is given to expert practice as a source for theory to one in which too little attention is given to the "imagined ideal." I fear the pendulum and long for the praxis—where theories, whatever their origin, are allowed to play back and forth between the real world of practice and the reflective world of theory so that each equally shapes the other and both are scholarly. In fact, Benner's work documents that this approach can make major contributions to nursing and nursing education.

Maintenance learning is referred to throughout this book as training. It consists of the first three types of learning (Chapter 4), which are item, directive, and rationale. These types are necessary but not sufficient to help students become the critical-thinking nurses necessary to make context-free decisions required as expert nurses in the technological jungle of modern health care.

Training (maintenance learning) does not provoke scholarship, and it does not support creative thinking. To do that requires a different type of teaching altogether—a kind of teaching that helps students with what Botkin et al. define as innovative learning. Innovative learning is defined by them as problem formulating and clustering. They say:

> Its main attributes are integration, synthesis, and the broadening of horizons. It operates in open situations or open systems. Its meaning derives from dissonance among contexts. It leads to critical questioning of conventional assumptions behind traditional thoughts and actions, focusing on necessary changes. Its values are not constant, but rather shifting. Innovative learning advances our thinking by reconstructing wholes, not by fragmenting reality. (p. 43)

This is the essence of university education for nurses. Although major strides have been taken under the behaviorist model, this model has not been able legitimately to encompass the kinds of approaches necessary to critical thinking. Critical thinking is not behaviorally assessed so easily; attempts to push that proverbial round peg into the square hole have resulted in largely moving into the illegitimate curriculum, and often it is really in the null curriculum . . . everyone thinking it is there, but it is not there at all. Nurses who can think critically can, if given sufficient numbers, change the whole health care system in ways that are of great benefit to the people.

A more personal and, therefore, to many a very important reason for critical thinking nurses is the very milieu of current health care. The high levels of technology, the severity of illness, and the critical nature of timing in interventions make the critical-thinking, expert clinician a significant factor in survival. The complexities of modern health care in homes, nursing homes, clinics, and hospitals mandates an educated nurse.

Human Caring

Since quite early in our history, nursing education has emphasized acquiring skills and using tools to do *things* to, for, and with people. However, since the emphasis was on doing things, as mentioned earlier, the people (subjects) became objects. They were referred to in our language as "cases," "the appendectomy," "room 459," and "problems." The whole emphasis on problem solving and "identifying the problems" arise from an emphasis on care as solving "problems." Use of this instrumentalist view of care leaves nurses feeling guilty, useless, or ineffectual when the "problem" does not get solved. When care itself is the goal, no such conflicts arise. Furthermore, the transition to patients being the "problem" was an easy one to make. This objectification of subject fitted the training mode well. However, there has been movement away from making objects of people, as nurses became more aware of the disservice to and discount of clients inherent in this. Teachers, as well as all nurses, moved to change their language and the attitudes reflected by the language.

One of the factors influencing this improvement has been the movement of nursing education into institutions of higher education. Both associate of arts and baccalaureate degree programs have used the educational setting to work with students in developing sensitivity and responsiveness to human vulnerability that so often accompanies experiences with health issues and problems. However, nursing educators, assuring themselves that nursing was an "applied" science, set about devising courses of study prerequisite to the nursing major that were science oriented. This was reinforced by our effort to be professionally recognized by our closest colleagues, physicians. These two factors, plus others, cast us in the role of health care providers that base our work primarily in the biological and physical sciences. Based upon the assumption that we were an "applied" science and the desire to be recognized by other academics and by physicians as worthy colleagues, we loaded our curricula with such subjects as anatomy and physiology, microbiology, physics, histology, cellular physiology, pathology, pathophysiology, genetics, and bacteriology. The obvious outcomes of this were nurses who were junior physicians who worked primarily with etiology, diagnosis, and treatment of diseases and the care directly related to that.

The nonnursing subjects that were selected as prerequisites were based in a Descartian dualism that denies the organismic (holistic) nature of humans. Furthermore, the traditional science set forced our research methods into a narrow focus on Comtean-type positivism and other quantitative methods. Only recently has nursing research recognized the value of qualitative research and the unlimited creativity of combining all types of methods into unique approaches to the special problems of nursing care and of the people requiring that care. In attempting to achieve colleagueship and recognition by forsaking our own human orientation and addressing primarily the biological sciences, we have continued to graduate large numbers of novice nurses who are primarily mechanistic and largely technical in their orientation—in doing this, we have deemphasized our unique place in the health care scheme.

Watson, in her book *Nursing: Human Science and Human Care* (1988), gives leadership to the view that nursing is a human science and, as such, that we acknowledge the following ideas:

1. There is anomaly between the organismic concept of person in medicine and traditional psychology and the concept of person as a whole referred to in nursing.

2. There is a strain between the study of person as *whole* (and human responses) and the process of nursing care and the traditional reductionistic assumptions of natural science, basic sciences and biomedical sciences.

3. Nursing is a relatively young discipline, dating back to the mid-to-late-19th century; hence, it is susceptible to the temptation to follow the rule of the older natural sciences, without raising important philosophical, epistemological, ethical, and scientific questions relevant to the study of nursing and nursing phenomena (p. 15).

It is worth reiterating here that she summarizes her view by saying a human science context is based upon the following:

- A philosophy of human freedom, choice, responsibility.
- A biology and psychology of holism (nonreducible persons interconnected with others and nature).
- An epistemology that allows not only for empirics, but for advancement of esthetics, ethical values, intuition, and process discovery.
- An ontology of time and space.

- A context of interhuman events, processes, and relationships.
- A scientific world view that is open. (p. 16)

It is such a view that supports this curriculum development paradigm.

Without attention to nursing as human science with its own unique contribution, its own meanings, attention to its own ethics, epistemology, and esthetics, and with new teaching modes to help students to learn the art and science of nursing, academia has diminished itself. Our content must interweave the humanities and the sciences in humanistic ways that consider the multiplicity and complexity of human beings in their varying contexts so that nursing is fundamentally transformed by academia to fulfill its mission in human health and illness.

Paterson and Zderad (1988) speak about the impact on nursing care that the arts and the humanities can make:

> When arts and humanities are included in nursing education programs, it is for their humanizing effects. Traditionally they have been recognized as having a civilizing influence. So in nursing they are seen as supporting the elements of humaneness and humanitarianism. Furthermore, they are a necessary antidote for the depersonalization that accompanies scientific technology and mechanization. . . . They stimulate imaginative creativity. They broaden a person's perspective of the human situation, of man in his world. For instance, depictions of suffering man or of other aspects of the human condition that are found in poetry, drama, or literature are far more descriptive and much closer to reality than those given in typical textbooks.
>
> Current nursing practice reflects the educational preparation of nurses that is weighted heavily with scientific courses and the methodology of positivistic science. Arts and humanities are a necessary complement. Science aims at universals and the discovery of general laws; art reveals the uniqueness of the individual. While science strives for quantification, art is more concerned with quality. Strict conformance to methodology and replicability are prized in scientific studies, whereas freedom and uniqueness of style reign in art. Science, forever updating itself, opens the nurse's eyes to constant change and innovation; the classics promote a sense of the unchanging and lasting in man's world. Science may provide the nurse with knowledge on which to base her decision, but it remains for the arts and humanities to direct the nurse toward examination of value underlying her practice. (p. 87)

The further humanization of nursing through increasing the arts and humanities courses in the collegiate nursing schools and through altering the kinds of uses teachers help students to make of these knowledges and understandings is central to this paradigm.

This humanization leads inevitably to the central purpose of nursing, which is to provide *care* to humans who are *experiencing* health problems. This can be contrasted to medicine, whose central mission is to provide treatment and cure. Awareness of this caring mission is growing and is reflected in the literature, in professional conferences and meetings, in the research, and in the philosophy of nursing. Awareness, however, is not enough. Under the present behaviorist paradigm, caring and its inescapable ethical dimension is a misfit. Returning to the metaphor, faculties spend large amounts of time trying to fit the round peg of caring into the square hole of measurable objectives.

Caring and its ethical dimension must pervade all of nursing. Caring, like other aspects of nursing, does not lend itself well to the behaviorist paradigm. It requires a curriculum-development model that makes legitimate and central the caring mission—the caring mandate—that is the heritage of all nurses. This paradigm makes caring central by legitimizing contextual learning, which is the learning of the culture of the field. For nursing this is a culture of caring. It also makes caring central by stressing the teacher–student–expert nurse interactions that are based in real-world paradigm experiences that are essential to living the caring legacy successfully. This will influence the humanistic, compassionate *treatment* of patients in health care agencies and will change the quality of nursing care.

The drive for status and recognition has not worked and will not work. Styles (1982) calls for us to establish our own criteria for professionalism and not attend to those imposed by other professions, since they are not appropriate to nursing's differing role in society. Nightingale enjoined us to listen to the voices from within, not to those from without. If we truly listen, then higher education can change the nature of nursing practice.

To that end, the American Association of Colleges of Nursing (1986) conducted a study to identify the "Essentials of College and University Education for Nursing." They listed the values, attitudes, and personal qualities of the nurse as a professional person. Under *values*, they listed such things as altruism, esthetics, equality, freedom, human dignity, justice, and truth. Under *attitude*, they listed caring, commitment, appreciation, acceptance, self-esteem, tolerance, confidence, hope, openness, consideration, empathy, trust, courage, objectivity, inquisitiveness, and reflection. Under *personal qualities,* they listed accountable, compassionate, perseverant, creative, imaginative, assertive, fair, independent, self-directive, self-disciplined, humane, kind, respectful, sensitive, integrity, moral, authentic, honest, and rational. These are all marks of the educated person and are readily discernible as important for nurses who deal with people at their most crucial and vulnerable times. It is also apparent that these characteristics cannot be developed in students through a behavioral-objectives-laden training mode and that graduates cannot practice to their full ability under the restrictive laws currently governing nursing practice in most states. It is also apparent that practice settings will need to alter their perceptions of nurses' roles and functions in order to provide the context for this more professional practice. Furthermore, nurses with a science-laden background will not be as likely to reflect these qualities as those with a more humanizing academic background. Styles (1982) speaks to this point:

> Despite our periodic raillery about the word "nursing" and the perceived stigma attached to this designation, our occupation is well named. Nursing is nurturing, nourishing, fostering, caring. Nursing is caring: both the attitude and the activity. Nursing is caring by promoting health and self-reliance for all. Nursing is caring for those who need to be nurtured in relation to their health status, wherever, as long, and as frequently as they need it, until that need is removed or revised by recovery, independence, or death. This caring responds to needs ranging broadly between the extremes of information and incentive for maintaining wellness to emotional support and technical assistance for sustaining life and providing comfort. As nurses, our MOTIVATION is *caring;* our SERVICES are *caring* and *managing;* our fundamental TOOL is *knowledge,* both tacit and explicit; the PRODUCT of these services is *health*—its maintenance and restoration to the highest possible level of attainment—and physical and psychological *comfort.*
>
> It [nursing] is comprehensive in that caring in all health states and in all settings is all encompassing; pivotal in that in primary care, as well as in nursing-intensive institutions, nursing manages or coordinates the variety of caring services around the patient. Nursing *does* encircle the entire clinical (as broadly defined) landscape in health, of which nursing and other professions occupy respective parts, and nursing should occupy the total sociopolitical landscape in health, of which others occupy the whole, or nearly so. (pp. 232–233)

Styles also predicts that "nursing will become the dominant force in the health care scene" (p. 233). That nursing is caring, there is no doubt; with the present behaviorist-scientific emphasis, however, nurses have limited opportunities to learn caring. If these possibilities are to become manifest realities, then the behaviorist paradigm that pervades both education and practice must be relegated to its proper and minor role and humanistic-caring paradigms must replace them. This curriculum-development model is designed to aid in that mission.

Ethical Advocacy

The road to ethical advocacy has not been a smooth one. Traditionally modern nursing arose through Florence Nightingale, whose experience in the Crimea was a military one. She was thwarted at every turn by Dr. Hall, Chief of Medical Staff for the British Expeditionary Force. Despite staggering statistics[2] regarding casualties suffered by the British Army in the Crimea, not by wounds, but by contagious diseases, (dysentery, typhoid, and cholera) contracted in the hospitals, the medical officers regarded Florence Nightingale as an outsider, an intruder, a meddling woman, and they drew together to defend, justify and protect themselves, and hide their bungling. In spite of this, the tradition of loyalty and an ethic of obedience became part of nursing's bones. Nightingale never betrayed Hall to the press, to the soldiers, or to the authorities. It was only in her letters that we know from her how difficult things were. However, others spoke out and the improved conditions were witness enough. But the military metaphor of bureaucracy, commanders, obedience, and loyalty, mixed with the family metaphor of physician–father, nurse–mother, and patient–child, was the dominant ethical force in nursing up until the late 1940s or early 1950s.

Slowly, the ethic altered to that of primary loyalty to the patient. This, as much as any other force, may account for the traditional opposition of physicians to the education of nurses. The change in ethic accompanied the change of nursing education primarily from hospital

---

[2] It has been estimated that three-quarters of all the casualties suffered by the British Army in the Crimean War were the result of unsanitary conditions. Nightingale found the water supplies contaminated by rotting horse carcasses, the medical supplies still on ships or not present at all, no blankets in the freezing temperatures of Russian winter, latrines clogged, and men who lay dying without care in their own excrement. Yet Dr. Hall viewed nurses as intruders who would "pamper" the men (Woodham-Smith, 1951).

schools to colleges, from places of great physician control to places of little physician control. It therefore became possible to teach the ethic of patient advocacy.

With a switch from behaviorist models of education and care to human caring models, the ethics of care rises to new heights. In behaviorist schools, however, the culture of nursing is usually taught through the hidden curriculum—it is a silent, unaware enculturation, and, therefore, change is slow. In the educative-caring paradigm, contextual learning (Chapter 4) provides for inclusion of enculturation into the legitimate curriculum. Through this legitimization, learning activities can center on the ethics of care as central to nursing. Change can be more rapid, and choices are more available regarding the nursing culture to be emphasized when such content has a legitimate place among the types of learning.

Nurses are caught in a bind in modern health care. A bind that places them in between the technology and skill that now enables many to live who would formerly have died, and the message is that if we cannot help the patient be cured, then our mission is to help them die. Gadow (1988) confronts this ethical dilemma:

> The ethical differences between care and cure are felt more poignantly by nurses than by any other professionals. This is made dramatically clear to me each time I receive a call from the intensive care unit for an ethics consultation on a patient around whom three groups typically are doing battle: the medical team who hope and press for cure; a family who on the patient's behalf desires release from treatment; and nurses who in the meantime—and in the middle—are committed to caring, despite the fact that theirs may be an infinite commitment without foreseeable aim or end, if the patient is able neither to die nor to recover. Without any direction in which to point their caring—either recovery or death with dignity—they are morally adrift. "Why am I doing this?" is the cry of the nurse caught in this situation. (p. 5)

Gadow holds that care itself is the moral end; it needs no other goal, either cure or death. She proposes that care "is the commitment to alleviating another's vulnerability" (pp. 6–7). If perceived this way, then cure that requires intervention has as an inevitable consequence the increasing, at least temporarily, of vulnerability. Care, therefore, is for Gadow the higher ethic. She says that when cure is the standard, then care becomes nothing more than a means toward that end. Care cannot be a means but must be an end in itself. Therefore, it is in the ethics of care that nursing finds its moral impetus.

Many factors have merged to make it possible for nursing to acknowledge, research, proclaim, and practice its ethic of care: the women's movement, the professionalization of nursing, significant changes in the knowledge of the public and their consequent intense interest in care, and the expanding education of nurses . . . expanding in the sense that it can violate the artificial boundaries imposed by behaviorism, empiricism, technology, and logic. It is new educational paradigms that will enable nursing to find its new ethic—paradigms that stress the legitimization of the contextual aspects of nursing—that provide interactive methodologies that allow learning to center on the real experiences of nurses with patients whose only need is for care. This is a crucial ethic, for, as mentioned earlier in the chapter, the problems that confront the health care system are aging, chronicity, and AIDS, all problems that mandate an ethic of care.

BENEFITS FOR NURSES, NURSING, AND SOCIETY

At the beginning of this book, I offered 10 things that any alternative paradigm must accomplish to be able to "graduate the skilled, compassionate scholar-clinicians necessary for the remaining years of the 20th century and the beginning of the new millennium." It is posited that to be effective, the alternative paradigm must accomplish things made difficult or impossible by the currently used behaviorist paradigm. These are worth recapitulating:

1. It must liberate both students and faculty from the authoritarian restraints of empiricist/behaviorist models as represented by specified behavioral objectives and the teacher roles and functions necessitated by those objectives.

2. It must acknowledge students as equal partners in the educational enterprise so that it restructures the way faculty and students relate to each other.

3. It must define curriculum as interactions between and among teachers and students with the intent that learning take place.

4. It must facilitate the structuring of learning differently so that the learner is actively engaged in scholarly pursuits, and through this it must support abandoning the dominance of lecture in nursing education.

5. It must help faculty humanize the educational process so that the curriculum is not dominated and driven by a surfeit of content.

6. It must support an alliance of students, teachers, and clinicians in the educational enterprise.

7. It must restructure the focus of learning so that experiences are clinically grounded.

8. It must provide practical guidelines to faculty without restricting individuality, creativity, and style.

9. It must acknowledge the wide variety of ways of knowing, and it must legitimize those things that are not empirically verifiable.

10. It must eliminate the education-based class and caste system in nursing by acknowledging and valuing the contributions of all nurses and by making higher levels of nursing education more easily accessible.

These represent the crux of this paradigm; they sum up the values, the methods, the models, and the mission of the humanist-educative model. Although the model offers no "rules" and no real road maps, what it offers is a few models and some guidelines. What it offers most is possibilities: possibilities for teachers, students, and staff to collaborate so that not only does the public benefit but nursing itself does, both as persons and as a profession. It offers the promise of liberating oppressive relationships between teachers and students. It offers the opportunity to make learning lived experience that is analyzed, reflected upon, synthesized, and understood. It offers alliances instead of opposition. It promises theory as lived curriculum and curriculum as lived theory. It tenders freedom for individuality, creativity, style, and multiple ways of knowing. It legitimizes intuition, caring, and morality, and it supports making baccalaureate and higher degrees accessible to nurses who hold diploma and associate of arts degrees. Finally, it provides a framework within which nursing can move to the nursing doctorate as the truly professional degree.

It is necessary at this point to ask the following questions: When and under what circumstances will the effect of an educational paradigm shift be felt by the public? What kinds of factors influence the ability of higher education in nursing to improve the quality of nursing care in the workplace? Naturally the first problem is having a graduate who is qualitatively different from graduates from nonacademic institutions; but once this problem has been addressed, as has been done here, what then? For answers to that, we must look to the workplace.

One aspect of the issue is having a critical mass of graduates that are qualitatively different. When that will occur is anyone's guess. In fact, how many constitute a critical mass is not a simple question. It cannot be answered quantitatively. There must be enough nurses graduated under a humanistic-educative paradigm to provide a strong support system both in the workplace and in the profession itself. Without such a support system, individuals will have a difficult time making definitive changes. Humans are herding animals, and the herding instinct is one of "average," of a desire to be like others . . . thus enculturation into the profession continues to take place after graduation and is controlled by those who most influence the novice nurse through approval and reinforcements both on a peer and authority levels. For changes to occur, a critical mass is essential. Nursing management positions, supervisors, and clinical specialists must be part of the critical mass.

Furthermore, valuing the contribution that practicing expert nurses can make in the education of nurses is essential. To be successful, these nurses must be included in the educational enterprise in ways that integrate classroom and clinical teaching. However, we cannot create a dichotomy by having expert nurses teach clinical courses and educators teach classroom courses. This would limit the potential for classroom learning based on active involvement in simulated paradigm experiences, cause an eventual discount by students of the importance of what can be learned in classrooms, and could cause a competitive rift between practice and education that would harm the whole educational enterprise. Ways must be found to integrate and include both expert clinicians and educators so that practice and classrooms make for living, growing, and animation of the practical and theoretical in a harmonious marriage.

Another strong factor in the impact of such a paradigm shift in higher education on practice is the socially approved modes of nursing care delivery. The physician is the gatekeeper to the whole health care system in most societies and is dominant in all matters of health care, even those matters unique to nursing and not dependent upon medical expertise. This is antithetical to the professional practice of nurses. Without clearer legal discrimination regarding the rights of nurses to make independent judgments about nursing's own domain of care, no amount of higher education will progress too far in altering the quality of care received. However, higher education will help us know how to influence legislation that will make more sense for the health problems of society and permit nurses to provide the care they know so well how to give and that research validates in its effectiveness.

In an age of continued, accelerated medical engineering and technology, the temptation to concentrate nursing care on the machines instead of the person is ever present. It is axiomatic that the goal of academics, that is, higher education in nursing, must be for creativity; for helping patients find meaning in their suffering, illness, and pain; and for helping them with their health experiences in ways compatible with states of being that are health-positive, health-seeking, and health-acting. Professionalism deals with values, colleagueship, discourse, symbolism, judgments, risks, caring, and care that is discriminating, creative, critical, theory based and theory creating, individualized, and contextual rather than rule driven. This requires a large degree of professional autonomy.

The chicken/egg question arises here. Which must happen first: Must the workplace change, or must the graduate change? It is a recip-rocal situation. The workplace cannot change substantively until there is a critical mass of the truly educated nurse, and the mass of truly educated nurses cannot be maximally effective without changes in the workplace. Reverby (1987) casts the problem in wide social terms. She, with other feminists, suggests that what women want is autonomy with connectedness. She says:

> In the case of nursing this will require the creation of the conditions under which it is possible to value caring and to understand that the empowerment of others does not have to involve self-immolation. To achieve this, nurses will have to create a new political under-standing for the basis of caring and find ways to gain the power to implement it. Nursing can do much within itself to bring this about . . . but nurses cannot do it alone. The dilemma of nursing is too tied into the broader problems of gender and class in our society to be solved solely by the political efforts of one occupa-tional group.
>
> Nor are nurses alone in benefiting from such an effort. If nurs-ing can create the vision of autonomy and altruism as linked quali-ties, and achieve the power to forge this unity, all of us have much to gain. Nursing has always been a much conflicted metaphor in our culture, reflecting all the ambivalence we give to the meaning of womanhood. Perhaps in the future it can give this metaphor, and ultimately caring, new value in all our lives. (p. 207)

As Reverby says, it is a social problem, not simply a nursing one, but nurses must attempt to solve it and to draw society into that work. The work has begun. Restructuring nursing education is one contribution to the greater whole. Without the truly educated nurse, the probability of capturing society's attention to the problems decreases.

Nursing has suffered a predicament that is part of the problem of larger society—the sacrifice of education for preparation for earning a living. Somehow, if we are not to fail society at this important juncture of its history, we must succeed in remarrying education and professional preparation.

The truly educated are an endangered group. Those who come to understand the inconstancy of the gods or fates through Odysseus and Oedipus; loyalty and faith through Penelope; remorse through Othello; vanity through Ozymandias; frustration through Cassandra; aging through Lear; terror through Dante; fear through *Moby Dick;* and the intertwining of suffering, loneliness, and love through Silas Marner and Quasimodo; those who understand that evil can triumph over good through studying Iago's malevolently successful plotting; and those who see society's injustice toward women in the suffering of Hester Prynne and toward the poor in Oliver Twist are not usually found among health care providers. In fact, it is rare to find them at all. Many people spend their lives being schooled, yet few are educated to find their solace in Tintern Abbey's ode to love, remembrance, and beauty; their peace of mind in a Mozart quartet; and their perspective on society's values in Alice's adventures in Wonderland. Who can bring to every day living the examples of courage, fortitude, love, wonder, and hope gleaned through a thousand eyes of a thousand imaginations as well as see the messages in the struggles of the Curies, Semmelweiss, Michelangelo, Van Gogh, Galileo, and Sojourner Truth? There are far too few who understand the deeper meaning of a sense of purpose and commitment that can be gleaned from Ghandi and Martin Luther King and who have learned from Nat Turner to understand how dependence and oppression can kindle anger and destruction; who can learn about injustice from Dred Scott, Alfred Dreyfus, and Leo Frank, and about society's indifference from the deaths of 9 million people in Nazi crematoriums. The truly educated take their map for living from the facts of history as well as fiction, poetry, philosophy, art, and music, and know that the difference between history and classical literature may be tenuous but the lessons are all valid, although often contradictory, richly textured, and cannot be expressed in the pithy, three-frames-at-a-time exploits of a wonderful, stupid penguin named Opus, no matter how satiric.

A humanities education can give nurses the tools to cope with the pain, helplessness, hopelessness, loneliness, joy, relief, and the day-to-day grind encountered in the world of the health vulnerable. A humanities background cannot teach them to use those tools, but it can supply them. It must be one of the main tasks of nursing curricula to teach the use of these tools.

It is my hope that this book will give nursing educators at least two things: the courage to examine how vital a liberal arts/humanities base is for nursing education and the incentive to restructure nursing education itself in such a way as to liberate both teachers and students while using paradigm experiences that engage students' total lives in learning to use the tools so richly supplied in the arts and humanities in order that the result will be a graduate more richly endowed for living, more capable of enlightened care, and more scholarly in pursuit of knowledge and understanding. It is my hope that in this age where science has given more humans the ability to live out their full life spans, nursing can help people achieve a high-enough quality of life for those additional years so that every day is not a test of endurance and courage but has in it some love, affection, joy, pleasure, and a sense of usefulness. It is my hope that in this age where technology makes hospitalization possible for only the very ill and makes discharges abrupt and rapid, nursing can ease that transition, help families cope with these very ill persons in the home safely, and speed recovery when it is possible, and comfort and integration when it is not. It is my hope, not so much that we meet the current nursing shortage crises with more nurses—although that would be a worthy goal—but that we have better nurses. It is my hope that through these changes in nursing education, nursing will be better able to help society through a period in history that, because of accumulated successes and failures, has left little room for error, and courts not only the destruction of the world but also the loss of that which is the highest in ethical value—the ability for caring. And, finally, it is my hope that because of this better educated, more skilled, more liberated, more socially conscious, more ethical, more politically competent, and more caring nurse, we can be a force in reshaping the health care system so that all the people are served with dignity and compassion.

REFERENCES

American Association of Colleges of Nursing. (1986). *Essentials of college and university education for professional nursing, final report.* Washington, DC: American Association of Colleges of Nursing.

Benner, P., & Wrubel, J. (1989). *The primacy of caring, stress and coping in health and illness.* Menlo Park, CA: Addison-Wesley.

Gadow, S. (1988). Covenant without cure: Letting go and holding on in chronic illness. In J. J. Watson & M. Ray (Eds.), *The ethics of care and the ethics of cure: Synthesis in chronicity.* New York: National League for Nursing.

Maraldo, P. (1989). *Executive director wire.* New York: National League for Nursing.

Mesce, D. (1989, March 16). Blacks' life expectancy drops further. The Associated Press, *Savannah Morning News.*

National Nursing Accrediting Service. (1949). *Manual of accrediting educational programs in nursing.* New York: Author.

Paterson, J., & Zderad, L. (1988). *Humanistic nursing.* New York: National League for Nursing.

Reverby, S. (1987). *Ordered to care, the dilemma of American nursing, 1850–1945.* New York: Cambridge University Press.

Selby, T., & Cizmek, C. (1989, March) Nurse supply, demand reach all-time high. *The American Nurse,* 1.

Styles, M. (1982). *On nursing, toward a new endowment.* St. Louis: C. V. Mosby.

Watson, J. (1988). *Nursing: The philosophy and science of caring.* Boulder, CO: Colorado Associated University Press.

Watson, J. (1989). *Human caring: A public agenda.* Paper presented for Wingspread Conference: Knowledge about Care and Caring.

Woodham-Smith, C. (1951). *Florence Nightingale.* New York: McGraw-Hill.

12

The Future-in-the-Making: Creating the New Age

Jean Watson

This book would not be complete without discussion of the future-in-the-making, as both imagined, through the transformative thinking in this book, and realized, through actual happenings in a given setting. For example, as part of the philosophical, moral, and social action initiatives in Colorado, the University of Colorado School of Nursing, along with a number of formal clinical affiliates, are shaping a new future for nursing. Aside from the philosophical and concrete discussions and calls for action outlined in this text, the ability of nursing to come of age for a new era is dependent upon a few courageous systems taking the lead with transformative thinking and action, both in education and clinical practice.

In Colorado, the model-in-the-making seeks to integrate a transformative philosophy of human caring in nursing education with restructured clinical practice roles in the health care delivery system. Such efforts are a result of renewed partnerships, in the form of formal collaborative programs and official relationships, between clinical care agencies and the University of Colorado School of Nursing. This formal collaborative model for professional nursing includes multiple activities such as the clinical teaching associate model (Phillips & Kaempfer, 1987), research-based nursing practice (Keefe, Pepper, & Stoner,

1988), practitioner-teacher positions, and shared research and educator positions.

In addition to these educator, clinician, researcher roles and activities, formal inter-institutional administrative links also have been established. For example, the directors and vice presidents of nursing in the collaborating clinical agencies serve as formal members of the Dean's Council in the University School of Nursing and hold formal positions as assistant or associate deans for clinical nursing affairs in the designated institution. These administrative positions are by dean, chancellor, and regental appointment, which serves to stabilize and formalize the university and clinical agency relationship. Other emerging arrangements include agency-based clinical faculty, some of whom are university school of nursing funded while others are funded by the respective clinical agency. These funding arrangements are part of the formal collaborative *education–service agreements* to *merge values and actions* in order to jointly shape, transform, and restructure professional nursing education, research, and clinical practice.

Such joint efforts are now beginning to shape new professional options and opportunities for nursing by simultaneously impacting both education and practice at their roots. In uniting education and service in new configurations, commonly held assumptions are bringing about a merger of professional values. For example, there is a shared acknowledgement between the educational program and the formal collaborating clinical agencies that nursing is the health profession of unmet expectation. There is the belief that, as both education and practice unite to professionalize nursing and all its missions, nursing will be able to more fully actualize its societal commitment to human caring, healing, and health. Thus, nursing will be increasingly capable of solving some of the current problems in the health care system.

SOCIAL ACTION POLICY POSITIONS

Other general points for consideration influencing nursing's future include the following social action policy positions and assumptions (Watson, 1988, 1989):

- The health care delivery system of the future will be a multifaceted, complex system of choices, both in traditional and nontraditional settings.

- Hospitals will continue to decline and eventually will accommodate only the most severely and acutely ill, and/or hospitals will radically redefine their role in the delivery of health care into the community.

- Home care, family-oriented personalized care, and self-care will continue to increase as the population becomes older, better informed, more responsible, and more assertive with respect to their own health care needs.

- A better use of nursing capabilities to provide health and illness care to the public will go a long way toward containing cost without limiting access or sacrificing quality (while also providing professional personnel to respond to the changing caring, healing, and health needs of society).

- The general public and business communities will become aware of steps that can be taken so the public can more fully benefit from the expert caring and health services that nurses can provide.

SIMULTANEOUSLY RESTRUCTURING EDUCATION AND PRACTICE

In order to move forward with these shared assumptions and social policy initiatives, the educational and clinical practice worlds of nursing will have to continue to unite in simultaneously restructuring nursing education and professional clinical care.

For example (Watson, 1989), all nursing capabilities and expert knowledge in health, healing, and human caring will need to be maximized and utilized differently, thus:

- There is the need to create and utilize advanced prepared nurses as patient-centered-caring experts and caring managers and coordinators who can interface between the traditional system and personal caring, healing and health needs of patients and families, thereby positioning nursing to be directly accountable to patients for continuous health and human caring needs.

- Nurses need to be included as covered caregivers and nurse-run clinics and care facilities need to be included in all insurance plans, with direct payment for nursing services.

- Professional practice and admitting privileges need to be initiated for qualified professional nurses in hospitals and other agencies, including joint practice privileges with physicians, pharmacists, and other health professionals.

- Professional nursing education and comprehensive professional nursing practice must continue to be upgraded to attract the best and brightest into progressive programs; this upgrading includes restructured curricula to ensure compassion, caring, ethics, technocure clinical competence with accountability, responsibility, and autonomy necessary to fill the void of health and human caring quality, access, and cost containment.

- Major leading schools of nursing, with formal collaborative clinical agency partnerships, must provide a full continuum of educational and clinical progression for nurses, from *technical*, (Associate degree, AD), to *beginning entry professional* (Baccalaureate degree, BSN), practice roles, to *advanced, autonomous professional practitioners of human caring nursing* (Nursing Doctorate, ND). The ND thus becomes the clinical nurse of the future with the appropriate preprofessional background (i.e., liberal arts degree), and complete professional preparation (i.e., postbaccalaureate clinical doctorate), who is prepared for autonomous practice roles as an expert in human caring, healing, and health and prepared as a professional patient-centered caring practitioner, manager, and coordinator.

- Nursing demonstration projects of expert human caring, healing, and health, with a mix of nurses with different levels of preparation, must be jointly initiated to test out and demonstrate quality, efficiency, and cost effectiveness in the provision of health services; these models need to be replicated in hospitals and other agencies across the country, in collaboration with academic health science center schools of nursing and other major leading nursing programs.

REDEFINING THE NURSE OF THE FUTURE

In order to implement these social action initiatives in education and practice, the nurse of the future has to be redefined from being a first-level employee of the medical system to an autonomous professional qualified to practice the latest advanced knowledge, skills, and ethics of compassion and caring, health and healing. This preparation has to combine additional advanced clinical decision-making competencies and advanced clinical practice skills in health promotion and self-care, including traditional and new, advanced caring and healing modalities. In other words, the comprehensively prepared professional nurse of the future must be clinically adept in clinical, ethical, and system decision making associated with interpretation, coordination, management, and delivery of direct care across settings. This comprehensive delivery, coordination, and management of expert human caring, healing, and health will occur in the midst of biotechnology and computer technology, but within the context of individual patients' and families personal human caring and health needs. Direct care and caring that will promote healing and self-care, regardless of medical condition or illness diagnosis, and regardless of setting becomes the comprehensive professional role of the future nurse. As a result, the nurse of the future is an expert in human caring who is directly accountable to society—one prepared as a full health professional who works collaboratively across settings within a continuous care model, as an equal member of the interdisciplinary health team.

THE POSTBACCALAUREATE NURSING DOCTORATE IN HUMAN CARING, HEALING, AND HEALTH

In order to actualize the dreams and destiny of nursing in the ancient tradition of caring, healing, and health, and also be responsive to the transformative events in education and clinical practice, and future health policy directions, the complete educational model for nursing must be concerned with educating the *whole* person. However, the educational model must also prepare a professional practitioner of human caring, healing, and health. Thus, the future proposed for professional education in nursing will follow a general liberal arts foundation and be postbaccalaureate in nature.

As a result, the proposed preferred, terminal comprehensive, clinical professional degree (versus the beginning professional entry level baccalaureate degree, or the technical associate degree) will be the nursing doctorate, the ND. The following are the proposed components of the educational base for this program: (Watson, 1988):

- A more extensive liberal arts foundation that focuses on understanding of and appreciation for cultural diversity and on the human subjective dimensions of health–illness, caring, healing experiences, and needs.
- Preparation in critical thinking and advanced problem solving, contributing to clinical judgments, and independent decision making.

- Core knowledge underpinning biomedical science, social behavioral sciences, and organization/system management theory and practice.

- Extensive preparation in philosophical and ethical decision-making skills based on ethics of human caring, which addresses health policy, and contextual, compassionate, relational, ethical dilemmas, as well as knowledge of the traditional rationalistic approach to principled biomedical ethics and traditional health policy positions.

- Exploration of the contextual value-laden relationship theory that is associated with human caring and healing transactions, emphasizing self-care and more autonomous decision-making processes.

- A curriculum based on human science and nursing theory that incorporates the latest research and practice knowledge of human caring, healing, and health, and emphasizes the relationship between human and system caring approaches and health/healing outcomes.

The ND, the PhD, and the MSN

The doctor of philosophy (PhD) will continue as the predominate and preeminent research and theory degree. The master's degree (MSN) in nursing will be consolidated into newly defined specialities of nursing and health and caring needs of specific populations. Some nursing master's programs will decline or become highly intense, highly specialized, subspecialty postgraduate clinical programs that somewhat model clinical fellowships in medicine.

The emerging comprehensive *professional nursing practice (versus research) doctoral degree* is, therefore, the postbaccalaureate ND degree. Moreover, the ND model that offers the full continuum of professional education and professional practice, while providing clinical career advancement for experienced nurses (for example, from AD to ND), will help the professional retain and revitalize existing practitioners.

At the same time, the ND program must attract a new generation of educated men and women into nursing and prepare them as full health and human caring professionals. In the model proposed, ND prepared nurses will interact with other health professionals on an equal footing as acknowledged experts in health, healing, and caring practices, and allow the profession to come of age for a new and timeless role.

Summary Description of the ND

The nursing doctorate (ND) is a postbaccalaureate advanced educational and clinical program for comprehensive professional nursing practice. The ND is professionally accountable to society for nursing's broad mission of human caring, healing, and health. Thus, the ND is prepared to be directly accountable to patients and families for continuous health, healing, and human caring needs, across clinical settings. The ND provides the interface between and among hospitals and other care agencies, including home and clinic care. The ND regulates and monitors the highest level of professional care between and among multiple health personnel; coordinates, educates, counsels, and advises the patient and family regarding different treatment protocols. The ND personalizes complex, acute, and chronic health care needs, including symptom management, demystifying the medical world, and instructing patients on how to optimize self-care and inner healing resources, including better use of the traditional health (medical) system. Finally, the ND is an advanced nurse practitioner who is a clinical expert in human caring, health, and healing knowledge and skills, a specialist in complex care management, self-care, and health promotion practices.

Educationally, the ND is distinguished by a general liberal arts preprofessional background, a postbaccalaureate advanced professional program of new and expanding nurse practitioner skills, and a human caring, healing, health promotion philosophy inclusive of theories and practices. Advanced practitioner skills include technocure and computer-based interventions. However, more extensive preparation in philosophical and ethical decision-making skills, based on nursing ethics and nursing theories of human caring, also are essential.

Clinically, the ND is distinguished by practice expertise in human caring, health, and healing, the patient-centered complex care-coordination-management role, and broad health care system competencies and advanced practitioner skills. In addition, graduates will be familiar with both traditional and new human caring practice modalities that incorporate natural healing approaches and esthetic-based approaches, such as therapeutic touch, visualization, imagery, music, movement, and other expressive modalities that potentiate self-care and coping and healing.

In this way, the ND will acquire and verify professional nursing skills within the context of human caring values, theories, and knowledge that are mutually supported and reinforced in both the educational and practice world. Such efforts lead to radical restructuring of teaching–learning, curriculum, and professional socialization and practice activities. Such changes allow nursing to come of age for a new era but in a context that restores nursing to its ancient roots while actualizing the metaparadigm of Florence Nightingale as well as contemporary nursing visions.

Implementation of ND as Collaborative Partnership

Implementation of the ND model can occur through a renewed partnership between and among schools of nursing and collaborating clinical agencies. For example, in Colorado, several local collaborative community hospitals have begun a corporate sponsorship program with the University of Colorado School of Nursing. The program underway allows the school of nursing to admit a new cohort of postbaccalaureate prepared students into an accelerated nursing program that is the precursor of a pilot ND. This new partnership and shared alliance between the University of Colorado School of Nursing and clinical agencies, within the established infrastructure of the collaborative framework discussed, creates both an operational and financial model for simultaneously restructuring professional nursing education and clinical practice roles. Together the nurse of the future as well as society gets the best of both worlds, while restoring and redefining, but also transforming nursing's professional health, healing, and caring role in society.

REFERENCES

Keefe, M., Pepper, G., & Stoner, M. (1988). Toward research-based nursing practice: The Denver collaborative research network. *Applied Nursing Research, 1*(3), 109–115.

Phillips, S., & Kaempfer, S. (1987). Clinical teaching associate model: Implementation in a community hospital setting. *Journal of Professional Nursing, 3*, 165–175.

Watson, J. (1988). Human caring as moral context for nursing education. *Nursing and Health Care, 9*(8), 423–425.

Watson, J. (1989). ND Materials prepared for University of Colorado School of Nursing\Center for Human Caring Visiting Board.

Appendixes

Appendix I

CRITERIA FOR TEACHER–STUDENT INTERACTIONS
CRITERIA FOR LEARNING ACTIVITIES

Teacher–Student Interactions Criteria

A. Creativity

   1. Teacher accepts and encourages the student to develop creative approaches to the subject matter (Hicks, 1979–1980; Torrance, 1981)
   2. Teacher acknowledges student's creative contributions to the class, to the subject matter, and to the discipline (Torrance, 1981)
   3. Teacher exhibits the general attitude that all students can show creativity (Torrance, 1981)
   4. Teacher uses self as a positive force to produce an atmosphere that fosters creativity (Krupey, 1982; Stenhouse, 1975; Torrance, 1981)

B. Style of presence

   5. Teacher is accessible for the purpose of an interactive critique of the student's work (Jacobson, 1983; Potamianos & Crilly, 1980; Stenhouse, 1975)
   6. Teacher demonstrates enthusiasm and a positive attitude toward student and subject matter (Krupey, 1982; Potamianos & Crilly, 1980)
   7. Teacher is open and nondefensive with student (Miron, 1983; Potamianos & Crilly, 1980)
   8. Teacher displays an appropriate sense of humor (Miron, 1983; Potamianos & Crilly, 1980)
   9. Teaching style encourages student participation (Chickering, 1969; Torrance, 1981)

10. Teacher asks many questions and interacts with the student around the answers while preserving the student's dignity (Noddings, 1984; Torrance, 1981; Sandefur & Adams, 1976)

11. Teacher shares student's feelings of excitement, joy, frustration, etc. (Noddings, 1984; Torrance, 1981)

12. Teacher takes an active interest and provides encouragement to student (Meredith & Ogasawara, 1981)

13. Teacher assists student to feel comfortable with their differences (Torrance, 1981)

C. Reciprocal interactions

14. Teacher–student interactions provide teacher and student with intellectual stimulation that requires disciplined thinking about subject area (Jacobson, 1983; Krupey, 1982; Noddings, 1984; Stenhouse, 1975)

15. Teacher–student interactions are frequent and friendly (Chickering, 1969; Meredith & Ogasawara, 1981)

16. Teacher–student interactions occur in diverse situations which call for varied roles (Beirs, 1986; Chickering, 1969)

17. Teacher–student interactions require responsibility on part of student and teacher to maintain a relationship conducive to learning (Noddings, 1984)

18. Teacher provides a climate that communicates a valuing of caring and concern as the moral imperative of nursing (Bevis, 1988; Griffith & Bakanauska, 1983; Noddings, 1984; Watson, 1985)

D. Contextual, syntactical, and inquiry learning

19. Teacher engages student in activities that develop cognitive structures and positive affective responses (Doll, 1979; Low, 1980; Rosner & Howey, 1982)

20. Teacher provides a positive milieu that is conducive to activities that promote learning, i.e., discussion, small group work, confrontation, etc. (Sandefur & Adams, 1976)

21. Teacher readily demonstrates expertise in the subject matter (Krupey, 1982; Mueller, Roach, & Malone, 1971; Potamianos & Crilly, 1980; Scheck & Bizio, 1977)

22. Teacher helps student to develop own meaningful ways of knowing and thinking processes (Eisner, 1985; Hicks, 1979–1980)

23. Teacher and student select goals that are important and may not be behaviorally measured (Peters, 1973; Raths, 1971; Stenhouse, 1975)

24. Teacher and student shared responsibility for critiquing student's work is more valued than the assigning of grades (Stenhouse, 1975)

25. Teacher–student interactions assist student in deriving meanings from the learning experiences (Eisner, 1985; Noddings, 1984)

26. Teacher–student interactions raise issues and questions about the subject matter that require the student to use a variety of heuristics (Botkin, Elmandjra, & Malitza, 1979; Stenhouse, 1975)

27. Teacher listens to a range of views carefully and uses questions to elicit amplification of issues, rather than arguing against opponents or attempting to resolve differences (Noddings, 1984; Stenhouse, 1975)

28. Teacher encourages student to reflect upon professional life experiences in relation to the subject matter (Benner, 1984; Botkin, Elmandjra, & Malitza, 1979; Noddings, 1984)

29. Teacher reacts in a constructively critical manner to the student's work, refining, and developing standards and stressing a sense of scholarliness (Raths, 1971; Stenhouse, 1975)

Learning Experiences Criteria

A. Introduction

1. Requires the student be actively involved in learning (Dewey, 1902; Raths, 1971)

2. Necessitates that the student become responsible for own learning (Dewey, 1902; Sandefur & Adams, 1976)

3. Structures for training or educative goals as appropriate to the subject matter inherent in the experience (Botkin, Elmandjra, & Malitza, 1979; Broudy, 1982; Peters, 1973; Stenhouse, 1975)

4. Identifies the type of encounter the student is to have with the subject matter (Burton, 1962; Eisner, 1985)

5. Requires an exploration of the context in which problems/issues exist and are understood (Bevis, 1988; Benner, 1984; Broudy, 1982)

6. Makes clear the critique of the student's work is the valued part of the learning process (Stenhouse, 1975)

B. Working phase

7. Creates a cognitive dissonance that requires the student to engage in educative heuristics such as reflection, incubation, dialogue, debate, imagining, hypothesizing, to approach the resolution of the dissonance (Bevis, 1988; Dewey, 1933; Eisner, 1985; Metcalf, 1963; Stenhouse, 1983)

8. Requires the student to practice creative approaches to the subject matter (Hicks, 1979–1980; Torrance, 1981)

9. Uses writing to encourage students to perceive, create, reflect, represent, and inquire (Torrance, 1981; Weimer, 1988)

10. Structures activities so that the student discovers solutions, alternatives, consequences, etc., for self (Hanley, Whitla, Moo, & Walter, 1970; Raths, 1971)

11. Requires the student to use a variety of methods of inquiry in order to find or create information, raise questions, etc. (Hanley, Whitla, Moo, & Walter, 1970; Stenhouse, 1975)

12. Requires the student to use a variety of theoretical frameworks from which to view issues/problems (Hanley, Whitla, Moo, & Walter, 1970; Stenhouse, 1975)

13. Engages the student in intellectual or higher thinking modes such as analyzing, critiquing, identifying and evaluating assumptions, inquiring into the nature of things, predicting, searching for patterns, engaging in praxis, viewing wholes, etc. (Benner, 1984; Bevis, 1988; Krishnamurti, 1953; MacDonald, 1974; Wang & Blumberg, 1983)

14. Makes clear that the student's ideas are dynamic and will evolve over time (Raths, 1971)

C. Culmination

15. Requires student to support and defend formulated propositions, postulates, and hypotheses (Hanley, Whitla, Moo, & Walter, 1970; Stenhouse, 1975)

16. Allows for interaction between the teacher and student around the many possible outcomes of the experience (Belenky, Clincky, Goldberg, & Tarule, 1986; Raths, 1971)

17. Promotes encounters with the artistic aspects of nursing such as meanings, relationships, context, patterns, and new insights (Benner, 1984; Eisner, 1985; MacDonald, 1974; Torrance, 1981)

18. Requires the student to use a variety of sources and rationales as evidence from which to draw conclusions (Hanley, Whitla, Moo, & Walter, 1970; Stenhouse, 1975)

D. Resolution

19. Provides an impetus that encourages student to synthesize what has been learned (Torrance, 1981; Wang & Blumberg, 1983)

20. Ensures that the interpretation of the quality of the student's work is guided by the teacher's understanding of the subject matter and is judged qualitatively in light of appropriate criteria. (Bevis, 1988; Stenhouse, 1975)

21. Guides exploration of how experience may enrich future career goals (Dewey, 1902; Torrance, 1981)

22. Allows for dialogue around finding meanings in experiences, such as making errors, acknowledging paradigm experiences, discovering diversity (Benner, 1984; Bevis, 1988; Diekelmann, 1986)

23. Allows the students to actively reflect upon the manner, quality, and patterns of change in their own intellectual growth (Bevis, 1988; Dewey, 1938; Metcalf, 1963; Noddings, 1984; Raths, 1971; Stenhouse, 1975)

REFERENCES

Belenky, M. F., Clinchy, B. M., Goldberger, N. R., & Tarule, J. M. (1986). *Women's ways of knowing.* New York: Basic Books.

Benner, P. (1984). *From novice to expert: Excellence and power in clinical nursing practice.* Menlo Park, CA: Addison-Wesley.

Botkin, J. W., Elmandjra, M., & Malitza, M. (1979). *No limits to learning.* Elmsford, NY: Pergamon Press.

Broudy, H. S. (1982). Challenge to the curriculum worker: Uses of knowledge. In W. H. Schubert & A. L. Schubert (Eds.), *Conceptions of curriculum knowledge: Focus on students and teachers* (pp. 3–8). University Park, PA: College of Education, The Pennsylvania State University.

Burton, W. H. (1962). *The guidance of learning activities.* New York: Appleton-Century-Crofts.

Chickering, A. W. (1969). *Education and identity.* San Francisco: Jossey-Bass.

Dewey, J. (1902). The child and the curriculum. In A. A. Bellack & H. H. Kliebard (Eds.), *Curriculum and evaluation* (pp. 175–178). Berkeley: McCutchan.

Diekelmann, N. (1986). *The curriculum as dialogue and meaning: An alternative model for the professional nursing curriculum.* Unpublished manuscript.

Doll, W. E. (1979). A structural view of curriculum. *Theory Into Practice, 18*(5), 336–348.

Eisner, E. (Ed.). (1985). *Learning and teaching the ways of knowing: Eighty-fourth yearbook of the national society for the study of education, part II.* Chicago: National Society for the Study of Education, Yearbook Committee and Associated Contributors.

Griffith, J. W., & Bakanauskas, A. J. (1983). Student-instructor relationships in nursing education. *Journal of Nursing Education, 22,* 104–107.

Hicks, L. P. (1979–1980, December/January). Abundance or richness in output: How can Webster's definition of productivity be applied to faculty? *Community and Junior College Journal,* 10–13.

Jacobson, C. R. (1983). *A look at graduate teaching at UND: Faculty perspectives* (Instructional Development Report No. ED 234 693 and HE 016 618). Grand Forks, ND: North Dakota University, Office of Instructional Development.

Krishnamurti, J. (1953). *Education and the significance of life.* San Francisco: Harper & Row.

Krupey, J. (1982). A gift for excellence: A Minnesota businessman believes outstanding teachers should be rewarded, so he does it. *American Education, 18*(4), 10–12.

Low, W. C. (1980). Changes in instructional development: The aftermath of an information processing takeover in psychology. *Journal of Instructional Development, 4,* 10–18.

MacDonald, J. B. (1974). A transcendental developmental ideology of education. In W. Pinar (Ed.), *Heightened consciousness, cultural revolution, and curriculum theory* (pp. 85–116). Berkeley: McCutchan.

Meredith, G. M., & Ogasawara, T. H. (1981). Scale for excellence in teaching award for teaching assistants. *Perceptual and Motor Skills, 53*(2), 633–634.

Miron, M. (1983). What makes a good teacher? *Higher Education in Europe, 8*(2), 45–53.

Mueller, R. H., Roach, P. J., & Malone, J. A. (1971). College students' views of the characteristics of an "ideal" professor. *Psychology in the Schools, 8,* 161–167.

Noddings, N. (1984). *Caring: A feminine approach to ethics and moral education.* Berkeley: University of California Press.

Peters, R. (1973). Must an educator have an aim? In R. Peters, *Authority, responsibility, and education* (pp. 83–85). London: George Allen and Unwin Ltd.

Potamianos, P., & Crilly, L. (1980, June). Grade "A" instructor: How do you know one when you see one? *NSPI Journal,* 24–27.

Raths, J. D. (1971). Teaching without specific objectives. *Educational Leadership, 28,* 714–720.

Rosner, F. C., & Howey, K. R. (1982). Construct validity in assessing teacher knowledge: New NTE inter-pretations. *Journal of Teacher Education, 33*(6), 7–12.

Sandefur, J. T., & Adams, R. A. (1976). An evaluation of teaching: An interim research report. *Journal of Teacher Education, 27*(1), 71–76.

Scheck, D. C., & Bizio, S. (1977). Students' perceptions of the ideal professor. *College Student Journal, 11,* 335–343.

Stenhouse, L. (1975). *An introduction to curriculum research and development.* New York: Holmes & Meier Pub. Inc.

Torrance, E. P. (1981). Predicting the creativity of elementary school children (1958–80)—and the teacher who "made a difference." *Gifted Child Quarterly, 25,* 55–62.

Wang, A. M., & Blumberg, P. (1983). A study on interaction techniques of nursing faculty in the clinical area. *Journal of Nursing Education, 22,* 144–151.

Watson, J. (1985). *Nursing: Human science and human care.* Norwalk, CT: Appleton-Century-Crofts.

Weimer, M. G. (1988). What should future teaching be like? *The Teaching Professor, 2*(2), 1–2.

Appendix II

EXAMPLES OF EDUCATIVE LEARNING ACTIVITIES

These are a few selected learning activities that reflect use of this paradigm and its principles to structure teaching in both the classroom and clinical areas in ways that meet the criteria. What is not reflected in these activities are the degree and extent to which the students were involved in setting up the course, selecting the topics, and collaborating in formulating them. Also, there is no detail here regarding the nature of the courses they were planned for, the sequencing of content/topics/ activities, and no clues about the curriculum in which they reside. There will be information regarding the level of curriculum for which they were planned (ADN, BSN, MSN, PhD).

EXAMPLE 1

Hospitalized Children with Respiratory Congestion

Level of the Student: Last quarter of the junior year.

Overview

It is midwinter, and there are a lot of children who have been hospitalized for a variety of upper respiratory diagnoses and complaints that result in symptoms like stridor, congestion, and fever. This time of year, there are seldom fewer than three children on the unit at once. It is important to see the similarities and differences among the children, the parents, the diseases, the symptomology, and the nursing care that is appropriate.

385

Goals

This learning activity is designed to help you get a comprehensive picture of the needs, problems, and care for these children and their families; help you find patterns, gain insights and determine the significance and meanings of what you perceive.

Directions

Preclinical. Read your textbook on respiratory disorders and their nursing care. Choose two articles from the library regarding respiratory problems in children that frequently require hospitalization. One must be a research article.

In Clinical. Choose any day you have time during the first 2 weeks of your time this quarter. Read the charts of at least four children with an acute respiratory disturbance. Spend some time with each child, and, if possible, at least one parent of each child.

While reading the chart, take careful note of the following: the lab work (CBC, nose and throat cultures, and x-rays); and other significant findings/diagnostic tests; the child's age, sibling placement, general health, and medical history. Note the medications, treatments, and general course of the disease to date. Read the nursing notes, the events that seem of significance to you, the times the temperature was taken and, if it was elevated, when. Make note if the URI has occurred to this child before and under what circumstances. Are there other accompanying problems (earache, sore throat, headache, rheumatic pains, etc.)?

Upon visiting the child, note the degree of variance in expected developmental level, the amount of anxiety or fear displayed, whether the child is alone or with someone and how long, how often, how affectionate the child is or how withdrawn, how the child responds to you, how active, how toxic the child appears, the energy level, the interactions with other children (if you have an opportunity to observe them), and interactions with parents. Note the general appearance of the child, weight, height, skin turgor, smell, eyes, breathing difficulty, and the condition of the chest when breathing. Listen to the child's breath sounds and describe them.

Spend at least 5 minutes with the parent(s). Talk with the parent(s) about what difficulties they feel they face as a result of this and other illnesses the child has had. Find out what the home is like. Use open-ended questions and listening noises. Find out (if they have other children) whether the other children have had similar problems.

If you see any significant similarities and differences in your children make special note. If there are any patterns among the children/ parents/home situation, make special note. Note any hunches, intuitions, and any insights or assumptions.

In Class. Bring your notes. Get into groups of three to four students and compare notes, similarities, differences, hunches, insights, and assumptions. *Take 20 minutes.* You are looking for patterns, general principles, similarities, and differences from the textbooks and articles you read. Prepare a report on the patterns, etc., for plenary session.

Plenary session will last 20 minutes.

EXAMPLE 2[1]

Georgia Southern College, Department of Nursing, Nursing 447: Nursing Issues

Level of the student: Senior Year
Learning Activity 2: Review of *AJN* as a Means of Providing a 20th Century Perspective on Nursing.

Overview. GSC has all of the *AJN* on microfilm. The *AJN* was born with the new century, and its first issue was published in January 1900. For many years it was the only nursing publication and for that and other reasons it remains the grand old dame of nursing publications and was chosen for this learning episode. Its format has changed through the years and through that alone one can perceive the changing self-image of nursing. On its pages virtually all of nursing's primary movers have left a trail of their thoughts about nursing's approach to its problems and issues. The very advertisements speak of the change in nursing's sanctioned way of being. The articles, letters to the editor, and regular features provide clues to nurses' perceptions of themselves, their workplace, their work roles, and their relationships to each other and other health providers. These pages give evidence of the origins

---

[1] This learning activity is modified from Georgia Southern College Department of Nursing. It is copyrighted, so please do not use without the permission of the college, and ensure that it is appropriately credited.

and development of our ethics, our development as a profession, our sense of power, the place of caring and compassion, and our relationship to patients. Our sisters and mothers speak to us across the decades and let us know how tenacious are old issues—they never seem to die, they just repeat themselves under different names, with different champions, and in different contexts.

It's all there for the perceptive student, exciting our imaginations, stirring our pride, lifting our spirits, laying bare our weaknesses, detailing our oppression, illustrating our courage, ingenuity, and perseverance, and, finally, charting our developmental processes. This learning activity is designed to help you gain insights into nursing's life during the twentieth century and will as no other activity can. You are a sleuth in the pages of history. GOOD HUNTING!

Goals. This learning activity is designed to help the student develop an appreciation of the history of nursing in the United States. Its intention is to help you recognize and understand some of the work done by nursing leaders and how their work laid the foundation for today. The overall ends-in-view are to help you develop a sense of nursing as a smoothly flowing stream and to perceive how the present is always situated in the context of the past and, therefore, to have an appreciation for the fact that unless the past is ever before us we cannot make adequate progress toward a chosen future.

Directions

Preclass. The class will be divided into groups. Each group will be given a number 0–9. If your group number is 0, you will peruse each year with a zero in it, if one, each year with a one in it, and so forth throughout the decades. Therefore, each group will peruse one whole year in each decade. As you examine the years assigned you, fill out the form provided for each of the assigned years. Make your sheets legible for it may be necessary for the rest of us to read them. Add as many sheets as necessary to complete the assignment. You will find the *AJN* microfilm in the microfilm section of the periodicals in the library. After these directions you will find some hints regarding what to look for that will help you get started.

Each student sign up one number (0–9) that is the last digit in a year. Depending upon the number in the course, have at least two students per digit. Try to distribute yourselves evenly.

In Class. We will walk through nursing in the twentieth century using the filled out forms. The topics developed as study guides are guides only and not intended to be limiting but exemplary only. Students are encouraged to discuss, share insights, inspirations, new awarenesses, or any sense of pattern, sequence, assumptions or their consequences with the class as we explore each decade.

Note: The following notes will help you survey the *AJN* and to fill out the forms provided. Please do not let these limit your insights.

1. *Advertisements.* Note and describe the types of advertisements. To what aspect of the reader do they attempt to appeal? What is the clothing like, what gimmicks are used to attract the reader? Are there job advertisements? When do they first appear? Are books advertised, hospital equipment, and pharmaceuticals? How are they presented? What comment on society, women, and nurses do these things make? Are there patterns that become apparent? What meanings do you find in these patterns?

2. *Articles, Topics, Authors, and Format.* See what were popular categories for articles. Who wrote them (physicians, nurses, allied health persons, etc.)? Note the trends up through the years in coauthorship of articles with nurses and physicians. What insight does a perusal of the articles provide for the cultural norms of nursing and society for the decade? What are the current events, the attitudes of nurses and the larger society toward women and nursing? Trace the expansion and change of roles and functions, such as preparing the food, taking blood pressures, giving medications, and the more modern functions such as reading and interpreting cardiac monitors. When did nurse practitioners, nurse anesthetists, and nurse-midwives come on the scene? Look at the pictures of model hospital units and patient care equipment. Note the changing credentials of the authors. Watch for the emergence of nursing theory and the shift in approach in articles.

3. *News, Features About Books or Book Reviews, Editorials, Letters to the Editor.* Through the years, the regular features changed names and topics several times. Skim through them. Read some and note how they changed through the years, the topics, the numbers and titles of the nursing organizations, and the wording of the obituaries. See the nurses off to two world wars and note the aftermath of war and the changes they brought about. When did "professionalism" first begin to be an

issue and what issues were addressed under that topic? Watch for nursing ethics and what changed about that, e.g., the appearance of the rights of patients and the change in the focus of nurses from loyalty to the physician and employing agency to loyalty and advocacy for the patient.

4. *Overall Impressions.*   What kinds of patterns do you see in nursing events? What has been its place in society over the years since 1900? What have been the main issues as reflected in your perusal? Looking through the eyes of the *AJN* what can you gather about:

a. Nursing as institutionalizing women's roles; nursing's place in society and nurse's relationship to physicians.
b. The values and ethics of nursing as an emerging profession.
c. Nurse's view of economic security, fringe benefits, politics, and power.
d. Licensure, education, academic legitimacy, higher education, interprofessional rivalry, and quality control.
e. Nursing history as it reflects U.S. history, values, and culture.
f. The role of frameworks, theory, concepts, research, and management.

EXAMPLE 3[2]

Georgia Southern College, Department of Nursing, Family Nurse Practitioner Master's Program

Rural primary care: Nursing problems caused by life style

Topic: Victomology across the life span

Learning activity: Caring for the abusive family

Overview.   Elder abuse, child abuse, the battered spouse, and neglect are forms of family abuse and violence that are a growing concern for society. Abuse is widespread in all socioeconomic and educational levels, and its consequences are devastating to family members.

---

[2] This learning activity is modified from Georgia Southern College Department of Nursing. It is copyrighted, so please do not use without the permission of the college and appropriate crediting.

Advertisements	Articles, Formats, Topics, & Authors	News, Obits, Book Reviews, Editorials, Letters to the Editor	Your Impressions & Insight, *e.g.*, View of Women, Cultural Norms, Implications, Assumptions, Nursing Reflecting American History and Culture, Work Role Relationships, Politics, Power, Meanings

Research is being conducted on the factors involved, and the data on domestic violence is becoming more reliable. However, the development of detection, treatment, or educational programs has not been widespread. The family nurse practitioner in primary care settings will encounter the abused family members. True caring requires a response. It is the purpose of this learning activity to examine the role of the FNP as it relates to ethical caring, legal liability for reporting abuse, using specific screening guidelines for diagnosing and evaluating suspected cases of abuse, looking at patterns, meanings, cultural conditions that support abuse, and to developing management protocols for working with abused clients. Additionally, the student will explore available community resources for the abused client and will determine if educational, preventive programs are conducted in the community.

Goals. It is the goal of this learning activity to help the caring nurse practitioner come to grips with the roles, commitments, ethics, collaborative practice, assessment parameters, and management protocols necessary to care for the abused family or individual.

Directions

Preclass. These are articles that will be helpful to you. You may read these or others of your choosing.

A. Elder Abuse

Fulmer, T., & Wetle, T. (1986). Elder abuse screening and intervention. *Nurse Practitioner, 11*(5), 33–38.

Johnson, D. (1981, Jan–Feb). Abuse of the elderly. *Nurse Practitioner,* 29–34.

B. Child Abuse

George, J. E., Quattrone, M. S., & Westville, J. D. (1988). Law and the emergency nurse reporting child abuse: Duties and dangers. *Journal of Emergency Nursing, 14*(1), 34–35.

Neff, J. A., & Scherb, B. J. (1988). Standardized care plans suspected abuse and neglect of children. *Journal of Emergency Nursing, 14*(1), 44–47.

Rhodes, A. M. (1987, Nov–Dec). Identifying and reporting child abuse. *MCN,* 399.

Kelley, S. J. (1988). Physical abuse of children: Recognition and reporting. *Journal of Emergency Nursing, 14*(2), 82–90.

Wong, D. L. (1987). False allegations of child abuse: The other side of the tragedy. *Pediatric Nursing, 13*(5), 329–333.

Katzman, E. M., & Roberts, J. I. (1987, Nov–Dec). No longer a silent partner. *MSN,* 383–388.

C. Spouse Abuse

Finley, B. (1981, Jul–Aug). Nursing process with the battered woman. *Nurse Practitioner,* 11–29.

Blair, K. A. (1986). The battered woman: Is she a silent victim? *Nurse Practitioner, 11*(6), 38–47.

Christie-Sealy, pp. 411–422.

D. Once you have completed your perusal of the literature, complete protocol parameter sheets; one for the abused elderly, one for the abused child, and one for the abused spouse.

E. Optional: There is a slide presentation available in the A-V lab entitled "Violence in the Family" if you choose to view.

In Class

You will be given two or three written simulated paradigm cases of abused and abusing families and individuals. These may be used or used to help the nurse to recall paradigm experiences in which abuse was a major factor. Read the simulated ones, share your own experiences:

1. Discuss them with the end-in-view of gaining insights regarding the role of abuse in society and its possible meanings for both abusers and abused.
2. Seek patterns in abusing/abused families and individuals and utilizing your discussions of own and others paradigm experiences, and current research and statistics, come to some conclusions regarding: the extent of family violence in our society, the ethical commitments of the caring nurse and the meaning of these things for your own practice.
3. Complete case study using protocol/management sheets.
4. Plenary session with presentation of student's work.

In Practicum

1. Generate the assessment parameters for screening suspected cases of elder, child, and spouse abuse.
2. Create a management protocol which includes treatment, support, and preventive strategies for the abused elderly, child, and spouse.
3. Assess a family for characteristics indicative of potential/existing abuse.
4. Collaborate with community resources and educational programs to meet the needs of abused clients and their families.
5. Survey your community for resources and agencies which respond to abused clients. Complete the agency data form on these agencies. Add these to your Community Resource Notebook.

Protocol/Management Sheet

1. Define the problem (include such items as social support absence, assertive/dominance issues, ethical issues)
2. Etiology (common causes: personal, social, community, ethnic)
3. Subjective/objective signs/symptoms
4. Desired goals
5. Plan/management
6. Consultation/referral
7. Follow-up

Permission Credits

Excerpts from page 15 of *Women's Ways of Knowing, the Development of Self, Voice, and Mind*, by Mary Field Belenky, Blythe McVicker Clinchy, Nancy Rule Goldberger, and Jill Mattuck Tarule, copyright © 1986 by Basic Books, Inc., reprinted with permission of the publishers.

Excerpts from pages xviii–xix and 40 of *From Novice to Expert: Excellence and Power in Clinical Nursing Practice*, by P. Benner, copyright © 1984 by Addison-Wesley Publishing Company, reprinted with permission of the publisher.

Excerpt from page 398 of *The Primacy of Caring, Stress, and Coping in Health and Illness*, by P. Benner, copyright © 1988 by Addison-Wesley Publishing Company, reprinted with permission of the publisher.

Excerpts from page 5 of *The Primacy of Caring*, by P. Benner and J. Wrubel, copyright © 1989 by Addison-Wesley Publishing Company, reprinted with permission of the publisher.

Excerpts from pages 4, 21, and 43 of *No Limits to Learning: Bridging the Human Gap*, by J. Botkin, M. Elmandjra, and M. Malitza, copyright © 1979 by Pergamon Press Publishing Company, reprinted with permission of the publisher.

Excerpt from page 3 of *Social Foundations for Education*, by G. Counts, copyright © 1934 by Scribner, reprinted with permission of the publisher.

Excerpt from page 362 "Educational Objectives: Help or Hinderance," by E. Eisner, in J. Gress and D. Purpel (Editors) *Curriculum, An Introduction to the Field*, copyright © 1978 by McCutchan Publishing Corporation, reprinted with permission of the publisher.

Excerpts from pages 3 and 5 of *The Conditions of Learning*, Second Edition, by Robert M. Gagne, copyright © 1970 by Holt, Rinehart and Winston, Inc., reprinted with permission of the publisher.

Excerpt from pages 2–8 of "The Aims of Education," by H. Gray, copyright © 1988, *The University of Chicago Magazine*, reprinted with permission of the publisher.

Excerpt from page 19 of "Water from Rock, Tomatoes from Sand," by L. Hazelton, in *Quest*, vol. 3, no. 5, copyright © 1979 by Human Kinetics Publishers, reprinted with permission of the publisher.

Excerpt from page 246 of "Curricular Objectives and Evaluation: A Reassessment," by H. Kliebard, in *The High School Journal*, vol. 5, 241–247, copyright © 1968 by University of North Carolina Press, reprinted with permission of the publisher.

Excerpt from page 201 of *Foundations of Education*, by G. Kneller, copyright © 1971 by John Wiley & Sons, Inc., reprinted with permission of the publisher.

Excerpt from page 50 of "Structural Analysis in Sociology," by R.K. Merton, in P. Blau (Editor) *Approaches to the Study of Social Structure*, copyright © 1975 by Free Press, reprinted with permission of the publisher.